The New
Complete Book of
FOOD

Second Edition

The New Complete Book of

FOOD

Second Edition

A Nutritional, Medical, and Culinary Guide

CAROL ANN RINZLER

Introduction by Jane E. Brody
Foreword by Manfred Kroger, Ph.D.

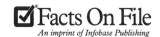

Facts On File
An imprint of Infobase Publishing

The New Complete Book of Food, Second Edition

Facts On File, Inc.
An imprint of Infobase Publishing, Inc.
132 West 31st Street
New York NY 10001

Library of Congress Cataloging-in-Publication Data
Rinzler, Carol Ann.
The new complete book of food : a nutritional, medical, and culinary guide / Carol Ann Rinzler; introduction by Jane E. Brody ; foreword by Manfred Kroger.—2nd ed.
    p. cm.
Includes bibliographical references and index.
ISBN-13: 978-0-8160-7710-6 (hardcover : alk. paper)
ISBN-10: 0-8160-7710-X (hardcover : alk. paper)
1. Food. 2. Nutrition. I. Title.
TX353.R525 2009
641.3—dc22   2008029255

Facts On File books are available at special discounts when purchased in bulk quantities for businesses, associations, institutions, or sales promotions. Please call our Special Sales Department in New York at (212) 967-8800 or (800) 322-8755.

You can find Facts On File on the World Wide Web at http://www.factsonfile.com

Text design by Evelyn Horovicz

Printed in the United States of America

MP KT 10 9 8 7 6 5 4 3 2

This book is printed on acid-free paper and contains 30 percent postconsumer recycled content.

This book is for
Phyllis Westberg,
who made it work;
Laurie Likoff and
James Chambers,
who made it real;
my husband, Perry Luntz,
who made it possible—
and, with my gratitude,
for Alex Bekker, M.D.;
Abraham Chachoua, M.D.;
and Raymonda Rastegar, M.D.,
who made Perry possible.

Contents

Introduction

You've no doubt heard of food for thought, food for love, food for strength, health food, healing food, soul food, brain food, and the like. For as long as people have inhabited this planet, edibles have been imbued with all sorts of attributes beyond satisfying hunger and sustaining life. And in many cases, popular notions about the powers of various foods and beverages have been documented by modern scientific investigations that have demonstrated, for example, the soothing qualities of chicken soup for sufferers of the common cold, and the antibiotic properties of garlic.

Then there are the newer discoveries not rooted in folklore, among them the protection against cancer afforded by vegetables and fruits rich in the carotenoid pigments and the cancer-blockers found in members of the cabbage family; the cholesterol-lowering ability of apples, barley, beans, garlic, and oats; the heart-saving qualities of fish and alcohol (in moderate amounts), and the antidiabetic properties of foods rich in dietary fiber.

But while thinking of food as preventive or cure, it is important not to lose sight of its basic values: to provide needed nutrients and a pleasurable eating experience while satisfying hunger and thirst.

In *The New Complete Book of Food* Carol Ann Rinzler has put it all together, providing a handy, illuminating guide for all who shop, cook, and eat. It is a "must have" for all those who want to get the very most out of the foods they eat, as well as avoid some inevitable dietary and culinary pitfalls. Ms. Rinzler tells you how to derive the maximum nutritive value from the foods you buy and ingest, with handy tips on how to select, store, prepare, and in some cases serve foods to preserve their inherent worth and avoid their risks. For example, in preparing bean sprouts, you'll be cautioned to eat them within a few days of purchase and to cook them minimally to get the most food value from this vitamin C-rich food. You'll appreciate the importance of variety and moderation in your diet when you discover that broccoli, which possesses two cancer-preventing properties, also can inhibit thyroid hormone if consumed in excess.

You will also recognize that not all wholesome foods are good for all folks. Sometimes a health condition will render a food unsuitable for you. For example, beans might be restricted for those with gout and certain greens may be limited for those who must stick to a low-sodium diet. Then too, there are possible interactions—both adverse and advantageous—between certain foods and nutrients or medications. For example, citrus fruits are recommended accompaniments for iron-rich vegetables and meats since the vitamin C in the fruits enhances the absorption of iron. Those taking anticoagulant medication are advised to avoid excessive amounts of green leafy vegetables since the vitamin K in these foods may reduce the effectiveness of the drug.

You'll learn what happens to foods when they are cooked at home or processed in factories. Want to avoid olive-drab green vegetables? Steam them quickly or, better yet, cook them in the microwave with a tiny bit of water to bypass the discoloring action of acids on the green pigment chlorophyll. You'll also get the full story on methods of preserving milk—from freezing and drying to evaporating and ultrapasteurizing—that should relieve any anxieties you may have about the safety and healthfulness of processed milk.

In short, this is a book no self-respecting eater should be without. It can serve as a lifetime reference for all interested in a safe and wholesome diet.

Jane E. Brody
Personal Health Columnist
The New York Times

Foreword

A Google search will verify that Carol Ann Rinzler has become a major food/nutrition writer over the years. I am constantly impressed by the quality of her work and delighted that she emphasizes science-based facts instead of the lore and half-baked truths that are so rampant when it comes to food and diet and the way they affect health and disease. There are far too few accredited experts to invest time and effort in "communicating" to the public the results of the findings in their field. So it is up to others to do that job, and with this book Ms. Rinzler shows again that she is up to that challenge.

The New Complete Book of Food is a well-ordered and well-documented compendium of useful and factual data on what is found in the proverbial pantry of humankind. In its 113 chapters the reader will find encyclopedic information on individual species, such as apples, bananas, carrots, dates, and so on, and on pluralistic items, such as distilled spirits, fish, game meat, cultured milk, poultry, and vegetable oils. Most foods covered are true agricultural products, but manufactured items are also described, notably beer, cheese, coffee, gelatin, sugar, wine, and wheat cereals.

The author is very systematic in displaying each entry. Primary emphasis is on nutrition, followed by household and culinary aspects, and then up-to-date medical information, complete with references. General readers may want to browse and pick; professionals, such as food scientists, nutritionists, dieticians, chefs, and medical practitioners, will consult this book for specific data they may need at a critical time. For example, how should a food be properly purchased, stored, and processed? What happens during cooking or other processing? Which is the most nutritious way to serve a food? And what are a food's medical or other benefits and its possible adverse reactions?

Health-conscious readers should value this handbook as much as *The Merck Manual of Medical Information*. If it behooves us to know how the human body functions, it is equally important to know about the food that goes into it. Indeed, there is much in this book that would pass as effective food-safety education. And the home economist/economizer or frugal gourmet will find ample advice on stretching the food dollar.

Manfred Kroger, Ph.D.
Professor of Food Science Emeritus, The Pennsylvania State University;
Scientific Editor, *Comprehensive Reviews in Food Science and Food Safety*;
Science Communicator, Institute of Food Technologists

Preface

As new studies and observations constantly alter our understanding of how what we eat affects our bodies, tracking the evolving rules of good nutrition becomes ever more challenging.

For example, eight years ago, when Facts On File published the first edition of *The New Complete Book of Food,* it was commonly accepted that

- ◆ a high-fiber diet could reduce the risk of colon cancer,
- ◆ beta-carotene, a yellow pigment in deep orange and dark green vegetables, would protect against cancer of the throat and lungs,
- ◆ fruit juice was healthful for kids—in fact, the more the better, and
- ◆ folic acid, a B vitamin, might lower the odds of suffering a second heart attack.

Today, none of these four beliefs are considered to be true. In the years between editions of this book, nutrition researchers have discovered that how much fiber you eat does not affect your risk of colon cancer; beta-carotene makes plant foods look good but is almost certainly not protective; fruit juice is loaded with sugar and too much is, well, too much; folic acid does lower the risk of birth defects but doesn't influence the chances of a second coronary event.

Another major change in nutrition science is how we measure the specific amounts of the various nutrients we require to maintain optimum health. Eight years ago, food scientists commonly used the term recommended dietary allowance (RDA) to signify healthful quantities of vitamins, minerals, and other nutrients such as protein, fat, carbohydrates, and dietary fiber. Today, a new umbrella term—dietary reference intake (DRI)—includes three different measurements:

- ◆ The *Recommended Dietary Allowance (RDA)* is a scientifically established daily level of a nutrient known to meet the nutritional needs of as many as 98 percent of healthy individuals. One example of an RDA is the 90 mg per day of vitamin C recommended for healthy adult males.
- ◆ The *Adequate Intake (AI)* is a daily quantity assigned to nutrients for which there is not yet enough evidence to establish

an RDA. One example of an AI is the 1,200 mg per day of calcium recommended for healthy adult women older than 50.

◆ The *Tolerable Upper Intake Level (UL)* is the largest amount of a nutrient that can be taken each day that is considered safe for virtually all individuals of a specific age or gender. One example of a UL is the 10,000 IU per day of vitamin A considered the highest amount adults may consume on a daily basis.

However, it is wise to note that RDAs, AIs, and ULs, like many newly discovered links between food and health, are works in progress, subject to revision. Yes, the current adult UL for vitamin A is 10,000 IU per day, but some studies strongly suggest that taking as little as half that amount over long periods of time may increase the risk of osteoporosis in older people.

As a result, updating this book for a second edition that includes what's new, or, rather, newest, has meant not only following the studies, surveys and reports, but also keeping an eye open for the stray fact that pops up in totally unexpected place. For example, in July 2008 when my husband had blood drawn for testing before surgery, Michael-Angelo Cassa, the registered nurse who drew the sample, had a stack of pamphlets on his desk describing a connection between food allergies and latex allergy. Food and latex linked? Who knew? Now, thanks to Mr. Cassa and his handy pamphlets, I do—and so do you.

Think of a grapefruit. Think of an aspirin. Now think how similar they are.

Both can make you feel better: the aspirin by relieving a headache, the grapefruit by curing (or preventing) scurvy, a disease caused by a deficiency in vitamin C. Both have side effects (the aspirin may make your stomach bleed; the grapefruit may set off allergic sensitivity). Both interact with drugs (the aspirin with "blood-thinners," the grapefruit with—aspirin).

In fact, they're both health products.

There's nothing new in that, of course. Food has always been used as medicine. Ancient Romans sterilized wounds with wine. Ancient Egyptians used honey to speed healing. Aztecs regarded chocolate as an aphrodisiac. Jewish grandmothers cured colds with chicken soup. Italian grandmothers used olive oil liberally to keep their brood in trim.

What is new is that today we understand the science behind the folk remedy. Wine sterilizes with alcohol. Hydrophilic ("water loving") honey sops up liquids, kills bacteria, and nourishes new cell growth. Chocolate's methylxanthine stimulants (caffeine, theophylline, theobromine) are mood elevators. Steam from chicken soup (and the hot liquid itself) stimulates a flow of natural secretions to clear the nasal passages. Pasta has fiber and B vitamins, and olive oil is rich in heart-healthy monounsaturated fatty acids. In short, what was once folklore is now nutritional good sense. And that's the point of this book.

What You Will Find in This Book

The information in this book is organized into a series of entries arranged in alphabetical order. Most foods are described individually, but some are so similar in composition and effects that they are grouped together. For example, chives, leeks, scallions, and shallots are all grouped under ONIONS. So, if you don't find the food you are looking for as an individual entry, check the index.

Each entry begins with a *nutritional profile* summarizing the nutrient content of the food—energy (calories), protein, fat, carbohydrates, dietary fiber, sodium, and vitamins and minerals—based on data from the United States Department of Agriculture (USDA) National Nutrient Database for Standard Reference. NOTE: The *major vitamin contribution* and *major mineral contribution* subheadings tell you which vitamins and minerals are most prominent in the food being discussed but not necessarily whether the food provides significant amounts of the nutrient. For example, the most prominent vitamins in fresh garlic are vitamin C and thiamine (vitamin B_1), but we eat so little garlic that it's not considered a good source of these nutrients.

DEFINING LOW, MODERATE & HIGH

Energy value (calories per serving).

In a varied diet, a food that has less than 50 calories per 3.5 oz. (100-g) serving is *low* in calories. A food with 50 to 250 calories per serving is *moderate*. One with more than 250 calories per serving is *high*.

Proteins

A food that derives less than 5 percent of its calories from protein is *low* in protein. A food that derives 5 to 20 percent of its calories from proteins is *moderate*. A food that derives more than 20 percent of its calories from proteins is *high*.

Fat

Foods that derive less than 30 percent of their calories from fat are *low* in fat. Foods that derive 30 to 50 percent of their calories from fat are *moderate*. Foods that derive more than 50 percent of their calories from fat are *high*. NOTE: Fats have nine calories per gram, so a food with 30 percent of its calories from fat has about three grams fat per 100 calories. A food with 50 percent of its calories from fat has six grams fat per 100 calories. Food and Drug Administration (FDA) regulations permit any food product with less than three grams fat per serving, regardless of the total number of calories, to be labeled "low fat." The amount of fat given in the *nutritional profiles* is the total fat content, including saturated, polyunsaturated, and monounsaturated fatty acids.

Saturated fat

A food with less than 1 gram saturated fat per serving is *low;* one to two grams saturated fat per serving is *moderate;* more than two grams saturated fat per serving is *high*.

Cholesterol

A food that provides less than 20 milligrams of cholesterol per serving is *low* in cholesterol. A food that provides 20 to 150 milligrams per serving is *moderate*. A food that provides more than 150 milligrams per serving is *high*.

Carbohydrates

A food that derives less than 20 percent of its calories from carbohydrates—sugars, starch, and dietary fiber—is *low* in carbohydrates. A food that derives 20 to 60 percent of its calories from carbohydrates is *moderate*. A food that derives more than 60 percent of its calories from carbohydrates is *high*.

Dietary fiber

A food with less than 1 gram fiber per serving is *low* in fiber. A food with one to two grams fiber per serving is *moderate* in fiber. A food with two to five grams fiber per serving is *high*. A food with more than five grams fiber per serving is *very high*. *NOTE:* Except where noted, a serving of fiber is one-half cup.

Sodium

A food with less than 50 milligrams sodium per serving is *low* in sodium. A food with 50 to 125 milligrams sodium per serving is *moderate*. A food with more than 125 milligrams sodium per serving is *high*.

About the nutrients in this food is a more detailed nutritional guide. What kinds of fiber does the food contain? Are its fats primarily saturated fatty acids or unsaturated ones? Does it have high quality proteins, with sufficient amounts of all the essential amino acids, or are its proteins "limited," with insufficient amounts of one or more essential amino acids? Does the food contain antinutrients, such as the avidin in raw egg white that inactivates the nutrient biotin? Does it contain naturally occurring toxins such as solanine, the nerve poison in the green parts of potatoes or tomatoes? You'll find the answers to this kind of question here. By the way, you will often see the term "RDA" in any discussion of vitamins minerals, and other nutrients. The letters stand for *recommended dietary allowance*, the amount of the nutrient the National Research Council believes sufficient to prevent the onset of deficiency diseases (such as the vitamin C deficiency disease scurvy) in healthy people. IU, another nutritional abbreviation, stands for *international units*, a term used to describe quantities of vitamins A and D.

Unless otherwise noted, the RDAs (recommended dietary allowances) and AIs (adequate intakes) listed in this section are for healthy adults, men and women ages 19 to 50. The amounts of the nutrients and the percentages of the RDAs are rounded to one decimal place. That is, an amount of a nutrient or a percentage of the RDA that equals 0.45 or 1.45 will be shown, respectively, as 0.5 or 1.5.

The following two charts give you the RDAs and AIs for several important vitamins and minerals.

Vitamins
Recommended Dietary Allowances For Healthy Adults (2006)

Age (Years)	Vitamin A (RE*/IU)	Vitamin D (mcg/IU)	Vitamin E (alpha-TE)	Vitamin K (mcg)	Vitamin C (mg)
Males					
19–24	900/2,970	5/200	15	120	90
25–50	900/2,970	5/200	15	120	90
51–70	900/2,970	10/400	15	120	90
71+	900/2,970	15/600	15	120	90
Females					
19–24	700/2,310	5/200	15	90	75
25–50	700/2,310	5/200	15	90	75
51–70	700/2,310	10/400	15	90	75
71+	700/2,310	15/600	15	90	75

Age (Years)	Thiamin (Vitamin B_1) (mg)	Riboflavin (Vitamin B_2) (mg)	Niacin (mcg/NE**)	Vitamin B_6 (mg)	Folate (mcg)
Males					
19–24	1.2	1.3	16	1.3	400
25–50	1.2	1.3	16	1.3	400
51–70	1.2	1.3	16	1.7	400
71+	1.2	1.1	16	1.7	400
Females					
19–24	1.1	1.1	14	1.3	400
25–50	1.1	1.1	14	1.3	400
51–70	1.1	1.1	14	1.5	400
71+	1.1	1.1	14	1.5	400

Age (Years)	Pantothenic acid (mg)	Biotin (mcg)	Choline (mg)
Males			
19–24	5	30	550
25–50	5	30	550
51–70	5	30	550
71+	5	30	550

* Retinol equivalent; ** Niacin equivalent

Age (Years)	Pantothenic acid (mg)	Biotin (mcg)	Choline (mg)
Females			
19–24	5	30	425
25–50	5	30	425
51–70	5	30	425
71+	5	30	425

Major Minerals
Recommended Dietary Allowances For Healthy Adults (2006)

Age (Years)	Calcium (mg)	Phosphorus (mg)	Magnesium (mg)	Iron (mg)	Zinc (mg)	Iodine (mg)	Selenium (mg)
Males							
19–30	1,000	700	400	8	11	150	55
31–50	1,000	700	420	8	11	150	55
51–70	1,200	700	420	8	11	150	55
71+	1,200	700	420	8	11	150	55
Females							
19–30	1,000	700	310	18	8	150	55
31–50	1,000	700	320	18	8	150	55
51–70	1,000/1,500*	700	320	8	8	150	55
71+	1,000/1,500*	700	320	8	8	150	55

* The higher figure is for women taking postmenopausal estrogen supplements.

Source: Food and Nutrition Board, Institute of Medicine, National Academies of Science. Available online. URL: www.iom.edu/Object.File/Master/21/372/0.pdf.

Knowing *the most nutritious way to serve this food* can improve the quality of your meals. For example, the proteins in beans are limited in several amino acids abundant in grains. And vice versa. Serving beans and grains together "completes" their proteins, a clear nutritional bonus.

If you have a medical problem or are on a special diet, you should know about *diets that may restrict or exclude this food*. Remember: this list is only a guide. For more detailed personal advice, always check with your doctor.

Shopping smart requires you to pick the freshest, safest products when *buying this food*. You already know the basics (e.g., avoid yellowed lettuce). Here's the chemistry (e.g., as lettuce ages, its green chlorophyll fades, allowing its yellow carotenoid pigments to show through).

At home, your challenge is to keep food fresh. Some foods need to be refrigerated, others can be safely stashed in any cool, dry cabinet. Some require more than one method. Take tomatoes, for example. Vine-ripened ones not yet completely red will get juicier and tastier after a few days at room temperature. Artificially ripened ones (the "hard ripe" variety) will rot before they soften. Sort out the facts under *storing this food.*

Ready to eat? Then it's time to begin *preparing this food.* This section tells you how to handle food you are about to cook or serve. With the pertinent science, of course. For example: we tear greens at the very last minute to keep them crisp—and to prevent the loss of vitamin C when torn cells release the anti-C enzyme ascorbic acid oxidase. We beat egg whites in a copper bowl because copper ions flaking off the surface stabilize the egg foam. We slice raw onions under running water to dilute sulfur compounds that make our eyes water.

What happens when you cook this food? Lots. Heating crystallizes sugars and proteins to form a flavorful crust. Aroma molecules move more quickly to produce enticing aromas. Pigments combine with oxygen or other chemicals, turning brown or olive drab. These reactions are familiar; here's the "how" and "why."

And there's the question of *how other kinds of processing affect this food.* Processing often changes a food's texture, and it may alter the nutritional value. Defrosted frozen potatoes and carrots are usually mushy; canned vegetables have less vitamin C. Sometimes, processing even makes food potentially hazardous: Dried fruit treated with sulfur compounds may be life-threatening to people sensitive to sulfites.

This leads quite naturally to the *medical uses and/or benefits* of food. The information in this section comes from sources current as the book is written, but research in this area is so new and expanding so rapidly that it must always be regarded as a work in progress rather than a final conclusion. What you read here is a guide, not the last word. Ditto for *adverse effects associated with this food* and *food/drug interactions.*

In some entries you may find a series of asterisks (* * *) at one or more headings. The asterisks mean that right now, we may not be aware of information pertaining to the category for this food.

When you are done, I hope you come away with a larger store of information about your favorite foods and guidelines for evaluating them as individual health products, just like the medicines on your drugstore shelf.

Remember the grapefruit. Remember the aspirin. Remember how similar they are.

Carol Ann Rinzler

MEASUREMENTS USED IN THIS BOOK

RDA = recommended dietary allowance
g = gram
mg = milligram
mcg = microgram
1 gram = 1,000 milligrams
= 1,000,000 micrograms
IU = international unit
l = liter

ml = milliliter
1 liter = 1,000 milliliters
oz = ounce
1 ounce (solid) = 28 grams
1 ounce (liquid) = 30 milliliters

A Note to the Reader

The material in this book regarding the medical benefits or side effects of certain foods and the possible interactions between food and drugs is drawn from sources current at the time the book was written. It is for your information only and should never be substituted for your own doctor's advice or used without his or her consent. Your doctor, the person most familiar with your medical history and current health, is always the person best qualified to advise you on medical matters, including the use or avoidance of specific foods. Please note also that the adverse effects attributed to some of the foods listed here may not happen to everyone who eats the food or every time the food is served, another reason your own doctor is your best guide to your personal nutritional requirements.

Apples

Nutritional Profile

Energy value (calories per serving): *Low*
Protein: *Low*
Fat: *Low*
Saturated fat: *Low*
Cholesterol: *None*
Carbohydrates: *High*
Fiber: *High*
Sodium: *Low (fresh or dried fruit)*
      High (dried fruit treated with sodium sulfur compounds)
Major vitamin contribution: *Vitamin C*
Major mineral contribution: *Potassium*

About the Nutrients in This Food

Apples are a high-fiber fruit with insoluble cellulose and lignin in the peel and soluble pectins in the flesh. Their most important vitamin is vitamin C.

One fresh apple, 2.5 inches in diameter, has 2.4 g dietary fiber and 4.6 mg vitamin C (6 percent of the RDA for a woman, 5 percent of the RDA for a man).

The sour taste of all immature apples (and some varieties, even when ripe) comes from malic acid. As an apple ripens, the amount of malic acid declines and the apple becomes sweeter.

Apple seeds contain amygdalin, a naturally occurring cyanide/sugar compound that degrades into hydrogen cyanide. While accidentally swallowing an apple seed once in a while is not a serious hazard for an adult, cases of human poisoning after eating apple seeds have been reported, and swallowing only a few seeds may be lethal for a child.

The Most Nutritious Way to Serve This Food

Fresh and unpared, to take advantage of the fiber in the peel and preserve the vitamin C, which is destroyed by the heat of cooking.

Diets That May Restrict or Exclude This Food

Antiflatulence diet (raw apples)
Low-fiber diet

Buying This Food

Look for: Apples that are firm and brightly colored: shiny red Macintosh, Rome, and red Delicious; clear green Granny Smith; golden yellow Delicious.

Avoid: Bruised apples. When an apple is damaged the injured cells release polyphenoloxidase, an enzyme that hastens the oxidation of phenols in the apple, producing brownish pigments that darken the fruit. It's easy to check loose apples; if you buy them packed in a plastic bag, turn the bag upside down and examine the fruit.

Storing This Food

Store apples in the refrigerator. Cool storage keeps them from losing the natural moisture that makes them crisp. It also keeps them from turning brown inside, near the core, a phenomenon that occurs when apples are stored at warm temperatures. Apples can be stored in a cool, dark cabinet with plenty of circulating air.

   Check the apples from time to time. They store well, but the longer the storage, the greater the natural loss of moisture and the more likely the chance that even the crispest apple will begin to taste mealy.

Preparing This Food

Don't peel or slice an apple until you are ready to use it. When you cut into the apple, you tear its cells, releasing polyphenoloxidase, an enzyme that darkens the fruit. Acid inactivates polyphenoloxidase, so you can slow the browning (but not stop it completely) by dipping raw sliced and/or peeled apples into a solution of lemon juice and water or vinegar and water or by mixing them with citrus fruits in a fruit salad. Polyphenoloxidase also works more slowly in the cold, but storing peeled apples in the refrigerator is much less effective than immersing them in an acid bath.

What Happens When You Cook This Food

When you cook an unpeeled apple, insoluble cellulose and lignin will hold the peel intact through all normal cooking. The flesh of the apple, though, will fall apart as the pectin in its cell walls dissolves and the water inside its cells swells, rupturing the cell walls and turning the apples into applesauce. Commercial bakers keep the apples in their apple pies firm by treating them with calcium; home bakers have to rely on careful timing. To prevent baked apples from melting into mush, core the apple and fill the center with sugar or raisins to absorb the moisture released as the apple cooks. Cutting away a circle of peel at the top will allow the fruit to swell without splitting the skin.

Red apple skins are colored with red anthocyanin pigments. When an apple is cooked, the anthocyanins combine with sugars to form irreversible brownish compounds.

How Other Kinds of Processing Affect This Food

Juice.   Apple juice comes in two versions: "cloudy" (unfiltered) and "clear" (filtered). Cloudy apple juice is made simply by chopping or shredding apples and then pressing out and straining the juice. Clear apple juice is cloudy juice filtered to remove solid particles and then treated with enzymes to eliminate starches and the soluble fiber pectin. Since 2000, following several deaths attributed to unpasteurized apple juice contaminated with *E. coli* O157: H7, the FDA has required that all juices sold in the United States be pasteurized to inactivate harmful organisms such as bacteria and mold. *Note*: "Hard cider" is a mildly alcoholic beverage created when natural enzyme action converts the sugars in apple juice to alcohol; "non-alcohol cider" is another name for plain apple juice.

Drying.   To keep apple slices from turning brown as they dry, apples may be treated with sulfur compounds that may cause serious allergic reactions in people allergic to sulfites.

Medical Uses and/or Benefits

As an antidiarrheal.   The pectin in apple is a natural antidiarrheal that helps solidify stool. Shaved raw apple is sometimes used as a folk remedy for diarrhea, and purified pectin is an ingredient in many over-the-counter antidiarrheals.

Lower cholesterol levels.   Soluble fiber (pectin) may interfere with the absorption of dietary fats, including cholesterol. The exact mechanism by which this occurs is still unknown, but one theory is that the pectins in the apple may form a gel in your stomach that sops up fats and cholesterol, carrying them out of your body as waste.

Potential anticarcinogenic effects.   A report in the April 2008 issue of the journal *Nutrition* from a team of researchers at the University of Kaiserslautern, in Germany, suggests that several natural chemicals in apples, including butyrate (produced naturally when the pectin in apples and apple juice is metabolized) reduce the risk of cancer of the colon by nourishing and protecting the mucosa (lining) of the colon.

Adverse Effects Associated with This Food

Intestinal gas.   For some children, drinking excess amounts of apple juice produces intestinal discomfort (gas or diarrhea) when bacteria living naturally in the stomach ferment the sugars in the juice. To reduce this problem, the American Academy of Pediatrics recommends that children ages one to six consume no more than four to six ounces of fruit juice a day; for children ages seven to 18, the recommended serving is eight to 12 ounces a day.

Cyanide poisoning.   See *About the nutrients in this food.*

Sulfite allergies (dried apples).   See *How other kinds of processing affect this food.*

Food/Drug Interactions

Digoxin (Lanoxicaps, Lanoxin).   Pectins may bind to the heart medication digoxin, so eating apples at the same time you take the drug may reduce the drug's effectiveness.

Apricots

Nutritional Profile

Energy value (calories per serving): *Low*
Protein: *Moderate*
Fat: *Low*
Saturated fat: *Low*
Cholesterol: *None*
Carbohydrates: *High*
Fiber: *High*
Sodium: *Low (fresh or dried fruit)*
        High (dried fruit treated with sodium sulfur compounds)
Major vitamin contribution: *Vitamin A*
Major mineral contribution: *Iron*

About the Nutrients in This Food

Apricots are a good source of dietary fiber with insoluble cellulose and lignin in the skin and soluble pectins in the flesh. The apricot's creamy golden color comes from deep yellow carotenes (including beta-carotene) that make the fruit a good source of vitamin A. Apricots also have vitamin C and iron.

One apricot has 0.7 g dietary fiber, 674 IU vitamin A (21 percent of the RDA for a woman, 23 percent of the RDA for a man), and 3.5 mg vitamin C (5 percent of the RDA for a woman, 4 percent of the RDA for a man). Two dried apricot halves provide 0.6 g dietary fiber, 252 IU vitamin A (11 percent of the RDA for a woman, 8 percent of the RDA for a man), no vitamin C, and 2 mg iron (11 percent of the RDA for a woman, 25 percent of the RDA for a man).

The bark, leaves, and inner stony pit of the apricot all contain amygdalin, a naturally occurring compound that degrades to release hydrogen cyanide (prussic acid) in your stomach. Apricot oil, treated during processing to remove the cyanide, is marked FFPA to show that it is "free from prussic acid." Cases of fatal poisoning from apricot pits have been reported, including one in a three-year-old girl who ate 15 apricot kernels (the seed inside the pit). Extract of apricot pits, known medically as Laetrile, has been used by some alternative practitioners to treat cancer on the theory that the cyanide in amygdalin is released only when it comes in contact with beta-glucuronidase, an enzyme common to tumor cells. Scientifically designed tests of amygdalin have not shown this to be true. Laetrile is illegal in the United States.

The Most Nutritious Way to Serve This Food

Ounce for ounce, dried apricots are richer in nutrients and fiber than fresh ones.

Diets That May Restrict or Exclude This Food

Low-fiber diet
Low-potassium diet
Low-sodium diet (dried apricots containing sodium sulfide)

Buying This Food

Look for: Firm, plump orange fruit that gives slightly when you press with your thumb.

Avoid: Bruised apricots. Like apples and potatoes, apricots contain polyphenoloxidase, an enzyme that combines with phenols in the apricots to produce brownish pigments that discolor the fruit. When apricots are bruised, cells are broken, releasing the enzyme so that brown spots form under the bruise.

Avoid apricots that are hard or mushy or withered; all are less flavorsome than ripe, firm apricots, and the withered ones will decay quickly.

Avoid greenish apricots; they are low in carotenes and will never ripen satisfactorily at home.

Storing This Food

Store ripe apricots in the refrigerator and use them within a few days. Apricots do not lose their vitamin A in storage, but they are very perishable and rot fairly quickly.

Preparing This Food

When you peel or slice an apricot, you tear its cells walls, releasing polyphenoloxidase, an enzyme that reacts with phenols in the apricots, producing brown compounds that darken the fruit. Acids inactivate polyphenoloxidase, so you can slow down this reaction (but not stop it completely) by dipping raw sliced and/or peeled apricots into a solution of lemon juice or vinegar and water or by mixing them with citrus fruits in a fruit salad. Polyphenoloxidase also works more slowly in the cold, but storing peeled apricots in the refrigerator is much less effective than an acid bath.

To peel apricots easily, drop them into boiling water for a minute or two, then lift them out with a slotted spoon and plunge them into cold water. As with tomatoes, this works because the change in temperature damages a layer of cells under the skin so the skin slips off easily.

What Happens When You Cook This Food

Cooking dissolves pectin, the primary fiber in apricots, and softens the fruit. But it does not change the color or lower the vitamin A content because carotenes are impervious to the heat of normal cooking.

How Other Kinds of Processing Affect This Food

Juice.   Since 2000, following several deaths attributed to unpasteurized apple juice contaminated with *E. coli* O157:H7, the FDA has required that all juices sold in the United States be pasteurized to inactivate harmful organisms such as bacteria and mold.

Drying.   Five pounds of fresh apricots produce only a pound of dried ones. Drying removes water, not nutrients; ounce for ounce, dried apricots have 12 times the iron, seven times the fiber, and five times the vitamin A of the fresh fruit. Three and a half ounces of dried apricots provide 12,700 IU vitamin A, two and a half times the full daily requirement for a healthy adult man, and 6.3 mg of iron, one-third the daily requirement for an adult woman. In some studies with laboratory animals, dried apricots have been as effective as liver, kidneys, and eggs in treating iron-deficiency anemia.

To keep them from turning brown as they dry, apricots may be treated with sulfur dioxide. This chemical may cause serious allergic reactions, including anaphylactic shock, in people who are sensitive to sulfites.

Medical Uses and/or Benefits

* * *

Adverse Effects Associated with This Food

Sulfite allergies.   See *How other kinds of processing affect this food.*

Food/Drug Interactions

* * *

Artichoke, Globe

Nutritional Profile

Energy value (calories per serving): *Low*

Protein: *Moderate*

Fat: *Low*

Saturated fat: *Low*

Cholesterol: *None*

Carbohydrates: *High*

Fiber: *Low*

Sodium: *Moderate to high*

Major vitamin contribution: *Vitamin C*

Major mineral contribution: *Potassium*

About the Nutrients in This Food

Globe artichokes are prickly plants with partly edible leaves enclosing a tasty "heart." Their most important nutrients are vitamin C and iron.

One medium boiled artichoke has 10.3 g dietary fiber, 8.9 mg vitamin C (12 percent of the RDA for a woman, 10 percent of the RDA for a man), and 0.7 mg iron (4 percent of the RDA for a woman, 9 percent of the RDA for a man).

One-half cup artichoke hearts has 7.2 g dietary fiber, 6.2 mg vitamin C (8 percent of the RDA for a woman, 7 percent of the RDA for a man), and 0.5 mg iron (3 percent of the RDA for a woman, 6 percent of the RDA for a man).

Raw globe artichokes contain an enzyme that interferes with protein digestion; cooking inactivates the enzyme.

The Most Nutritious Way to Serve This Food

Cooked.

Diets That May Restrict or Exclude This Food

* * *

Buying This Food

Look for: Compact vegetables, heavy for their size. The leaves should be tightly closed, but the color changes with the season—bright green in the spring, olive green or bronze in the winter if they have been exposed to frost.

Avoid: Artichokes with yellowed leaves, which indicate the artichoke is aging (the chlorophyll in its leaves has faded so the yellow carotenes underneath show through).

Storing This Food

Do   refrigerate fresh globe artichokes in plastic bags.

Do   refrigerate cooked globe artichokes in a covered container if you plan to hold them longer than a day or two.

Preparing This Food

Cut off the stem. Trim the tough outer leaves. Then plunge the artichoke, upside down, into a bowl of cold water to flush out debris. To remove the core, put the artichoke upside down on a cutting board and cut out the center. Slicing into the base of the artichoke rips cell walls and releases polyphenoloxidase, an enzyme that converts phenols in the vegetable to brown compounds that darken the "heart" of the globe. To slow the reaction, paint the cut surface with a solution of lemon juice or vinegar and water.

What Happens When You Cook This Food

Chlorophyll, the green plant pigment, is sensitive to acids. When you heat a globe artichoke, the chlorophyll in its green leaves reacts with acids in the artichoke or in the cooking water, forming brown pheophytin. The pheophytin, plus yellow carotenes in the leaves, can turn a cooked artichoke's leaves bronze. To prevent this reaction, cook the artichoke very quickly so there is no time for the chlorophyll to react with the acid, or cook it in lots of water to dilute the acids, or cook it with the lid off the pot so that the volatile acids can float off into the air.

How Other Kinds of Processing Affect This Food

Canning.   Globe artichoke hearts packed in brine are higher in sodium than fresh artichokes. Artichoke hearts packed in oil are much higher in fat.

Freezing.   Frozen artichoke hearts are comparable in nutritional value to fresh ones.

Medical Uses and/or Benefits

Anti-inflammatory action.   In 2006, a report in the *Journal of the Pharmaceutical Society of Japan* suggested that cynarin might be beneficial in lowering blood levels of cholesterol and that cynaropicrin, a form of cynarin found in artichoke leaves, might act as an anti-inflammatory agent, protecting the skin from sun damage, improving liver function, and reducing the effects of stress-related gastritis.

Reduced levels of cholesterol.   In 2008, researchers at the University of Reading (United Kingdom) published a report in the journal *Phytomedicine* detailing the results of a 150-person study suggesting that an over-the-counter herbal supplement containing extract of globe artichoke leaf lowers cholesterol in healthy people with moderately raised cholesterol readings. In the study, 75 volunteers were given 1,280 mg of the herbal supplement each day for 12 weeks; a control group got a placebo (a look-alike pill without the herbal supplement). At the end of the trial, those who took the artichoke leaf extract experienced an average 4.2 percent decrease in cholesterol levels, a result the researchers deemed "modest but significant."

Adverse Effects Associated with This Food

Contact dermatitis.   Globe artichokes contain essential oils that may cause contact dermatitis in sensitive people.

Alterations in the sense of taste.   Globe artichokes contain cynarin, a sweet tasting chemical that dissolves in water (including the saliva in your mouth) to sweeten the flavor of anything you eat next.

Food/Drug Interactions

False-positive test for occult blood in the stool.   The guaiac slide test for hidden blood in feces relies on alphaguaiaconic acid, a chemical that turns blue in the presence of blood. Artichokes contain peroxidase, a natural chemical that also turns alphaguaiaconic acid blue and may produce a positive test in people who do not have blood in the stool.

Artichoke, Jerusalem

(Sunchoke)

Nutritional Profile

Energy value (calories per serving): *Low*
Protein: *Moderate*
Fat: *Low*
Saturated fat: *Low*
Cholesterol: *None*
Carbohydrates: *High*
Fiber: *High*
Sodium: *Moderate*
Major vitamin contribution: *Folate, vitamin C*
Major mineral contribution: *Potassium*

About the Nutrients in This Food

Jerusalem artichokes are the edible roots of a plant related to the American sunflower. They store carbohydrates as inulin, a complex carbohydrate (starch) made of units of fruit sugar (fructose). Right after the Jerusalem artichoke is dug up, it tastes bland and starchy. After it has been stored for a while, the starches turn to sugars, so the artichoke tastes sweet. Jerusalem artichokes are high in fiber with the B vitamin folate, vitamin C, and iron.

One-half cup raw sliced Jerusalem artichoke has one gram dietary fiber, 10 mcg folate (2.5 percent of the adult RDA), 3 mcg vitamin C (4 percent of the RDA for a woman, 3 percent of the RDA for a man), and 2.5 mg iron (14 percent of the RDA for a woman, 32 percent of the RDA for a man).

The Most Nutritious Way to Serve This Food

Sliced and served raw in salads or cooked as a vegetable side dish.

Diets That May Restrict or Exclude This Food

Low-sodium diet

Buying This Food

Look for: Firm clean roots with no soft or bruised patches.

Storing This Food

Refrigerate Jerusalem artichokes in plastic bags, covered containers or the vegetable crisper to protect their moisture and keep them fresh.

Preparing This Food

When you slice a Jerusalem artichoke, you tear cell walls, releasing polyphenoloxidase, an enzyme that converts phenols to brown compounds that darken the flesh. You can slow the reaction (but not stop it completely) by painting the cut surface with a solution of lemon juice or vinegar and water.

What Happens When You Cook This Food

In cooking, the starch granules in the Jerusalem artichoke absorb water, swell, and eventually rupture, softening the root and releasing the nutrients inside.

How Other Kinds of Processing Affect This Food

* * *

Medical Uses and/or Benefits

* * *

Adverse Effects Associated with This Food

Some people are unable to properly digest inulin, the carbohydrate in the Jerusalem artichoke. For them, eating this tuber raw may cause painful gas. Cooking breaks down inulin and improves digestibility.

Food/Drug Interactions

* * *

Asparagus

Nutritional Profile

Energy value (calories per serving): *Low*
Protein: *High*
Fat: *Low*
Saturated fat: *Low*
Cholesterol: *None*
Carbohydrates: *Moderate*
Fiber: *Moderate*
Sodium: *Low*
Major vitamin contribution: *Vitamin A, folate, vitamin C*
Major mineral contribution: *Potassium, iron*

About the Nutrients in This Food

Asparagus has some dietary fiber, vitamin A, and vitamin C. It is an excellent source of the B vitamin folate.

A serving of four cooked asparagus spears (½ inch wide at the base) has 1.2 g dietary fiber, 604 IU vitamin A (26 percent of the RDA for a woman, 20 percent of the RDA for a man), 4.5 mg vitamin C (6 percent of the RDA for a woman, 5 percent of the RDA for a man), and 89 mcg folate (22 percent of the RDA).

The Most Nutritious Way to Serve This Food

Fresh, boiled and drained. Canned asparagus may have less than half the nutrients found in freshly cooked spears.

Diets That May Restrict or Exclude This Food

Low-sodium diet (canned asparagus)

Buying This Food

Look for: Bright green stalks. The tips should be purplish and tightly closed; the stalks should be firm. Asparagus is in season from March through August.

Avoid: Wilted stalks and asparagus whose buds have opened.

Storing This Food

Store fresh asparagus in the refrigerator. To keep it as crisp as possible, wrap it in a damp paper towel and then put the whole package into a plastic bag. Keeping asparagus cool helps it hold onto its vitamins. At 32°F, asparagus will retain all its folic acid for at least two weeks and nearly 80 percent of its vitamin C for up to five days; at room temperature, it would lose up to 75 percent of its folic acid in three days and 50 percent of the vitamin C in 24 hours.

Preparing This Food

The white part of the fresh green asparagus stalk is woody and tasteless, so you can bend the stalk and snap it right at the line where the green begins to turn white. If the skin is very thick, peel it, but save the parings for soup stock.

What Happens When You Cook This Food

Chlorophyll, the pigment that makes green vegetables green, is sensitive to acids. When you heat asparagus, its chlorophyll will react chemically with acids in the asparagus or in the cooking water to form pheophytin, which is brown. As a result, cooked asparagus is olive-drab.

You can prevent this chemical reaction by cooking the asparagus so quickly that there is no time for the chlorophyll to react with acids, or by cooking it in lots of water (which will dilute the acids), or by leaving the lid off the pot so that the volatile acids can float off into the air.

Cooking also changes the texture of asparagus: water escapes from its cells and they collapse. Adding salt to the cooking liquid slows the loss of moisture.

How Other Kinds of Processing Affect This Food

Canning. The intense heat of canning makes asparagus soft, robs it of its bright green color, and reduces the vitamin A, B, and C content by at least half. (White asparagus, which is bleached to remove the green color, contains about 5 percent of the vitamin A in fresh asparagus.) With its liquid, canned asparagus, green or white, contains about 90 times the sodium in fresh asparagus (348 mg in 3.5 oz. canned against 4 mg in 3.5 oz. fresh boiled asparagus).

Medical Uses and/or Benefits

Lower risk of some birth defects. As many as two of every 1,000 babies born in the United States each year may have cleft palate or a neural tube (spinal cord) defect due to their mothers' not having gotten adequate amounts of folate during pregnancy. The RDA for folate is

400 mcg for healthy adult men and women, 600 mcg for pregnant women, and 500 mcg for women who are nursing. Taking folate supplements before becoming pregnant and through the first two months of pregnancy reduces the risk of cleft palate; taking folate through the entire pregnancy reduces the risk of neural tube defects.

Lower risk of heart attack.   In the spring of 1998, an analysis of data from the records for more than 80,000 women enrolled in the long-running Nurses' Health Study at Harvard School of Public Health/Brigham and Woman's Hospital, in Boston, demonstrated that a diet providing more than 400 mcg folate and 3 mg vitamin B_6 daily, from either food or supplements, more than twice the current RDA for each, may reduce a woman's risk of heart attack by almost 50 percent. Although men were not included in the analysis, the results are assumed to apply to them as well.

However, data from a meta-analysis published in the *Journal of the American Medical Association* in December 2006 called this theory into question. Researchers at Tulane University examined the results of 12 controlled studies in which 16,958 patients with preexisting cardiovascular disease were given either folic acid supplements or placebos ("look-alike" pills with no folic acid) for at least six months. The scientists, who found no reduction in the risk of further heart disease or overall death rates among those taking folic acid, concluded that further studies will be required to verify whether taking folic acid supplements reduces the risk of cardiovascular disease.

Adverse Effects Associated with This Food

Odorous urine.   After eating asparagus, we all excrete the sulfur compound methyl mercaptan, a smelly waste product, in our urine.

Food/Drug Interactions

Anticoagulants.   Asparagus is high in vitamin K, a vitamin manufactured naturally by bacteria in our intestines, an adequate supply of which enables blood to clot normally. Eating foods that contain this vitamin may interfere with the effectiveness of anticoagulants such as heparin and warfarin (Coumadin, Dicumarol, Panwarfin) whose job is to thin blood and dissolve clots.

Avocados

Nutritional Profile

Energy value (calories per serving): *Moderate*

Protein: *Low*

Fat: *High*

Saturated fat: *High*

Cholesterol: *None*

Carbohydrates: *Moderate*

Fiber: *High to very high*

Sodium: *Low*

Major vitamin contribution: *Vitamins A, folate, vitamin C*

Major mineral contribution: *Potassium*

About the Nutrients in This Food

The avocado is an unusual fruit because about 16 percent of its total weight is fat, primarily monounsaturated fatty acids. Like many other fruits, avocados are high in fiber (the Florida avocado is very high in fiber), a good source of the B vitamin folate, vitamin C, and potassium.

The edible part of half of one average size avocado (100 g/3.5 ounces) provides 6.7 g dietary fiber, 15 g fat (2.1 g saturated fat, 9.7 g monounsaturated fat, 1.8 g polyunsaturated fat), 81 mcg folate (20 percent of the RDA), 20 mg vitamin C (26 percent of the RDA for a woman, 22 percent for a man), and 485 mg potassium (the equivalent of one eight-ounce cup of fresh orange juice).

The edible part of one-half a Florida avocado (a.k.a. alligator pear) has eight grams dietary fiber, 13.5 g fat (2.65 g saturated fat), 81 mcg folate (41 percent of the RDA for a man, 45 percent of the RDA for a woman), 12 mg vitamin C (20 percent of the RDA), and 741 mg potassium, 50 percent more than one cup fresh orange juice.

Diets That May Exclude or Restrict This Food

Controlled-potassium diet

Low-fat diet

Buying This Food

Look for: Fruit that feels heavy for its size. The avocados most commonly sold in the U.S. are the Hass—a purple-black bumpy fruit that accounts for 85 percent of the avocados shipped from California—and the smooth-skinned Florida avocado ("alligator pear"). The California Avocado Commission lists several more on its Web site (http://www.avocado. org/about/varieties): the oval, midwinter Bacon; the pear-shaped, late-fall Fuerte; the Gwen, a slightly larger Hass; Pinkerton, pear-shaped with a smaller seed; the round summer Reed; and the yellow-green, pear-shaped Zutano.

Avoid: Avocados with soft dark spots on the skin that indicate damage underneath.

Storing This Food

Store hard, unripened avocados in a warm place; a bowl on top of the refrigerator will do. Avocados are shipped before they ripen, when the flesh is hard enough to resist bruising in transit, but they ripen off the tree and will soften nicely at home.

Store soft, ripe avocados in the refrigerator to slow the natural enzyme action that turns their flesh brown as they mature even when the fruit has not been cut.

Preparing This Food

When you peel or slice an avocado, you tear its cell walls, releasing polyphenoloxidase, an enzyme that converts phenols in the avocado to brownish compounds that darken the avocado's naturally pale green flesh. You can slow this reaction (but not stop it completely) by brushing the exposed surface of the avocado with an acid (lemon juice or vinegar). To store a cut avocado, brush it with lemon juice or vinegar, wrap it tightly in plastic, and keep it in the refrigerator—where it will eventually turn brown. Or you can store the avocado as guacamole; mixing it with lemon juice, tomatoes, onions, and mayonnaise (all of which are acidic) is an efficient way to protect the color of the fruit.

What Happens When You Cook This Food

* * *

How Other Kinds of Processing Affect This Food

* * *

Medical Uses and/or Benefits

Lower risk of some birth defects. As many as two of every 1,000 babies born in the United States each year may have cleft palate or a neural tube (spinal cord) defect due to their mothers' not having gotten adequate amounts of folate during pregnancy. The current RDA for folate is 180 mcg for a healthy woman and 200 mcg for a healthy man, but the FDA now recommends 400 mcg for a woman who is or may become pregnant. Taking folate supplements before becoming pregnant and through the first two months of pregnancy reduces the risk of cleft palate; taking folate through the entire pregnancy reduces the risk of neural tube defects.

Lower risk of heart attack. In the spring of 1998, an analysis of data from the records for more than 80,000 women enrolled in the long-running Nurses' Health Study at Harvard School of Public Health/Brigham and Woman's Hospital, in Boston, demonstrated that a diet providing more than 400 mcg folate and 3 mg vitamin B_6 daily, from either food or supplements, more than twice the current RDA for each, may reduce a woman's risk of heart attack by almost 50 percent. Although men were not included in the analysis, the results are assumed to apply to them as well.

However, data from a meta-analysis published in the *Journal of the American Medical Association* in December 2006 called this theory into question. Researchers at Tulane University examined the results of 12 controlled studies in which 16,958 patients with preexisting cardiovascular disease were given either folic acid supplements or placebos ("look-alike" pills with no folic acid) for at least six months. The scientists, who found no reduction in the risk of further heart disease or overall death rates among those taking folic acid, concluded that further studies will be required to ascertain whether taking folic acid supplements reduces the risk of cardiovascular disease.

Lower levels of cholesterol. Avocados are rich in oleic acid, a monounsaturated fat believed to reduce cholesterol levels.

Potassium benefits. Because potassium is excreted in urine, potassium-rich foods are often recommended for people taking diuretics. In addition, a diet rich in potassium (from food) is associated with a lower risk of stroke. A 1998 Harvard School of Public Health analysis of data from the long-running Health Professionals Study shows 38 percent fewer strokes among men who ate nine servings of high potassium foods a day vs. those who ate less than four servings. Among men with high blood pressure, taking a daily 1,000 mg potassium supplement—about the amount of potassium in one avocado—reduced the incidence of stroke by 60 percent.

Adverse Effects Associated with This Food

Latex-fruit syndrome. Latex is a milky fluid obtained from the rubber tree and used to make medical and surgical products such as condoms and protective latex gloves, as well as rubber bands, balloons, and toys; elastic used in clothing; pacifiers and baby-bottle nipples; chewing gum; and various adhesives. Some of the proteins in latex are allergenic, known to cause reactions ranging from mild to potentially life-threatening. Some of the proteins found naturally in latex also occur naturally in foods from plants such as avocados, bananas, chestnuts, kiwi fruit, tomatoes, and food and diet sodas sweetened with aspartame. Persons sensitive to these foods are likely to be sensitive to latex as well. NOTE: The National Institute of Health Sciences, in Japan, also lists the following foods as suspect: Almonds, apples, apricots, bamboo shoots, bell peppers, buckwheat, cantaloupe, carrots, celery, cherries, chestnuts, coconut, figs, grapefruit, lettuce, loquat, mangoes, mushrooms, mustard, nectarines, oranges, passion fruit, papaya, peaches, peanuts, peppermint, pineapples, potatoes, soybeans, strawberries, walnuts, and watermelon.

Food/Drug Interactions

MAO inhibitors.   Monoamine oxidase (MAO) inhibitors are drugs used as antidepressants or antihypertensives. They inhibit the action of enzymes that break down the amino acid tyramine so it can be eliminated from the body. Tyramine is a pressor amine, a chemical that constricts blood vessels and raises blood pressure. If you eat a food such as avocado that contains tyramine while you are taking an MAO inhibitor you cannot eliminate the pressor amine, and the result may be abnormally high blood pressure or a hypertensive crisis (sustained elevated blood pressure).

False-positive test for tumors.   Carcinoid tumors (which may arise from tissues in the endocrine system, the intestines, or the lungs) secrete serotonin, a natural chemical that makes blood vessels expand or contract. Because serotonin is excreted in urine, these tumors are diagnosed by measuring the levels of serotonin by-products in the urine. Avocados contain large amounts of serotonin; eating them in the three days before a test for an endocrine tumor might produce a false-positive result, suggesting that you have the tumor when in fact you don't. (Other foods high in serotonin are bananas, eggplant, pineapples, plums, tomatoes, and walnuts.)

Bananas

Nutritional Profile

Energy value (calories per serving): *Moderate*
Protein: *Low*
Fat: *Low*
Saturated fat: *Low*
Cholesterol: *None*
Carbohydrates: *High*
Fiber: *Moderate*
Sodium: *Low*
Major vitamin contribution: *B vitamins, vitamin C*
Major mineral contribution: *Potassium, magnesium*

About the Nutrients in This Food

A banana begins life with more starch than sugar, but as the fruit ripens
its starches turn to sugar, which is why ripe bananas taste so much better
than unripe ones.* The color of a banana's skin is a fair guide to its starch/
sugar ratio. When the skin is yellow-green, 40 percent of its carbohydrates
are starch; when the skin is fully yellow and the banana is ripe, only 8 percent of the carbohydrates are still starch. The rest (91 percent) have broken
down into sugars—glucose, fructose, sucrose, the most plentiful sugar in
the fruit. Its high sugar content makes the banana, in its self-contained
packet, a handy energy source.

Bananas are a high-fiber food with insoluble cellulose and lignin in
the tiny seeds and soluble pectins in the flesh. They are also a good source
of vitamin C and potassium.

One small (six-inch) banana or a half-cup of sliced banana has 2.6 g
dietary fiber and 8.8 mg vitamin C (12 percent of the RDA for a woman,
10 percent of the RDA for a man), plus 363 mg potassium.

The Most Nutritious Way to Serve This Food

Fresh and ripe. Green bananas contain antinutrients, proteins that inhibit
the actions of amylase, an enzyme that makes it possible for us to digest

---

* They are also more healthful. Green bananas contain proteins that inhibit amylase, an enzyme that makes it possible for us to digest complex carbohydrates.

starch and other complex carbohydrates. Raw bananas are richer in potassium than cooked bananas; heating depletes potassium.

Diets That May Restrict or Exclude This Food

* * *

Buying This Food

Look for: Bananas that will be good when you plan to eat them. Bananas with brown specks on the skin are ripe enough to eat immediately. Bananas with creamy yellow skin will be ready in a day or two. Bananas with mostly yellow skin and a touch of green at either end can be ripened at home and used in two or three days.

Avoid: Overripe bananas whose skin has turned brown or split open. A grayish yellow skin means that the fruit has been damaged by cold storage. Bananas with soft spots under the skin may be rotten.

Storing This Food

Store bananas that aren't fully ripe at room temperature for a day or two. Like avocados, bananas are picked green, shipped hard to protect them from damage en route and then sprayed with ethylene gas to ripen them quickly. Untreated bananas release ethylene naturally to ripen the fruit and turn its starches to sugar, but natural ripening takes time. Artificial ripening happens so quickly that there is no time for the starches to turn into sugar. The bananas look ripe but they may taste bland and starchy. A few days at room temperature will give the starches a chance to change into sugars.

Store ripe bananas in the refrigerator. The cold air will slow (but not stop) the natural enzyme action that ripens and eventually rots the fruit if you leave it at room temperature. Cold storage will darken the banana's skin, since the chill damages cells in the peel and releases polyphenoloxidase, an enzyme that converts phenols in the banana peel to dark brown compounds, but the fruit inside will remain pale and tasty for several days.

Preparing This Food

Do not slice or peel bananas until you are ready to use them. When you cut into the fruit, you tear its cell walls, releasing polyphenoloxidase, an enzyme that hastens the oxidation of phenols in the banana, producing brown pigments that darken the fruit. (Chilling a banana produces the same reaction because the cold damages cells in the banana peel.) You can slow the browning (but not stop it completely) by dipping raw sliced or peeled bananas into a solution of lemon juice or vinegar and water or by mixing the slices with citrus fruits in a fruit salad. Overripe, discolored bananas can be used in baking, where the color doesn't matter and their intense sweetness is an asset.

What Happens When You Cook This Food

When bananas are broiled or fried, they are cooked so quickly that there is very little change in color or texture. Even so, they will probably taste sweeter and have a more intense aroma than uncooked bananas. Heat liberates the volatile molecules that make the fruit taste and smell good.

How Other Kinds of Processing Affect This Food

Drying. Drying removes water and concentrates the nutrients and calories in bananas. Bananas may be treated with compounds such as sulfur dioxide to inhibit polyphenoloxidase and keep the bananas from browning as they dry. People who are sensitive to sulfites may suffer severe allergic reactions, including anaphylactic shock, if they eat these treated bananas.

Freezing. Fresh bananas freeze well but will brown if you try to thaw them at room temperature. To protect the creamy color, thaw frozen bananas in the refrigerator and use as quickly as possible.

Medical Uses and/or Benefits

Lower risk of stroke. Various nutrition studies have attested to the power of adequate potassium to keep blood pressure within safe levels. For example, in the 1990s, data from the long-running Harvard School of Public Health/Health Professionals Follow-Up Study of male doctors showed that a diet rich in high-potassium foods such as bananas, oranges, and plantain may reduce the risk of stroke. In the study, the men who ate the higher number of potassium-rich foods (an average of nine servings a day) had a risk of stroke 38 percent lower than that of men who consumed fewer than four servings a day. In 2008, a similar survey at the Queen's Medical Center (Honolulu) showed a similar protective effect among men and women using diuretic drugs (medicines that increase urination and thus the loss of potassium).

Improved mood. Bananas and plantains are both rich in serotonin, dopamine, and other natural mood-elevating neurotransmitters—natural chemicals that facilitate the transmission of impulses along nerve cells.

Potassium benefits. Because potassium is excreted in urine, potassium-rich foods are often recommended for people taking diuretics. In addition, a diet rich in potassium (from food) is associated with a lower risk of stroke. A 1998 Harvard School of Public Health analysis of data from the long-running Health Professionals Study shows 38 percent fewer strokes among men who ate nine servings of high potassium foods a day vs. those who ate less than four servings. Among men with high blood pressure, taking a daily 1,000 mg potassium supplement—about the amount of potassium in one banana—reduced the incidence of stroke by 60 percent.

Adverse Effects Associated with This Food

Digestive Problems.   Unripe bananas contain proteins that inhibit the actions of amylase, an enzyme required to digest starch and other complex carbohydrates.

Sulfite allergies.   See *How other kinds of processing affect this food.*

Latex-fruit syndrome.   Latex is a milky fluid obtained from the rubber tree and used to make medical and surgical products such as condoms and protective latex gloves, as well as rubber bands, balloons, and toys; elastic used in clothing; pacifiers and baby bottle-nipples; chewing gum; and various adhesives. Some of the proteins in latex are allergenic, known to cause reactions ranging from mild to potentially life-threatening. Some of the proteins found naturally in latex also occur naturally in foods from plants such as avocados, bananas, chestnuts, kiwi fruit, tomatoes, and food and diet sodas sweetened with aspartame. Persons sensitive to these foods are likely to be sensitive to latex as well. NOTE: The National Institute of Health Sciences, in Japan, also lists the following foods as suspect: Almonds, apples, apricots, bamboo shoots, bell peppers, buckwheat, cantaloupe, carrots, celery, cherries, chestnuts, coconut, figs, grapefruit, lettuce, loquat, mangoes, mushrooms, mustard, nectarines, oranges, passion fruit, papaya, peaches, peanuts, peppermint, pineapples, potatoes, soybeans, strawberries, walnuts, and watermelon.

Food/Drug Interactions

Monoamine oxidase (MAO) inhibitors.   Monoamine oxidase inhibitors are drugs used to treat depression. They inactivate naturally occurring enzymes in your body that metabolize tyramine, a substance found in many fermented or aged foods. Tyramine constricts blood vessels and increases blood pressure. If you eat a food containing tyramine while you are taking an MAO inhibitor, you cannot effectively eliminate the tyramine from your body. The result may be a hypertensive crisis. There have been some reports in the past of such reactions in people who have eaten rotten bananas or bananas stewed with the peel.

False-positive test for tumors.   Carcinoid tumors—which may arise from tissues of the endocrine system, the intestines, or the lungs—secrete serotonin, a natural chemical that makes blood vessels expand or contract. Because serotonin is excreted in urine, these tumors are diagnosed by measuring the levels of serotonin by-products in the urine. Bananas contain large amounts of serotonin; eating them in the three days before a test for an endocrine tumor might produce a false-positive result, suggesting that you have the tumor when in fact you don't. (Other foods high in serotonin are avocados, eggplant, pineapple, plums, tomatoes, and walnuts.)

Barley

See also Wheat Cereals.

Nutritional Profile*

Energy value (calories per serving): *Moderate*
Protein: *Moderate*
Fat: *Low*
Saturated fat: *Low*
Cholesterol: *None*
Carbohydrates: *High*
Fiber: *High*
Sodium: *Low*
Major vitamin contribution: *B vitamins, folate*
Major mineral contribution: *Iron, potassium*

About the Nutrients in This Food

Barley is a high-carbohydrate food, rich in starch and dietary fiber, particularly pectins and soluble gums, including beta-glucans, the fiber that makes cooked oatmeal sticky. The proteins in barley are incomplete, limited in the essential amino acid lysine. Barley is a good source of the B vitamin folate.

One-half cup cooked barley has 4.5 grams dietary fiber and 12.5 mg folate (3 percent of the RDA for healthy adults).

The Most Nutritious Way to Serve This Food

With a calcium-rich food and with a food such as legumes or meat, milk, or eggs that supplies the lysine barley is missing.

Diets That May Restrict or Exclude This Food

Gluten-free diet

Buying This Food

Look for: Clean, tightly sealed boxes or plastic bags. Stains indicate that something has spilled on the box and may have seeped through to contaminate the grain inside.

---

* Values are for pearled barley.

Storing This Food

Store barley in air- and moisture-proof containers in a cool, dark, dry cabinet. Well protected, it will keep for several months with no loss of nutrients.

Preparing This Food

Pick over the barley and discard any damaged or darkened grains.

What Happens When You Cook This Food

Starch consists of molecules of the complex carbohydrates amylose and amylopectin packed into a starch granule. When you cook barley in water, its starch granules absorb water molecules, swell, and soften. When the temperature of the liquid reaches approximately 140°F, the amylose and amylopectin molecules inside the granules relax and unfold, breaking some of their internal bonds (bonds between atoms on the same molecule) and forming new bonds between atoms on different molecules. The result is a network that traps and holds water molecules. The starch granules swell and the barley becomes soft and bulky. If you continue to cook the barley, the starch granules will rupture, releasing some of the amylose and amylopectin molecules inside. These molecules will attract and immobilize some of the water molecules in the liquid, which is why a little barley added to a soup or stew will make the soup or stew thicker.

The B vitamins in barley are water-soluble. You can save them by serving the barley with the liquid in which it was cooked.

How Other Kinds of Processing Affect This Food

Pearling. Pearled barley is barley from which the outer layer has been removed. Milling, the process by which barley is turned into flour, also removes the outer coating (bran) of the grain. Since most of the B vitamins and fiber are concentrated in the bran, both pearled and milled barley are lower in nutrients and fiber than whole barley.

Malting. After barley is harvested, the grain may be left to germinate, a natural chemical process during which complex carbohydrates in the grain (starches and beta-glucans) change into sugar. The grain, now called *malted barley,* is used as the base for several fermented and distilled alcohol beverages, including beer and whiskey.

Medical Uses and/or Benefits

To reduce cholesterol levels. The soluble gums and pectins in barley appear to lower the amount of cholesterol circulating in your blood. There are currently two theories to explain how this might work. The first theory is that the pectins form a gel in your stomach that sops up fats and keeps them from being absorbed by your body. The second is that bacteria living in your gut may feed on the beta-glucans in the barley to produce short-chain fatty acids that slow the natural production of cholesterol in your liver. Barley is very rich in beta-glucans; some strains have three times as much as oats. It also has tocotrienol, another chemical that mops up cholesterol.

Adverse Effects Associated with This Food

* * *

Food/Drug Interactions

* * *

Bean Sprouts

See also Beans.

Nutritional Profile

Energy value (calories per serving): *Low*
Protein: *High*
Fat: *Low*
Saturated fat: *Low*
Cholesterol: *None*
Carbohydrates: *High*
Fiber: *Moderate*
Sodium: *Low*
Major vitamin contribution: *B vitamins, folate, vitamin C*
Major mineral contribution: *Iron, potassium*

About the Nutrients in This Food

Because beans use stored starches and sugars to produce green shoots called sprouts, sprouted beans have less carbohydrate than the beans from which they grow. But bean sprouts are a good source of dietary fiber, including insoluble cellulose and lignin in leaf parts and soluble pectins and gums in the bean. The sprouts are also high in the B vitamin folate and vitamin C.

One-half cup raw mung bean sprouts has 1.2 mg dietary fiber, 31.5 mcg folate (8 percent of the RDA), and 7 mg vitamin C (9 percent of the RDA for a woman, 7 percent of the RDA for a man).

Raw beans contain anti-nutrient chemicals that inhibit the enzymes we use to digest proteins and starches; hemagglutinins (substances that make red blood cells clump together); and "factors" that may inactivate vitamin A. These chemicals are usually destroyed when the beans are heated. Sprouted beans served *with* the bean must be cooked before serving.

The Most Nutritious Way to Serve This Food

Cooked (see *Adverse effects associated with this food*).

Diets That May Restrict or Exclude This Food

Low-fiber, low-residue diet

Buying This Food

Look for: Fresh, crisp sprouts. The tips should be moist and tender. (The shorter the sprout, the more tender it will be.) It is sometimes difficult to judge bean sprouts packed in plastic bags, but you can see through to tell if the tip of the sprout looks fresh. Sprouts sold from water-filled bowls should be refrigerated, protected from dirt and debris, and served with a spoon or tongs, *not scooped up by hands.*

Avoid: Mushy sprouts (they may be decayed) and soft ones (they have lost moisture and vitamin C).

Storing This Food

Refrigerate sprouts in a plastic bag to keep them moist and crisp. If you bought them in a plastic bag, take them out and repack them in bags large enough that they do not crush each other. To get the most vitamin C, use the sprouts within a few days.

Preparing This Food

Rinse the sprouts thoroughly under cold running water to get rid of dirt and sand. Discard any soft or browned sprouts, then cut off the roots and cook the sprouts.

Do not tear or cut the sprouts until you are ready to use them. When you slice into the sprouts, you tear cells, releasing enzymes that begin to destroy vitamin C.

What Happens When You Cook This Food

Cooking destroys some of the heat-sensitive vitamin C in sprouts. To save it, steam the sprouts quickly, stir-fry them, or add them uncooked just before you serve the dish.

How Other Kinds of Processing Affect This Food

Canning. Vitamin C is heat-sensitive, and heating the sprouts during the canning process reduces their vitamin C content.

Medical Uses and/or Benefits

Lower risk of some birth defects. As many as two of every 1,000 babies born in the United States each year may have cleft palate or a neural tube (spinal cord) defect due to their mothers' not having gotten adequate amounts of folate during pregnancy. The RDA for folate is 400 mcg for healthy adult men and women, 600 mcg for pregnant women, and 500 mcg for women who are nursing. Taking folate supplements before becoming pregnant and continuing through the first two months of pregnancy reduces the risk of cleft palate; taking folate through the entire pregnancy reduces the risk of neural tube defects.

Lower risk of heart attack.   In the spring of 1998, an analysis of data from the records for more than 80,000 women enrolled in the long-running Nurses' Health Study at Harvard School of Public Health/Brigham and Woman's Hospital, in Boston, demonstrated that a diet providing more than 400 mcg folate and 3 mg vitamin B_6 daily, from either food or supplements, more than twice the current RDA for each, may reduce a woman's risk of heart attack by almost 50 percent. Although men were not included in the analysis, the results are assumed to apply to them as well. However, data from a meta-analysis published in the *Journal of the American Medical Association* in December 2006 called this theory into question. Researchers at Tulane University examined the results of 12 controlled studies in which 16,958 patients with preexisting cardiovascular disease were given either folic acid supplements or placebos ("look-alike" pills with no folic acid) for at least six months. The scientists, who found no reduction in the risk of further heart disease or overall death rates among those taking folic acid, concluded that further studies will be required to verify whether taking folic acid supplements reduces the risk of cardiovascular disease.

Adverse Effects Associated with This Food

Food poisoning: Reacting to an outbreak of *Salmonella* and *E. coli* O157:H7 food poisoning associated with eating raw alfalfa sprouts, the Food and Drug Administration issued a warning in 1998 and again in summer 1999, cautioning those at high risk of food-borne illness not to eat any raw sprouts. The high-risk group includes children, older adults, and people with a weakened immune system (for example, those who are HIV-positive or undergoing cancer chemotherapy). Tests conducted by the U.S. Department of Agriculture in 1999 suggest that irradiating raw sprouts and bathing them in an antiseptic solution at the processing plant may eliminate disease organisms and prolong the vegetable's shelf life; this remains to be proven.

Food Drug Interactions

* * *

Beans

(Black beans, chickpeas, kidney beans, navy beans, white beans)

See also Bean sprouts, Lentils, Lima beans, Peas, Soybeans.

Nutritional Profile

Energy value (calories per serving): *Moderate*
Protein: *High*
Fat: *Low*
Saturated fat: *Low*
Cholesterol: *None*
Carbohydrates: *High*
Fiber: *Very high*
Sodium: *Low*
Major vitamin contribution: *Vitamin B$_6$, folate*
Major mineral contribution: *Iron, magnesium, zinc*

About the Nutrients in This Food

Beans are seeds, high in complex carbohydrates including starch and dietary fiber. They have indigestible sugars (stachyose and raffinose), plus insoluble cellulose and lignin in the seed covering and soluble gums and pectins in the bean. The proteins in beans are limited in the essential amino acids methionine and cystine.[*] All beans are a good source of the B vitamin folate, and iron.

One-half cup canned kidney beans has 7.5 g dietary fiber, 65 mcg folate (15 percent of the RDA), and 1.6 mg iron (11 percent of the RDA for a woman, 20 percent of the RDA for a man).

Raw beans contain antinutrient chemicals that inactivate enzymes required to digest proteins and carbohydrates. They also contain factors that inactivate vitamin A and also hemagglutinins, substances that make red blood cells clump together. Cooking beans disarms the enzyme inhibitors and the anti-vitamin A factors, but not the hemagglutinins. However, the amount of hemagglutinins in the beans is so small that it has no measurable effect in your body.

---

[*] Soybeans are the only beans that contain proteins considered "complete" because they contain sufficient amounts of all the essential amino acids.

The Folate Content of ½ Cup Cooked Dried Beans

Bean	Folate (mcg)
Black beans	129
Chickpeas	191
Kidney beans canned	65
Navy beans	128
Pinto beans	147

Source: USDA Nutrient Database: www.nal.usda.gov/fnic/cgibin/nut_search.pl, *Nutritive Value of Foods,* Home and Gardens Bulletin No. 72 (USDA, 1989).

The Most Nutritious Way to Serve This Food

Cooked, to destroy antinutrients.

With grains. The proteins in grains are deficient in the essential amino acids lysine and isoleucine but contain sufficient tryptophan, methionine, and cystine; the proteins in beans are exactly the opposite. Together, these foods provide "complete" proteins.

With an iron-rich food (meat) or with a vitamin C-rich food (tomatoes). Both enhance your body's ability to use the iron in the beans. The meat makes your stomach more acid (acid favors iron absorption); the vitamin C may convert the ferric iron in beans into ferrous iron, which is more easily absorbed by the body.

Diets That May Restrict or Exclude This Food

Low-calcium diet
Low-fiber diet
Low-purine (antigout) diet

Buying This Food

Look for: Smooth-skinned, uniformly sized, evenly colored beans that are free of stones and debris. The good news about beans sold in plastic bags is that the transparent material gives you a chance to see the beans inside; the bad news is that pyridoxine and pyridoxal, the natural forms of vitamin B_6, are very sensitive to light.

Avoid: Beans sold in bulk. Some B vitamins, such as vitamin B_6 (pyridoxine and pyridoxal), are very sensitive to light. In addition, open bins allow insects into the beans, indicated by tiny holes showing where the bug has burrowed into or through the bean. If you choose to buy in bulk, be sure to check for smooth skinned, uniformly sized, evenly colored beans free of holes, stones, and other debris.

Storing This Food

Store beans in air- and moistureproof containers in a cool, dark cabinet where they are protected from heat, light, and insects.

Preparing This Food

Wash dried beans and pick them over carefully, discarding damaged or withered beans and any that float. (Only withered beans are light enough to float in water.)

Cover the beans with water, bring them to a boil, and then set them aside to soak. When you are ready to use the beans, discard the water in which beans have been soaked. Some of the indigestible sugars in the beans that cause intestinal gas when you eat the beans will leach out into the water, making the beans less "gassy."

What Happens When You Cook This Food

When beans are cooked in liquid, their cells absorb water, swell, and eventually rupture, releasing the pectins and gums and nutrients inside. In addition, cooking destroys antinutrients in beans, making them more nutritious and safe to eat.

How Other Kinds of Processing Affect This Food

Canning.   The heat of canning destroys some of the B vitamins in the beans. Vitamin B is water-soluble. You can recover all the lost B vitamins simply by using the liquid in the can, but the liquid also contains the indigestible sugars that cause intestinal gas when you eat beans.

Preprocessing.   Preprocessed dried beans have already been soaked. They take less time to cook but are lower in B vitamins.

Medical Uses and/or Benefits

Lower risk of some birth defects.   As many as two of every 1,000 babies born in the United States each year may have cleft palate or a neural tube (spinal cord) defect due to their mothers' not having gotten adequate amounts of folate during pregnancy. The current RDA for folate is 180 mcg for a woman and 200 mcg for a man, but the FDA now recommends 400 mcg for a woman who is or may become pregnant. Taking a folate supplement before becoming pregnant and continuing through the first two months of pregnancy reduces the risk of cleft palate; taking folate through the entire pregnancy reduces the risk of neural tube defects.

Lower risk of heart attack.   In the spring of 1998, an analysis of data from the records for more than 80,000 women enrolled in the long-running Nurses Health Study at Harvard School of Public Health/Brigham and Woman's Hospital in Boston demonstrated that a diet providing more than 400 mcg folate and 3 mg vitamin B_6 a day from either food or supplements, more than twice the current RDA for each, may reduce a woman's risk of heart attack by almost 50 percent. Although men were not included in the analysis, the results are assumed to apply to them as well. NOTE: Beans are high in B_6 as well as folate. Fruit, green leafy vegetables, whole grains, meat, fish, poultry, and shellfish are good sources of vitamin B_6.

To reduce the levels of serum cholesterol.　The gums and pectins in dried beans and peas appear to lower blood levels of cholesterol. Currently there are two theories to explain how this may happen. The first theory is that the pectins in the beans form a gel in your stomach that sops up fats and keeps them from being absorbed by your body. The second is that bacteria in the gut feed on the bean fiber, producing short-chain fatty acids that inhibit the production of cholesterol in your liver.

As a source of carbohydrates for people with diabetes.　Beans are digested very slowly, producing only a gradual rise in blood-sugar levels. As a result, the body needs less insulin to control blood sugar after eating beans than after eating some other high-carbohydrate foods (such as bread or potato). In studies at the University of Kentucky, a bean, whole-grain, vegetable, and fruit-rich diet developed at the University of Toronto enabled patients with type 1 diabetes (who do not produce any insulin themselves) to cut their daily insulin intake by 38 percent. Patients with type 2 diabetes (who can produce some insulin) were able to reduce their insulin injections by 98 percent. This diet is in line with the nutritional guidelines of the American Diabetes Association, but people with diabetes should always consult with their doctors and/or dietitians before altering their diet.

As a diet aid.　Although beans are high in calories, they are also high in bulk (fiber); even a small serving can make you feel full. And, because they are insulin-sparing, they delay the rise in insulin levels that makes us feel hungry again soon after eating. Research at the University of Toronto suggests the insulin-sparing effect may last for several hours after you eat the beans, perhaps until after the next meal.

Adverse Effects Associated with This Food

Intestinal gas.　All legumes (beans and peas) contain raffinose and stachyose, complex sugars that human beings cannot digest. The sugars sit in the gut and are fermented by intestinal bacteria which then produce gas that distends the intestines and makes us uncomfortable. You can lessen this effect by covering the beans with water, bringing them to a boil for three to five minutes, and then setting them aside to soak for four to six hours so that the indigestible sugars leach out in the soaking water, which can be discarded. Alternatively, you may soak the beans for four hours in nine cups of water for every cup of beans, discard the soaking water, and add new water as your recipe directs. Then cook the beans; drain them before serving.

Production of uric acid.　Purines are the natural metabolic by-products of protein metabolism in the body. They eventually break down into uric acid, sharp crystals that may concentrate in joints, a condition known as gout. If uric acid crystals collect in the urine, the result may be kidney stones. Eating dried beans, which are rich in proteins, may raise the concentration of purines in your body. Although controlling the amount of purines in the diet does not significantly affect the course of gout (which is treated with allopurinol, a drug that prevents the formation of uric acid crystals), limiting these foods is still part of many gout regimens.

Food/Drug Interactions

Monoamine oxidase (MAO) inhibitors. Monoamine oxidase inhibitors are drugs used to treat depression. They inactivate naturally occurring enzymes in your body that metabolize tyramine, a substance found in many fermented or aged foods. Tyramine constricts blood vessels and increases blood pressure. If you eat a food containing tyramine while you are taking an MAO inhibitor, you cannot effectively eliminate the tyramine from your body. The result may be a hypertensive crisis. Some nutrition guides list dried beans as a food to avoid while using MAO inhibitors.

Beef

Nutritional Profile*

Energy value (calories per serving): *Moderate*
Protein: *High*
Fat: *Moderate*
Saturated fat: *High*
Cholesterol: *Moderate*
Carbohydrates: *None*
Fiber: *None*
Sodium: *Low*
Major vitamin contribution: *B vitamins*
Major mineral contribution: *Iron, phosphorus, zinc*

About the Nutrients in This Food

Like fish, pork, poultry, milk, and eggs, beef has high-quality proteins, with sufficient amounts of all the essential amino acids. Beef fat is slightly more highly saturated than pork fat, but less saturated than lamb fat. All have about the same amount of cholesterol per serving.

Beef is an excellent source of B vitamins, including niacin, vitamin B_6, and vitamin B_{12}, which is found only in animal foods. Lean beef provides heme iron, the organic iron that is about five times more useful to the body than nonheme iron, the inorganic form of iron found in plant foods. Beef is also an excellent source of zinc.

One four-ounce serving of lean broiled sirloin steak has nine grams fat (3.5 g saturated fat), 101 mg cholesterol, 34 g protein, and 3.81 mg iron (21 percent of the RDA for a woman, 46 percent of the RDA for a man). One four-ounce serving of lean roast beef has 16 g fat (6.6 g saturated fat), 92 mg cholesterol, and 2.96 mg iron (16 percent of the RDA for a woman, 37 percent of the RDA for a man).

The Most Nutritious Way to Serve This Food

With a food rich in vitamin C. Ascorbic acid increases the absorption of iron from meat.

---

* These values apply to lean cooked beef.

Diets That May Restrict or Exclude This Food

Controlled-fat, low-cholesterol diet
Low-protein diet (for some forms of kidney disease)

Buying This Food

Look for: Fresh, red beef. The fat should be white, not yellow.

Choose lean cuts of beef with as little internal marbling (streaks of fat) as possible. The leanest cuts are flank steak and round steak; rib steaks, brisket, and chuck have the most fat. USDA grading, which is determined by the maturity of the animal and marbling in meat, is also a guide to fat content. U.S. prime has more marbling than U.S. choice, which has more marbling than U.S. good. All are equally nutritious; the difference is how tender they are, which depends on how much fat is present.

Choose the cut of meat that is right for your recipe. Generally, the cuts from the center of the animal's back—the rib, the T-Bone, the porterhouse steaks—are the most tender. They can be cooked by dry heat—broiling, roasting, pan-frying. Cuts from around the legs, the underbelly, and the neck—the shank, the brisket, the round—contain muscles used for movement. They must be tenderized by stewing or boiling, the long, moist cooking methods that break down the connective tissue that makes meat tough.

Storing This Food

Refrigerate raw beef immediately, carefully wrapped to prevent its drippings from contaminating other foods. Refrigeration prolongs the freshness of beef by slowing the natural multiplication of bacteria on the meat surface. Unchecked, these bacteria will convert proteins and other substances on the surface of the meat to a slimy film and change meat's sulfur-containing amino acids methionine and cystine into smelly chemicals called mercaptans. When the mercaptans combine with myoglobin, they produce the greenish pigment that gives spoiled meat its characteristic unpleasant appearance.

Fresh ground beef, with many surfaces where bacteria can live, should be used within 24 to 48 hours. Other cuts of beef may stay fresh in the refrigerator for three to five days.

Preparing This Food

Trim the beef carefully. By judiciously cutting away all visible fat you can significantly reduce the amount of fat and cholesterol in each serving.

When you are done, clean all utensils thoroughly with soap and hot water. Wash your cutting board, wood or plastic, with hot water, soap, and a bleach-and-water solution. For ultimate safety in preventing the transfer of microorganisms from the raw meat to other foods, keep one cutting board exclusively for raw meats, fish, and poultry, and a second one for everything else. Finally, don't forget to wash your hands.

What Happens When You Cook This Food

Cooking changes the appearance and flavor of beef, alters nutritional value, makes it safer, and extends its shelf life.

Browning meat after you cook it does not "seal in the juices," but it does change the flavor by caramelizing sugars on the surface. Because beef's only sugars are the small amounts of glycogen in the muscles, we add sugars in marinades or basting liquids that may also contain acids (vinegar, lemon juice, wine) to break down muscle fibers and tenderize the meat. (Browning has one minor nutritional drawback. It breaks amino acids on the surface of the meat into smaller compounds that are no longer useful proteins.)

When beef is cooked, it loses water and shrinks. Its pigments, which combine with oxygen, are denatured (broken into fragments) by the heat and turn brown, the natural color of well-done meat.

At the same time, the fats in the beef are oxidized. Oxidized fats, whether formed in cooking or when the cooked meat is stored in the refrigerator, give cooked meat a characteristic warmed-over flavor. Cooking and storing meat under a blanket of antioxidants—catsup or a gravy made of tomatoes, peppers, and other vitamin C-rich vegetables—reduces the oxidation of fats and the intensity of warmed-over flavor. Meat reheated in a microwave oven also has less warmed-over flavor.

An obvious nutritional benefit of cooking is the fact that heat lowers the fat content of beef by liquifying the fat so it can run off the meat. One concrete example of how well this works comes from a comparison of the fat content in regular and extra-lean ground beef. According to research at the University of Missouri in 1985, both kinds of beef lose mass when cooked, but the lean beef loses water and the regular beef loses fat and cholesterol. Thus, while regular raw ground beef has about three times as much fat (by weight) as raw ground extra-lean beef, their fat varies by only 5 percent after broiling.

To reduce the amount of fat in ground beef, heat the beef in a pan until it browns. Then put the beef in a colander, and pour one cup of warm water over the beef. Repeat with a second cup of warm water to rinse away fat melted by heating the beef. Use the ground beef in sauce and other dishes that do not require it to hold together.

Finally, cooking makes beef safer by killing *Salmonella* and other organisms in the meat. As a result, cooking also serves as a natural preservative. According to the USDA, large pieces of fresh beef can be refrigerated for two or three days, then cooked and held safely for another day or two because the heat of cooking has reduced the number of bacteria on the surface of the meat and temporarily interrupted the natural cycle of deterioration.

How Other Kinds of Processing Affect This Food

Aging. Hanging fresh meat exposed to the air, in a refrigerated room, reduces the moisture content and shrinks the meat slightly. As the meat ages enzymes break down muscle proteins, "tenderizing" the beef.

Canning. Canned beef does not develop a warmed-over flavor because the high temperatures in canning food and the long cooking process alter proteins in the meat so that they act as antioxidants. Once the can is open, however, the meat should be protected from oxygen that will change the flavor of the beef.

Curing.   Salt-curing preserves meat through osmosis, the physical reaction in which liquids flow across a membrane, such as the wall of a cell, from a less dense to a more dense solution. The salt or sugar used in curing dissolves in the liquid on the surface of the meat to make a solution that is more dense than the liquid inside the cells of the meat. Water flows out of the meat and out of the cells of any microorganisms living on the meat, killing the microorganisms and protecting the meat from bacterial damage. Salt-cured meat is much higher in sodium than fresh meat.

Freezing.   When you freeze beef, the water inside its cells freezes into sharp ice crystals that can puncture cell membranes. When the beef thaws, moisture (and some of the B vitamins) will leak out through these torn cell walls. The loss of moisture is irreversible, but some of the vitamins can be saved by using the drippings when the meat is cooked. Freezing may also cause freezer burn—dry spots left when moisture evaporates from the surface of the meat. Waxed freezer paper is designed specifically to hold the moisture in meat; plastic wrap and aluminum foil are less effective. NOTE: Commercially prepared beef, which is frozen very quickly at very low temperatures, is less likely to show changes in texture.

Irradiation.   Irradiation makes meat safer by exposing it to gamma rays, the kind of high-energy ionizing radiation that kills living cells, including bacteria. Irradiation does not change the way meat looks, feels or tastes, or make the food radioactive, but it does alter the structure of some naturally occurring chemicals in beef, breaking molecules apart to form new compounds called radiolytic products (RP). About 90 percent of RPs are also found in nonirradiated foods. The rest, called unique radiolytic products (URP), are found only in irradiated foods. There is currently no evidence to suggest that URPs are harmful; irradiation is an approved technique in more than 37 countries around the world, including the United States.

Smoking.   Hanging cured or salted meat over an open fire slowly dries the meat, kills microorganisms on its surface, and gives the meat a rich, "smoky" flavor that varies with the wood used in the fire. Meats smoked over an open fire are exposed to carcinogenic chemicals in the smoke, including a-benzopyrene. Meats treated with "artificial smoke flavoring" are not, since the flavoring is commercially treated to remove tar and a-benzopyrene.

Medical Uses and/or Benefits

Treating and/or preventing iron deficiency.   Without meat in the diet, it is virtually impossible for an adult woman to meet her iron requirement without supplements. One cooked 3.5-ounce hamburger provides about 2.9 mg iron, 16 percent of the RDA for an adult woman of childbearing age.

Possible anti-diabetes activity.   CLA may also prevent type 2 diabetes, also called adult-onset diabetes, a non-insulin-dependent form of the disease. At Purdue University, rats bred to develop diabetes spontaneously between eight and 10 weeks of age stayed healthy when given CLA supplements.

Adverse Effects Associated with This Food

Increased risk of heart disease.   Like other foods from animals, beef contains cholesterol and saturated fats that increase the amount of cholesterol circulating in your blood, raising your risk of heart disease. To reduce the risk of heart disease, the National Cholesterol Education Project recommends following the Step I and Step II diets.

The Step I diet provides no more than 30 percent of total daily calories from fat, no more than 10 percent of total daily calories from saturated fat, and no more than 300 mg of cholesterol per day. It is designed for healthy people whose cholesterol is in the range of 200–239 mg/dL.

The Step II diet provides 25–35 percent of total calories from fat, less than 7 percent of total calories from saturated fat, up to 10 percent of total calories from polyunsaturated fat, up to 20 percent of total calories from monounsaturated fat, and less than 300 mg cholesterol per day. This stricter regimen is designed for people who have one or more of the following conditions:

◆ Existing cardiovascular disease
◆ High levels of low-density lipoproteins (LDLs, or "bad" cholesterol) or low levels of high-density lipoproteins (HDLs, or "good" cholesterol)
◆ Obesity
◆ Type 1 diabetes (insulin-dependent diabetes, or diabetes mellitus)
◆ Metabolic syndrome, a.k.a. insulin resistance syndrome, a cluster of risk factors that includes type 2 diabetes (non-insulin-dependent diabetes)

Increased risk of some cancers.   According the American Institute for Cancer Research, a diet high in red meat (beef, lamb, pork) increases the risk of developing colorectal cancer by 15 percent for every 1.5 ounces over 18 ounces consumed per week. In 2007, the National Cancer Institute released data from a survey of 500,000 people, ages 50 to 71, who participated in an eight-year AARP diet and health study identifying a higher risk of developing cancer of the esophagus, liver, lung, and pancreas among people eating large amounts of red meats and processed meats.

Food-borne illness.   Improperly cooked meat contaminated with *E. coli* O157:H7 has been linked to a number of fatalities in several parts of the United States. In addition, meats contaminated with other bacteria, viruses, or parasites pose special problems for people with a weakened immune system: the very young, the very old, cancer chemotherapy patients, and people with HIV. Cooking meat to an internal temperature of 140°F should destroy *Salmonella* and *Campylobacter jejuni;* 165°F, the *E. coli* organism; and 212°F, *Listeria monocytogenes.*

Antibiotic sensitivity.   Cattle in the United States are routinely given antibiotics to protect them from infection. By law, the antibiotic treatment must stop three days to several weeks before the animal is slaughtered. Theoretically, the beef should then be free of antibiotic residues, but some people who are sensitive to penicillin or tetracycline may have an allergic reaction to the meat, although this is rare.

Antibiotic-resistant Salmonella and toxoplasmosis. Cattle treated with antibiotics may produce meat contaminated with antibiotic-resistant strains of *Salmonella,* and all raw beef may harbor ordinary *Salmonella* as well as *T. gondii,* the parasite that causes toxoplasmosis. Toxoplasmosis is particularly hazardous for pregnant women. It can be passed on to the fetus and may trigger a series of birth defects including blindness and mental retardation. Both *Salmonella* and the *T. gondii* can be eliminated by cooking meat thoroughly and washing all utensils, cutting boards, and counters as well as your hands with hot soapy water before touching any other food.

Decline in kidney function. Proteins are nitrogen compounds. When metabolized, they yield ammonia, which is excreted through the kidneys. In laboratory animals, a sustained high-protein diet increases the flow of blood through the kidneys, accelerating the natural age-related decline in kidney function. Some experts suggest that this may also occur in human beings.

Food/Drug Interactions

Tetracycline antibiotics (demeclocycline [Declomycin], doxycycline [Vibtamycin], methacycline [Rondomycin], minocycline [Minocin], oxytetracycline [Terramycin], tetracycline [Achromycin V, Panmycin, Sumycin]). Because meat contains iron, which binds tetracyclines into compounds the body cannot absorb, it is best to avoid meat for two hours before and after taking one of these antibiotics.

Monoamine oxidase (MAO) inhibitors. Meat "tenderized" with papaya or a papain powder can interact with the class of antidepressant drugs known as monoamine oxidase inhibitors. Papain meat tenderizers work by breaking up the long chains of protein molecules. One by-product of this process is tyramine, a substance that constructs blood vessels and raises blood pressure. MAO inhibitors inactivate naturally occurring enzymes in your body that metabolize tyramine. If you eat a food such as papain-tenderized meat, which is high in tyramine, while you are taking a MAO inhibitor, you cannot effectively eliminate the tyramine from your body. The result may be a hypertensive crisis.

Theophylline. Charcoal-broiled beef appears to reduce the effectiveness of theophylline because the aromatic chemicals produced by burning fat speed up the metabolism of theophylline in the liver.

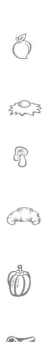

Beer

(Ale)

Nutritional Profile

Energy value (calories per serving): *Low*
Protein: *Moderate*
Fat: *None*
Saturated fat: *None*
Cholesterol: *None*
Carbohydrates: *High*
Fiber: *None*
Sodium: *Low*
Major vitamin contribution: *B vitamins*
Major mineral contribution: *Phosphorus*

About the Nutrients in This Food

Beer and ale are fermented beverages created by yeasts that convert the sugars in malted barley and grain to ethyl alcohol (a.k.a. "alcohol," "drinking alcohol").[*]

The USDA/Health and Human Services Dietary Guidelines for Americans defines one drink as 12 ounces of beer, five ounces of wine, or 1.25 ounces of distilled spirits. One 12-ounce glass of beer has 140 calories, 86 of them (61 percent) from alcohol. But the beverage—sometimes nicknamed "liquid bread"—is more than empty calories. Like wine, beer retains small amounts of some nutrients present in the food from which it was made.

---

[*] Because yeasts cannot digest the starches in grains, the grains to be used in making beer and ale are allowed to germinate ("malt"). When it is time to make the beer or ale, the malted grain is soaked in water, forming a mash in which the starches are split into simple sugars that can be digested (fermented) by the yeasts. If undisturbed, the fermentation will continue until all the sugars have been digested, but it can be halted at any time simply by raising or lowering the temperature of the liquid. Beer sold in bottles or cans is pasteurized to kill the yeasts and stop the fermentation. Draft beer is not pasteurized and must be refrigerated until tapped so that it will not continue to ferment in the container. The longer the shipping time, the more likely it is that draft beer will be exposed to temperature variations that may affect its quality—which is why draft beer almost always tastes best when consumed near the place where it was brewed.

The Nutrients in Beer (12-ounce glass)

Nutrients	Beer	%RDA
Calcium	17 mg	1.7
Magnesium	28.51 mg	7–9*
Phosphorus	41.1 mg	6
Potassium	85.7 mg	(na)
Zinc	0.06 mg	0.5–0.8*
Thiamin	0.02 mg	1.6–1.8*
Riboflavin	0.09 mg	7–8*
Niacin	1.55 mg	10
Vitamin B_6	0.17 mg	13
Folate	20.57 mcg	5

* the first figure is the %RDA for a man; the second, for a woman

Source: USDA Nutrient Database: www.nal.usda.gov/fnic/cgi-bin/nut_search.pl.

Diets That May Restrict or Exclude This Food

Bland diet
Gluten-free diet
Low-purine (antigout) diet

Buying This Food

Look for: A popular brand that sells steadily and will be fresh when you buy it.

Avoid: Dusty or warm bottles and cans.

Storing This Food

Store beer in a cool place. Beer tastes best when consumed within two months of the day it is made. Since you cannot be certain how long it took to ship the beer to the store or how long it has been sitting on the grocery shelves, buy only as much beer as you plan to use within a week or two.

Protect bottled beer and open bottles or cans of beer from direct sunlight, which can change sulfur compounds in beer into isopentyl mercaptan, the smelly chemical that gives stale beer its characteristic unpleasant odor.

When You Are Ready to Serve This Food

Serve beer only in absolutely clean glasses or mugs. Even the slightest bit of grease on the side of the glass will kill the foam immediately. Wash beer glasses with detergent, not soap, and let them drain dry rather than drying them with a towel that might carry grease from your hands to the glass. If you like a long-lasting head on your beer, serve the brew in tall, tapering glasses to let the foam spread out and stabilize.

For full flavor, serve beer and ales cool but not ice-cold. Very low temperatures immobilize the molecules that give beer and ale their flavor and aroma.

What Happens When You Cook This Food

When beer is heated (in a stew or as a basting liquid), the alcohol evaporates but the flavoring agents remain intact. Alcohol, an acid, reacts with metal ions from an aluminum or iron pot to form dark compounds that discolor the pot or the dish you are cooking in. To prevent this, prepare dishes made with beer in glass or enameled pots.

How Other Kinds of Processing Affect This Food

* * *

Medical Uses and/or Benefits

Reduced risk of heart attack. Data from the American Cancer Society's Cancer Prevention Study 1, a 12-year survey of more than 1 million Americans in 25 states, shows that men who take one drink a day have a 21 percent lower risk of heart attack and a 22 percent lower risk of stroke than men who do not drink at all. Women who have up to one drink a day also reduce their risk of heart attack. Numerous later studies have confirmed these findings.

Lower risk of stroke. In January 1999, the results of a 677-person study published by researchers at New York Presbyterian Hospital-Columbia University showed that moderate alcohol consumption reduces the risk of stroke due to a blood clot in the brain among older people (average age: 70). How the alcohol prevents stroke is still unknown, but it is clear that moderate use of alcohol is a key. Heavy drinkers (those who consume more than seven drinks a day) have a higher risk of stroke. People who once drank heavily, but cut their consumption to moderate levels, can also reduce their risk of stroke. Numerous later studies have confirmed these findings.

Lower cholesterol levels. Beverage alcohol decreases the body's production and storage of low-density lipoproteins (LDLs), the protein and fat particles that carry cholesterol into your arteries. As a result, people who drink moderately tend to have lower cholesterol levels and higher levels of high density lipoproteins (HDLs), the fat and protein particles that carry cholesterol out of the body. The USDA/Health and Human Services Dietary Guidelines for Americans defines moderation as two drinks a day for a man, one drink a day for a woman.

Stimulating the appetite. Alcoholic beverages stimulate the production of saliva and the gastric acids that cause the stomach contractions we call hunger pangs. Moderate amounts of alcoholic beverages, which may help stimulate appetite, are often prescribed for geriatric patients, convalescents, and people who do not have ulcers or other chronic gastric problems that might be exacerbated by the alcohol.

Dilation of blood vessels. Alcohol dilates the capillaries (the tiny blood vessels just under the skin), and moderate amounts of alcoholic beverages produce a pleasant flush that temporarily warms the drinker. But drinking is not an effective way to warm up in cold weather since the warm blood that flows up to the capillaries will cool down on the surface of your skin and make you even colder when it circulates back into the center of your body. Then an alcohol flush will make you perspire, so that you lose more heat. Excessive amounts of beverage alcohol may depress the mechanism that regulates body temperature.

Adverse Effects Associated with This Food

Increased risk of breast cancer. In 2008, scientists at the National Cancer Institute released data from a seven-year survey of more than 100,000 postmenopausal women showing that even moderate drinking (one to two drinks a day) may increase by 32 percent a woman's risk of developing estrogen-receptor positive (ER+) and progesterone-receptor positive (PR+) breast cancer, tumors whose growth is stimulated by hormones. No such link was found between consuming alcohol and the risk of developing ER-/PR- tumors (not fueled by hormones). The finding applies to all types of alcohol: beer, wine, and spirits.

Increased risk of oral cancer (cancer of the mouth and throat). Numerous studies confirm the American Cancer Society's warning that men and women who consume more than two drinks a day are at higher risk of oral cancer than are nondrinkers or people who drink less. Note: *The Dietary Guidelines for Americans* describes one drink as 12 ounces of beer, five ounces of wine, or 1.5 ounces of distilled spirits.

Increased risk of cancer of the colon and rectum. In the mid-1990s, studies at the University of Oklahoma suggested that men who drink more than five beers a day are at increased risk of rectal cancer. Later studies suggested that men and women who are heavy beer or spirits drinkers (but not those who are heavy wine drinkers) have a higher risk of colorectal cancers. Further studies are required to confirm these findings.

Fetal alcohol syndrome. Fetal alcohol syndrome is a specific pattern of birth defects—low birth weight, heart defects, facial malformations, and mental retardation—first recognized in a study of babies born to alcoholic women who consumed more than six drinks a day while pregnant. Subsequent research has found a consistent pattern of milder defects in babies born to women who consume three to four drinks a day or five drinks on any one occasion while pregnant. To date, there is no evidence of a consistent pattern of birth defects in babies born to women who consume less than one drink a day while pregnant, but two studies at Columbia University have suggested that as few as two drinks a week while pregnant may raise a woman's risk of miscarriage. ("One drink" means 12 ounces of beer, five ounces of wine, or 1.25 ounces of distilled spirits.)

Alcoholism. Alcoholism is an addiction disease, the inability to control one's alcohol consumption. It is a potentially life-threatening condition, with a higher risk of death by accident, suicide, malnutrition, or acute alcohol poisoning, a toxic reaction that kills by paralyzing body organs, including the heart.

Malnutrition. While moderate alcohol consumption stimulates appetite, alcohol abuse depresses it. In addition, an alcoholic may drink instead of eating. When an alcoholic does eat, excess alcohol in his/her body prevents absorption of nutrients and reduces the ability to synthesize new tissue.

Hangover. Alcohol is absorbed from the stomach and small intestine and carried by the bloodstream to the liver, where it is oxidized to acetaldehyde by alcohol dehydrogenase (ADH), the enzyme our bodies use to metabolize the alcohol we produce when we digest carbohydrates. The acetaldehyde is converted to acetyl coenzyme A and either eliminated from the body or used in the synthesis of cholesterol, fatty acids, and body tissues. Although individuals vary widely in their capacity to metabolize alcohol, on average, normal healthy adults can metabolize the alcohol in one quart of beer in approximately five to six hours. If they drink more than that, they will have more alcohol than the body's natural supply of ADH can handle. The unmetabolized alcohol will pile up in the bloodstream, interfering with the liver's metabolic functions. Since alcohol decreases the reabsorption of water from the kidneys and may inhibit the secretion of an antidiuretic hormone, they will begin to urinate copiously, losing magnesium, calcium, and zinc but retaining more irritating uric acid. The level of lactic acid in the body will increase, making them feel tired and out of sorts; their acid-base balance will be out of kilter; the blood vessels in their heads will swell and throb; and their stomachs, with linings irritated by the alcohol, will ache. The ultimate result is a "hangover" whose symptoms will disappear only when enough time has passed to allow their bodies to marshal the ADH needed to metabolize the extra alcohol in their blood.

Changes in body temperature. Alcohol dilates capillaries, tiny blood vessels just under the skin, producing a "flush" that temporarily warms the drinker. But drinking is not an effective way to stay warm in cold weather. Warm blood flowing up from the body core to the surface capillaries is quickly chilled, making you even colder when it circulates back into your organs. In addition, an alcohol flush triggers perspiration, further cooling your skin. Finally, very large amounts of alcohol may actually depress the mechanism that regulates body temperature.

Impotence. Excessive drinking decreases libido (sexual desire) and interferes with the ability to achieve or sustain an erection.

"Beer belly." Data from a 1995, 12,000 person study at the University of North Carolina in Chapel Hill show that people who consume at least six beers a week have more rounded abdomens than people who do not drink beer. The question left to be answered is which came first: the tummy or the drinking.

Food/Drug Interactions

Acetaminophen (Tylenol, etc.). The FDA recommends that people who regularly have three or more drinks a day consult a doctor before using acetaminophen. The alcohol/acetaminophen combination may cause liver failure.

Disulfiram (Antabuse). Taken with alcohol, disulfiram causes flushing, nausea, low blood pressure, faintness, respiratory problems, and confusion. The severity of the reaction generally depends on how much alcohol you drink, how much disulfiram is in your body, and how long ago you took it. Disulfiram is used to help recovering alcoholics avoid alcohol. (If taken with alcohol, metronidazole [Flagyl], procarbazine [Matulane], quinacrine [Atabrine], chlorpropamide (Diabinase), and some species of mushrooms may produce a mild disulfiramlike reaction.)

Anticoagulants. Alcohol slows the body's metabolism of anticoagulants (blood thinners) such as warfarin (Coumadin), intensifying the effect of the drugs and increasing the risk of side effects such as spontaneous nosebleeds.

Antidepressants. Alcohol may increase the sedative effects of antidepressants. Drinking alcohol while you are taking a monoamine oxidase (MAO) inhibitor is especially hazardous. MAO inhibitors inactivate naturally occurring enzymes in your body that metabolize tyramine, a substance found in many fermented or aged foods. Tyramine constricts blood vessels and increases blood pressure. If you eat a food containing tyramine while you are taking an MAO inhibitor, you cannot effectively eliminate the tyramine from your body. The result may be a hypertensive crisis. Ordinarily, fermentation of beer and ale does not produce tyramine, but some patients have reported tyramine reactions after drinking some imported beers. Beer and ale are usually prohibited to those using MAO inhibitors.

Aspirin, ibuprofen, ketoprofen, naproxen, and nonsteroidal anti-inflammatory drugs. Like alcohol, these analgesics irritate the lining of the stomach and may cause gastric bleeding. Combining the two intensifies the effect.

Insulin and oral hypoglycemics. Alcohol lowers blood sugar and interferes with the metabolism of oral antidiabetics; the combination may cause severe hypoglycemia.

Sedatives and other central nervous system depressants (tranquilizers, sleeping pills, antidepressants, sinus and cold remedies, analgesics, and medication for motion sickness). Alcohol intensifies sedation and, depending on the dose, may cause drowsiness, respiratory depression, coma, or death.

Beets

Nutritional Profile

Energy value (calories per serving): *Low*
Protein: *Moderate*
Fat: *Low*
Saturated fat: *Low*
Cholesterol: *None*
Carbohydrates: *High*
Fiber: *Moderate*
Sodium: *Moderate*
Major vitamin contribution: *Vitamin C*
Major mineral contribution: *Potassium*

About the Nutrients in This Food

Beets are roots, high-carbohydrate foods that provide sugars, starch, and small amounts of dietary fiber, insoluble cellulose in the skin, and soluble pectins in the flesh. Beets are also a good source of the B vitamin folate.

One-half cup cooked fresh beets has one gram of dietary fiber and 68 mcg folate (17 percent of the RDA).

The Most Nutritious Way to Serve This Food

Cooked, to dissolve the stiff cell walls and make the nutrients inside available.

Diets That May Restrict or Exclude This Food

Anti-kidney-stone diet
Low-sodium diet

Buying This Food

Look for: Smooth round globes with fresh, crisp green leaves on top.

Avoid: Beets with soft spots or blemishes that suggest decay underneath.

Storing This Food

Protect the nutrients in beets by storing the vegetables in a cool place, such as the vegetable crisper in your refrigerator. When stored, the beet root converts its starch into sugars; the longer it is stored, the sweeter it becomes.

Remove the green tops from beets before storing and store the beet greens like other leafy vegetables, in plastic bags in the refrigerator to keep them from drying out and losing vitamins (also see GREENS).

Use both beets and beet greens within a week.

Preparing This Food

Scrub the globes with a vegetable brush under cold running water. You can cook them whole or slice them. Peel before (or after) cooking.

What Happens When You Cook This Food

Betacyamin and betaxanthin, the red betalain pigments in beets, are water-soluble. (That's why borscht is a scarlet soup.) Betacyanins and betaxanthins turn more intensely red when you add acids; think of scarlet sweet-and-sour beets in lemon juice or vinegar with sugar. They turn slightly blue in a basic (alkaline) solution such as baking soda and water.

Like carrots, beets have such stiff cell walls that it is hard for the human digestive tract to extract the nutrients inside. Cooking will not soften the cellulose in the beet's cell walls, but it will dissolve enough hemicellulose so that digestive juices are able to penetrate. Cooking also activates flavor molecules in beets, making them taste better.

How Other Kinds of Processing Affect This Food

Canning. Beets lose neither their color nor their texture in canning.

Medical Uses and/or Benefits

Lower risk of some birth defects. As many as two of every 1,000 babies born in the United States each year may have cleft palate or a neural tube (spinal cord) defect due to their mothers' not having gotten adequate amounts of folate during pregnancy. The RDA for folate is 400 mcg for healthy adult men and women, 600 mcg for pregnant women, and 500 mcg for women who are nursing. Taking folate supplements before becoming pregnant and continuing through the first two months of pregnancy reduces the risk of cleft palate; taking folate through the entire pregnancy reduces the risk of neural tube defects.

Possible lower risk of heart attack. In the spring of 1998, an analysis of data from the records of more than 80,000 women enrolled in the long-running Nurses' Health Study at Harvard

School of Public Health/Brigham and Women's Hospital, in Boston, demonstrated that a diet providing more than 400 mcg folate and 3 mg vitamin B$_6$ daily, either from food or supplements, might reduce a woman's risk of heart attack by almost 50 percent. Although men were not included in the study, the results were assumed to apply to them as well.

However, data from a meta-analysis published in the *Journal of the American Medical Association* in December 2006 called this theory into question. Researchers at Tulane University examined the results of 12 controlled studies in which 16,958 patients with preexisting cardiovascular diseases were given either folic acid supplements or placebos ("look-alike" pills with no folic acid) for at least six months. The scientists, who found no reduction in the risk of further heart disease or overall death rates among those taking folic acid, concluded that further studies will be required to verify whether taking folic acid supplements reduces the risk of cardiovascular disease.

Adverse Effects Associated with This Food

Pigmented urine and feces. The ability to metabolize betacyanins and be taxanthins is a genetic trait. People with two recessive genes for this trait cannot break down these red pigments, which will be excreted, bright red, in urine. Eating beets can also turn feces red, but it will not cause a false-positive result in a test for occult blood in the stool.

Nitrosamine formation. Beets, celery, eggplant, lettuce, radishes, spinach, and collard and turnip greens contain nitrates that convert naturally into nitrites in your stomach—where some of the nitrites combine with amines to form nitrosamines, some of which are known carcinogens. This natural chemical reaction presents no known problems for a healthy adult. However, when these vegetables are cooked and left standing for a while at room temperature, microorganisms that convert nitrates to nitrites begin to multiply, and the amount of nitrites in the food rises. The resulting higher-nitrite foods may be dangerous for infants (see SPINACH).

Food/Drug Interactions

* * *

Blackberries

(Boysenberries, dewberries, youngberries)

Nutritional Profile

Energy value (calories per serving): *Low*
Protein: *Low*
Fat: *Low*
Saturated fat: *Low*
Cholesterol: *None*
Carbohydrates: *High*
Fiber: *Moderate*
Sodium: *Low*
Major vitamin contribution: *Vitamin A, vitamin C*
Major mineral contribution: *Calcium*

About the Nutrients in This Food

Blackberries have no starch but do contain sugars and dietary fiber, primarily pectin, which dissolves as the fruit matures. Unripe blackberries contain more pectin than ripe ones.

One-half cup fresh blackberries has 3.8 g dietary fiber, 15 mg vitamin C (20 percent of the RDA for a woman, 17 percent of the RDA for a man), and 18 mcg folate (5 percent of the RDA).

The Most Nutritious Way to Serve This Food

Fresh or lightly cooked.

Diets That May Exclude or Restrict This Food

* * *

Buying This Food

Look for: Plump, firm dark berries with no hulls. A firm, well-rounded berry is still moist and fresh; older berries lose moisture, which is why their skin wrinkles.

Avoid: Baskets of berries with juice stains or liquid leaking out of the berries. The stains and leaks are signs that there are crushed—and possibly moldy—berries inside.

Storing This Food

Cover berries and refrigerate them. Then use them in a day or two.

Do not wash berries before storing. The moisture collects in spaces on the surface of the berries that may mold in the refrigerator. Also, handling the berries may damage their cells, releasing enzymes that can destroy vitamins.

Preparing This Food

Rinse the berries under cool running water, then drain them and pick them over carefully to remove all stems and leaves.

What Happens When You Cook This Food

Cooking destroys some of the vitamin C in fresh blackberries and lets water-soluble B vitamins leach out. Cooked berries are likely to be mushy because the heat and water dissolve their pectin and the skin of the berry collapses. Cooking may also change the color of blackberries, which contain soluble red anthocyanin pigments that stain cooking water and turn blue in basic (alkaline) solutions. Adding lemon juice to a blackberry pie stabilizes these pigments; it is a practical way to keep the berries a deep, dark reddish blue.

How Other Kinds of Processing Affect This Food

Canning.   The intense heat used in canning fruits reduces the vitamin C content of blackberries. Berries packed in juice have more nutrients, ounce for ounce, than berries packed in either water or syrup.

Medical Uses and/or Benefits

Anticancer activity.   Blackberries are rich in anthocyanins, bright-red plant pigments that act as antioxidants—natural chemicals that prevent free radicals (molecular fragments) from joining to form carcinogenic (cancer-causing) compounds. Some varieties of blackberries also contain ellagic acid, another anticarcinogen with antiviral and antibacterial properties.

Adverse Effects Associated with This Food

Allergic reaction.   Hives and angioedema (swelling of the face, lips, and eyes) are common allergic responses to berries, virtually all of which have been known to trigger allergic reactions. According to the *Merck Manual,* berries are one of the 12 foods most likely to trigger classic food allergy symptoms. The others are chocolate, corn, eggs, fish, legumes (peas, lima beans, peanuts, soybeans), milk, nuts, peaches, pork, shellfish, and wheat (see WHEAT CEREALS).

Food/Drug Interactions

* * *

Blueberries

(Huckleberries)

Nutritional Profile

Energy value (calories per serving): *Low*
Protein: *Low*
Fat: *Low*
Saturated fat: *Low*
Cholesterol: *None*
Carbohydrates: *High*
Fiber: *Moderate*
Sodium: *Low*
Major vitamin contribution: *Vitamin C*
Major mineral contribution: *Calcium*

About the Nutrients in This Food

Blueberries have some protein and a little fat. They have no starch but do contain sugars and dietary fiber—primarily pectin, which dissolves as the fruit matures—and lignin in the seeds. (The difference between blueberries and huckleberries is the size of their seeds; blueberries have smaller ones than huckleberries.)

One-half cup fresh blueberries has 1.5 g dietary fiber and 9.5 mg. vitamin C (13 percent of the RDA for a woman, 11 percent of the RDA for a man).

The Most Nutritious Way to Serve This Food

Fresh, raw, or lightly cooked.

Diets That May Exclude or Restrict This Food

* * *

Buying This Food

Look for: Plump, firm dark-blue berries. The whitish color on the berries is a natural protective coating.

Avoid: Baskets of berries with juice stains or liquid leaking out of the berries. The stains and leaks are signs that there are crushed (and possibly moldy) berries inside.

Storing This Food

Cover berries and refrigerate them. Then use them in a day or two.

Do not wash berries before storing. The moisture increases the chance that they will mold in the refrigerator. Also, handling the berries can damage them, tearing cells and releasing enzymes that will destroy vitamins.

Do not store blueberries in metal containers. The anthocyanin pigments in the berries can combine with metal ions to form dark, unattractive pigment/metal compounds that stain the containers and the berries.

Preparing This Food

Rinse the berries under cool running water, then drain them and pick them over carefully to remove all stems, leaves, and hard (immature) or soft (over-ripe) berries.

What Happens When You Cook This Food

Cooking destroys some of the vitamin C in fresh blueberries and lets water-soluble B vitamins leach out. Cooked berries are likely to be mushy because heat dissolves the pectin inside.

Blueberries may also change color when cooked. The berries are colored with blue anthocyanin pigments. Ordinarily, anthocyanin-pigmented fruits and vegetables turn reddish in acids (lemon juice, vinegar) and deeper blue in bases (baking soda). But blueberries also contain yellow pigments (anthoxanthins). In a basic (alkaline) environments, as in a batter with too much baking soda, the yellow and blue pigments will combine, turning the blueberries greenish blue. Adding lemon juice to a blueberry pie stabilizes these pigments; it is a practical way to keep the berries a deep, dark reddish blue.

How Other Kinds of Processing Affect This Food

Canning and freezing. The intense heat used in canning the fruit or in blanching it before freezing reduces the vitamin C content of blueberries by half.

Medical Uses and/or Benefits

Anticancer activity. According to the U.S. Department of Agriculture, wild blueberries rank first among all fruits in antioxidant content; cultivated blueberries (the ones sold in most food markets) rank second. Antioxidants are natural chemicals that inactivate free radicals, molecule fragments that can link together to form cancer-causing compounds. Several animal studies attest to the ability of blueberries to inhibit the growth of specific cancers. For example, in 2005, scientists at the University of Georgia reported in the journal *Food Research International* that blueberry extracts inhibited the growth of liver cancer cells in laboratory settings. The following year, researchers at Rutgers University (in New Jersey) delivered data to the national meeting of the American Chemical Society from a study in which laboratory rats fed a diet supplemented with pterostilbene, another compound extracted from blueberries, had 57 percent fewer precancerous lesions in the colon than rats whose diet did not contain the supplement. The findings, however, have not been confirmed in humans.

Enhanced memory function. In 2008, British researchers at the schools of Food Biosciences and Psychology at the University of Reading and the Institute of Biomedical and Clinical Sciences at the Peninsula Medical School (England) reported that adding blueberries to one's normal diet appears to improve both long-term and short-term memory, perhaps because anthocyanins and flavonoids (water-soluble pigments in the berries) activate signals in the hippocampus, a part of the brain that controls learning and memory. If confirmed, the data would support the role played by diet in maintaining memory and brain function.

Urinary antiseptic. A 1991 study at the Weizmann Institute of Science (Israel) suggests that blueberries, like CRANBERRIES, contain a compound that inhibits the ability of *Escherichia coli,* a bacteria commonly linked to urinary infections, to stick to the wall of the bladder. If it cannot cling to cell walls, the bacteria will not cause an infection. This discovery lends some support to folk medicine, but how the berries work, how well they work, or in what "dosages" remains to be proven.

Adverse Effects Associated with This Food

Allergic reaction. Hives and angiodemea (swelling of the face, lips, and eyes) are common allergic responses to berries, virtually all of which have been reported to trigger these reactions. According to the *Merck Manual,* berries are one of the 12 foods most likely to trigger classic food allergy symptoms. The others are chocolate, corn, eggs, fish, legumes (peas, lima beans, peanuts, soybeans), milk, nuts, peaches, pork, shellfish, and wheat (see WHEAT CEREALS).

Food/Drug Interactions

* * *

Bread

Nutritional Profile

Energy value (calories per serving): *Moderate*
Protein: *Moderate*
Fat: *Low to moderate*
Saturated fat: *Low to high*
Cholesterol: *Low to high*
Carbohydrates: *High*
Fiber: *Moderate to high*
Sodium: *Moderate to high*
Major vitamin contribution: *B vitamins*
Major mineral contribution: *Calcium, iron, potassium*

About the Nutrients in This Food

All commercially made yeast breads are approximately equal in nutritional value. Enriched white bread contains virtually the same amounts of proteins, fats, and carbohydrates as whole wheat bread, although it may contain only half the dietary fiber (see FLOUR).

Bread is a high-carbohydrate food with lots of starch. The exact amount of fiber, fat, and cholesterol in the loaf varies with the recipe. Bread's proteins, from grain, are low in the essential amino acid lysine. The most important carbohydrate in bread is starch; all breads contain some sugar. Depending on the recipe, the fats may be highly saturated (butter or hydrogenated vegetable fats) or primarily unsaturated (vegetable fat).

All bread is a good source of B vitamins (thiamin, riboflavin, niacin), and in 1998, the Food and Drug Administration ordered food manufacturers to add folates—which protect against birth defects of the spinal cord and against heart disease—to flour, rice, and other grain products. One year later, data from the Framingham Heart Study, which has followed heart health among residents of a Boston suburb for nearly half a century, showed a dramatic increase in blood levels of folic acid. Before the fortification of foods, 22 percent of the study participants had a folic acid deficiency; after, the number fell to 2 percent.

Bread is a moderately good source of calcium, magnesium, and phosphorus. (Breads made with milk contain more calcium than breads made without milk.) Although bread is made from grains and grains contain phytic acid, a natural antinutrient that binds calcium ions into insoluble, indigestible compounds, the phytic acid is inactivated by enzyme action during leavening. Bread does not bind calcium.

All commercially made breads are moderately high in sodium; some contain more sugar than others. Grains are not usually considered a good source of iodine, but commercially made breads often pick up iodine from the iodophors and iodates used to clean the plants and machines in which they are made.

Homemade breads share the basic nutritional characteristics of commercially made breads, but you can vary the recipe to suit your own taste, lowering the salt, sugar, or fat and raising the fiber content, as you prefer.

The Most Nutritious Way to Serve This Food

As sandwiches, with cheese, milk, eggs, meat, fish, or poultry. These foods supply the essential amino acid lysine to "complete" the proteins in grains.

With beans or peas. The proteins in grains are deficient in the essential amino acids lysine and isoleucine and rich in the essential amino acids tryptophan, methionine, and cystine. The proteins in legumes (beans and peas) are exactly the opposite.

Diets That May Restrict or Exclude This Food

Gluten-free diet (excludes breads made with wheat, oats, rye, buckwheat and barley flour)
Lactose-free diet
Low-fiber diet (excludes coarse whole-grain breads)
Low-sodium diet

Buying This Food

Look for: Fresh bread. Check the date on closed packages of commercial bread.

Storing This Food

Store bread at room temperature, in a tightly closed plastic bag (the best protection) or in a breadbox. How long bread stays fresh depends to a great extent on how much fat it contains. Bread made with some butter or other fat will keep for about three days at room temperature. Bread made without fat (Italian bread, French bread) will dry out in just a few hours; for longer storage, wrap it in foil, put it inside a plastic bag, and freeze it. When you are ready to serve the French or Italian bread, you can remove it from the plastic bag and put the foil-wrapped loaf directly into the oven.

Throw away moldy bread. The molds that grow on bread may produce carcinogenic toxins.

Do not store fresh bread in the refrigerator; bread stales most quickly at temperatures just above freezing. The one exception: In warm, humid weather, refrigerating bread slows the growth of molds.

When You Are Ready to Serve This Food

Use a serrated knife to cut bread easily.

What Happens When You Cook This Food

Toasting is a chemical process that caramelizes sugars and amino acids (proteins) on the surface of the bread, turning the bread a golden brown. This chemical reaction, known both as the browning reaction and the Maillard reaction (after the French chemist who first identified it), alters the structure of the surface sugars, starches, and amino acids. The sugars become indigestible food fiber; the amino acids break into smaller fragments that are no longer nutritionally useful. Thus toast has more fiber and less protein than plain bread. However, the role of heat-generated fibers in the human diet is poorly understood. Some experts consider them inert and harmless; others believe they may be hazardous.

How Other Kinds of Processing Affect This Food

Freezing. Frozen bread releases moisture that collects inside the paper, foil, or plastic bag in which it is wrapped. If you unwrap the bread before defrosting it, the moisture will be lost and the bread will be dry. Always defrost bread in its wrappings so that it can reabsorb the moisture that keeps it tasting fresh.

Drying. Since molds require moisture, the less moisture a food contains, the less likely it is support mold growth. That is why bread crumbs and Melba toast, which are relatively moisture-free, keep better than fresh bread. Both can be ground fine and used as a toasty-flavored thickener in place of flour or cornstarch.

Medical Uses and/or Benefits

A lower risk of some kinds of cancer. In 1998, scientists at Wayne State University in Detroit conducted a meta-analysis of data from more than 30 well-designed animal studies measuring the anti-cancer effects of wheat bran, the part of grain with highest amount of the insoluble dietary fibers cellulose and lignin. They found a 32 percent reduction in the risk of colon cancer among animals fed wheat bran; now they plan to conduct a similar meta-analysis of human studies. Breads made with whole grain wheat are a good source of wheat bran. NOTE: The amount of fiber per serving listed on a food package label shows the total amount of fiber (insoluble and soluble).

Early in 1999, however, new data from the long-running Nurses Health Study at Brigham Women's Hospital/Harvard University School of Public Health showed that women who ate a high-fiber diet had a risk of colon cancer similar to that of women who ate a low fiber diet. Because this study contradicts literally hundreds of others conducted over the past 30 years, researchers are awaiting confirming evidence before changing dietary recommendations.

Calming effect.   Mood is affected by naturally occurring chemicals called neurotransmitters that facilitate transmission of impulses between brain cells. The amino acid tryptophan amino acid is the most important constituent of serotonin, a "calming" neurotransmitter. Foods such as bread, which are high in complex carbohydrates, help move tryptophan into your brain, increasing the availability of serotonin.

Adverse Effects Associated with This Food

Allergic reactions and/or gastric distress.   Bread contains several ingredients that may trigger allergic reactions, aggravate digestive problems, or upset a specific diet, among them gluten (prohibited on gluten-free diets); milk (prohibited on a lactose- and galactose-free diet or for people who are sensitive to milk proteins); sugar (prohibited on a sucrose-free diet); salt (controlled on a sodium-restricted diet); and fats (restricted or prohibited on a controlled-fat, low-cholesterol diet).

Food/Drug Interactions

* * *

Broccoli

Nutritional Profile

Energy value (calories per serving): *Low*
Protein: *High*
Fat: *Low*
Saturated fat: *Low*
Cholesterol: *None*
Carbohydrates: *Moderate*
Fiber: *Very high*
Sodium: *Low*
Major vitamin contribution: *Vitamin A, folate, vitamin C*
Major mineral contribution: *Calcium*

About the Nutrients in This Food

Broccoli is very high-fiber food, an excellent source of vitamin A, the B vitamin folate, and vitamin C. It also has some vitamin E and vitamin K, the blood-clotting vitamin manufactured primarily by bacteria living in our intestinal tract.

One cooked, fresh broccoli spear has five grams of dietary fiber, 2,500 IU vitamin A (108 percent of the RDA for a woman, 85 percent of the RDA for a man), 90 mcg folate (23 percent of the RDA), and 130 mg vitamin C (178 percent of the RDA for a woman, 149 percent of the RDA for a man).

The Most Nutritious Way to Serve This Food

Raw. Studies at the USDA Agricultural Research Center in Beltsville, Maryland, show that raw broccoli has up to 40 percent more vitamin C than broccoli that has been cooked or frozen.

Diets That May Restrict or Exclude This Food

Antiflatulence diet
Low-fiber diet

Buying This Food

Look for: Broccoli with tightly closed buds. The stalk, leaves, and florets should be fresh, firm, and brightly colored. Broccoli is usually green; some varieties are tinged with purple.

Avoid: Broccoli with woody stalk or florets that are open or turning yellow. When the green chlorophyll pigments fade enough to let the yellow carotenoids underneath show through, the buds are about to bloom and the broccoli is past its prime.

Storing This Food

Pack broccoli in a plastic bag and store it in the refrigerator or in the vegetable crisper to protect its vitamin C. At 32°F, fresh broccoli can hold onto its vitamin C for as long as two weeks.

Keep broccoli out of the light; like heat, light destroys vitamin C.

Preparing This Food

First, rinse the broccoli under cool running water to wash off any dirt and debris clinging to the florets. Then put the broccoli, florets down, into a pan of salt water (1 tsp. salt to 1 qt. water) and soak for 15 to 30 minutes to drive out insects hiding in the florets. Then cut off the leaves and trim away woody section of stalks. For fast cooking, divide the broccoli up into small florets and cut the stalk into thin slices.

What Happens When You Cook This Food

The broccoli stem contains a lot of cellulose and will stay firm for a long time even through the most vigorous cooking, but the cell walls of the florets are not so strongly fortified and will soften, eventually turning to mush if you cook the broccoli long enough.

Like other cruciferous vegetables, broccoli contains mustard oils (isothiocyanates), natural chemicals that break down into a variety of smelly sulfur compounds (including hydrogen sulfide and ammonia) when the broccoli is heated. The reaction is more intense in aluminum pots. The longer you cook broccoli, the more smelly compounds there will be, although broccoli will never be as odorous as cabbage or cauliflower.

Keeping a lid on the pot will stop the smelly molecules from floating off into the air but will also accelerate the chemical reaction that turns green broccoli olive-drab.

Chlorophyll, the pigment that makes green vegetables green, is sensitive to acids. When you heat broccoli, the chlorophyll in its florets and stalk reacts chemically with acids in the broccoli or in the cooking water to form pheophytin, which is brown. The pheophytin turns cooked broccoli olive-drab or (since broccoli contains some yellow carotenes) bronze.

To keep broccoli green, you must reduce the interaction between the chlorophyll and the acids. One way to do this is to cook the broccoli in a large quantity of water, so the acids will be diluted, but this increases the loss of vitamin C.* Another alternative is to leave the lid off the pot so that the hydrogen atoms can float off into the air, but this allows the smelly sulfur compounds to escape, too. The best way is probably to steam the broccoli quickly with very little water, so it holds onto its vitamin C and cooks before there is time for reaction between chlorophyll and hydrogen atoms to occur.

How Other Kinds of Processing Affect This Food

Freezing. Frozen broccoli usually contains less vitamin C than fresh broccoli. The vitamin is lost when the broccoli is blanched to inactivate catalase and peroxidase, enzymes that would otherwise continue to ripen the broccoli in the freezer. On the other hand, according to researchers at Cornell University, blanching broccoli in a microwave oven—two cups of broccoli in three tablespoons of water for three minutes at 600–700 watts—nearly doubles the amount of vitamin C retained. In experiments at Cornell, frozen broccoli blanched in a microwave kept 90 percent of its vitamin C, compared to 56 percent for broccoli blanched in a pot of boiling water on top of a stove.

Medical Uses and/or Benefits

Protection against some cancers. Naturally occurring chemicals (indoles, isothiocyanates, glucosinolates, dithiolethiones, and phenols) in Brussels sprouts, broccoli, cabbage, cauliflower, and other cruciferous vegetables appear to reduce the risk of some forms of cancer, perhaps by preventing the formation of carcinogens in your body or by blocking cancer-causing substances from reaching or reacting with sensitive body tissues or by inhibiting the transformation of healthy cells to malignant ones.

All cruciferous vegetables contain sulforaphane, a member of a family of chemicals known as isothiocyanates. In experiments with laboratory rats, sulforaphane appears to increase the body's production of phase-2 enzymes, naturally occurring substances that inactivate and help eliminate carcinogens. At the Johns Hopkins University in Baltimore, Maryland, 69 percent of the rats injected with a chemical known to cause mammary cancer developed tumors vs. only 26 percent of the rats given the carcinogenic chemical plus sulforaphane.

To get a protective amount of sulforaphane from broccoli you would have to eat about two pounds a week. But in 1997, Johns Hopkins researchers discovered that broccoli seeds and three-day-old broccoli sprouts contain a compound converted to sulforaphane when the seed and sprout cells are crushed. Five grams of three-day-old sprouts contain as much sulphoraphane as 150 grams of mature broccoli.

---

* Broccoli will lose large amounts of vitamin C if you cook it in water that is cold when you start. As it boils, water releases oxygen that would otherwise destroy vitamin C, so you can cut the vitamin loss dramatically simply by letting the water boil for 60 seconds before adding the broccoli.

Vision protection.   In 2004, the Johns Hopkins researchers updated their findings on sulfora-phane to suggest that it may also protect cells in the eyes from damage due to ultraviolet light, thus reducing the risk of macular degeneration, the most common cause of age-related vision loss.

Lower risk of some birth defects.   Up to two or every 1,000 babies born in the United States each year may have cleft palate or a neural tube (spinal cord) defect due to their mothers' not having gotten adequate amounts of folate during pregnancy. The current RDA for folate is 180 mcg for a woman, 200 mcg for a man, but the FDA now recommends 400 mcg for a woman who is or may become pregnant. Taking a folate supplement before becoming pregnant and continuing through the first two months of pregnancy reduces the risk of cleft palate; taking folate through the entire pregnancy reduces the risk of neural tube defects. Broccoli is a good source of folate. One raw broccoli spear has 107 mcg folate, more than 50 percent of the RDA for an adult.

Possible lower risk of heart attack.   In the spring of 1998, an analysis of data from the records for more than 80,000 women enrolled in the long-running Nurses' Health Study at Harvard School of Public Health/Brigham and Women's Hospital, in Boston, demonstrated that a diet providing more than 400 mcg folate and 3 mg vitamin B_6 daily, either from food or supple-ments, might reduce a woman's risk of heart attack by almost 50 percent. Although men were not included in the study, the results were assumed to apply to them as well.

However, data from a meta-analysis published in the *Journal of the American Medical Association* in December 2006 called this theory into question. Researchers at Tulane Univer-sity examined the results of 12 controlled studies in which 16,958 patients with preexisting cardiovascular disease were given either folic acid supplements or placebos ("look-alike" pills with no folic acid) for at least six months. The scientists, who found no reduction in the risk of further heart disease or overall death rates among those taking folic acid, concluded that further studies will be required to ascertain whether taking folic acid supplements reduces the risk of cardiovascular disease.

Possible inhibition of the herpes virus.   Indoles, another group of chemicals in broccoli, may inhibit the growth of some herpes viruses. In 2003, at the 43rd annual Interscience Confer-ence on Antimicrobial Agents and Chemotherapy, in Chicago, researchers from Stockholm's Huddinge University Hospital, the University of Virginia, and Northeastern Ohio University reported that indole-3-carbinol (I3C) in broccoli stops cells, including those of the herpes sim-plex virus, from reproducing. In tests on monkey and human cells, I3C was nearly 100 percent effective in blocking reproduction of the HSV-1 (oral and genital herpes) and HSV-2 (genital herpes), including one strain known to be resistant to the antiviral drug acyclovir (Zovirax).

Adverse Effects Associated with This Food

Enlarged thyroid gland.   Cruciferous vegetables, including broccoli, contain goitrin, thio-cyanate, and isothiocyanate, chemical compounds that inhibit the formation of thyroid hormones and cause the thyroid to enlarge in an attempt to produce more. These chemicals, known collectively as goitrogens, are not hazardous for healthy people who eat moderate amounts of cruciferous vegetables, but they may pose problems for people who have thyroid problems or are taking thyroid medication.

False-positive test for occult blood in the stool. The guaiac slide test for hidden blood in feces relies on alphaguaiaconic acid, a chemical that turns blue in the presence of blood. Broccoli contains peroxidase, a natural chemical that also turns alphaguaiaconic acid blue and may produce a positive test in people who do not actually have blood in the stool.

Food/Drug Interactions

Anticoagulants Broccoli is rich in vitamin K, the blood-clotting vitamin produced naturally by bacteria in the intestines. Consuming large quantities of this food may reduce the effectiveness of anticoagulants (blood thinners) such as warfarin (Coumadin). One cup of drained, boiled broccoli contains 220 mcg vitamin K, nearly four times the RDA for a healthy adult.

Brussels Sprouts

Nutritional Profile

Energy value (calories per serving): *Low*
Protein: *High*
Fat: *Low*
Saturated fat: *Low*
Cholesterol: *None*
Carbohydrates: *High*
Fiber: *High*
Sodium: *Low*
Major vitamin contribution: *Vitamin A, folate, vitamin C*
Major mineral contribution: *Potassium, iron*

About the Nutrients in This Food

Brussels sprouts are high in dietary fiber, especially insoluble cellulose and lignan in the leaf ribs. They are also a good source of vitamin A and vitamin C.

One-half cup cooked fresh brussels sprouts has three grams of dietary fiber, 1,110 IU vitamin A (48 percent of the RDA for a woman, 37 percent of the RDA for a man), 47 mcg folate (16 percent of the RDA), and 48 mg vitamin C (64 percent of the RDA for a woman, 53 percent of the RDA for a man).

Brussels sprouts also contain an antinutrient, a natural chemical that splits the thiamin (vitamin B_1) molecule so that it is no longer nutritionally useful. This thiamin inhibitor is inactivated by cooking.

The Most Nutritious Way to Serve This Food

Fresh, lightly steamed to preserve the vitamin C and inactivate the antinutrient.

Diets That May Restrict or Exclude This Food

Antiflatulence diet
Low-fiber diet

Buying This Food

Look for: Firm, compact heads with bright, dark-green leaves, sold loose so that you can choose the sprouts one at a time. Brussels sprouts are available all year round.

Avoid: Puffy, soft sprouts with yellow or wilted leaves. The yellow carotenes in the leaves show through only when the leaves age and their green chlorophyll pigments fade. Wilting leaves and puffy, soft heads are also signs of aging.

Avoid sprouts with tiny holes in the leaves through which insects have burrowed.

Storing This Food

Store the brussels sprouts in the refrigerator. While they are most nutritious if used soon after harvesting, sprouts will keep their vitamins (including their heat-sensitive vitamin C) for several weeks in the refrigerator.

Store the sprouts in a plastic bag or covered bowl to protect them from moisture loss.

Preparing This Food

First, drop the sprouts into salted ice water to flush out any small bugs hiding inside. Next, trim them. Remove yellow leaves and leaves with dark spots or tiny holes, but keep as many of the darker, vitamin A–rich outer leaves as possible. Then, cut an X into the stem end of the sprouts to allow heat and water in so that the sprouts cook faster.

What Happens When You Cook This Food

Brussels sprouts contain mustard oils (isothiocyanates), natural chemicals that break down into a variety of smelly sulfur compounds (including hydrogen sulfide and ammonia) when the sprouts are heated, a reaction that is intensified in aluminum pots. The longer you cook the sprouts, the more smelly compounds there will be. Adding a slice of bread to the cooking water may lessen the odor; keeping a lid on the pot will stop the smelly molecules from floating off into the air.

But keeping the pot covered will also increase the chemical reaction that turns cooked brussels sprouts drab. Chlorophyll, the pigment that makes green vegetables green, is sensitive to acids. When you heat brussels sprouts, the chlorophyll in their green leaves reacts chemically with acids in the sprouts or in the cooking water to form pheophytin, which is brown. The pheophytin turns cooked brussels sprouts olive or, since they also contain yellow carotenes, bronze.

To keep cooked brussels sprouts green, you have to reduce the interaction between chlorophyll and acids. One way to do this is to cook the sprouts in a lot of water, so the acids will be diluted, but this increases the loss of vitamin C.* Another alternative is to leave the lid off the pot so that the hydrogen atoms can float off into the air, but this allows the smelly sulfur compounds to escape, too. The best solution is to steam the sprouts quickly in very little water, so they retain their vitamin C and cook before there is time for reaction between chlorophyll and hydrogen atoms to occur.

How Other Kinds of Processing Affect This Food

Freezing. Frozen brussels sprouts contain virtually the same amounts of vitamins as fresh boiled sprouts.

Medical Uses and/or Benefits

Protection against cancer. Naturally occurring chemicals (indoles, isothiocyanates, glucosinolates, dithiolethiones, and phenols) in brussels sprouts, broccoli, cabbage, cauliflower and other cruciferous vegetables appear to reduce the risk of some cancers, perhaps by preventing the formation of carcinogens in your body or by blocking cancer-causing substances from reaching or reacting with sensitive body tissues or by inhibiting the transformation of healthy cells to malignant ones.

All cruciferous vegetables contain sulforaphane, a member of a family of chemicals known as isothiocyanates. In experiments with laboratory rats, sulforaphane appears to increase the body's production of phase-2 enzymes, naturally occurring substances that inactivate and help eliminate carcinogens. At Johns Hopkins University in Baltimore, Maryland, 69 percent of the rats injected with a chemical known to cause mammary cancer developed tumors vs. only 26 percent of the rats given the carcinogenic chemical plus sulforaphane.

In 1997, the Johns Hopkins researchers discovered that broccoli seeds and three-day-old broccoli sprouts contain a compound converted to sulforaphane when the seed and sprout cells are crushed. Five grams of three-day-old broccoli sprouts contain as much sulforaphane as 150 grams of mature broccoli. The sulforaphane levels in other cruciferous vegetables have not yet been calculated.

Lower risk of some birth defects. Up to two or every 1,000 babies born in the United States each year may have cleft palate or a neural tube (spinal cord) defect due to their mothers' not having gotten adequate amounts of folate during pregnancy. NOTE: The current RDA for folate is 180 mcg for a woman and 200 mcg for a man, but the FDA now recommends

---

* Brussels sprouts will lose as much as 25 percent of their vitamin C if you cook them in water that is cold when you start. As it boils, water releases oxygen that would otherwise destroy vitamin C. You can cut the vitamin loss dramatically simply by letting the water boil for 60 seconds before adding the sprouts.

400 mcg for a woman who is or may become pregnant. Taking a folate supplement before becoming pregnant and continuing through the first two months of pregnancy reduces the risk of cleft palate; taking folate through the entire pregnancy reduces the risk of neural tube defects.

Possible lower risk of heart attack.   In the spring of 1998, an analysis of data from the records for more than 80,000 women enrolled in the long-running Nurses' Health Study at Harvard School of Public Health/Brigham and Women's Hospital, in Boston, demonstrated that a diet providing more than 400 mcg folate and 3 mg vitamin B_6 daily, either from food or supplements, might reduce a woman's risk of heart attack by almost 50 percent. Although men were not included in the study, the results were assumed to apply to them as well.

However, data from a meta-analysis published in the *Journal of the American Medical Association* in December 2006 called this theory into question. Researchers at Tulane University examined the results of 12 controlled studies in which 16,958 patients with preexisting cardiovascular disease were given either folic acid supplements or placebos ("look-alike" pills with no folic acid) for at least six months. The scientists, who found no reduction in the risk of further heart disease or overall death rates among those taking folic acid, concluded that further studies will be required to verify whether taking folic acid supplements reduces the risk of cardiovascular disease.

Vision protection.   In 2004, the Johns Hopkins researchers updated their findings on sulforaphane to suggest that it may also protect cells in the eyes from damage due to ultraviolet light, thus reducing the risk of macular degeneration, the most common cause of age-related vision loss.

Adverse Effects Associated with This Food

Enlarged thyroid gland (goiter).   Cruciferous vegetables, including brussels sprouts, contain goitrin, thiocyanate, and isothiocyanate. These chemicals, known collectively as goitrogens, inhibit the formation of thyroid hormones and cause the thyroid to enlarge in an attempt to produce more. Goitrogens are not hazardous for healthy people who eat moderate amounts of cruciferous vegetables, but they may pose problems for people who have a thyroid condition or are taking thyroid medication.

Intestinal gas.   Bacteria that live naturally in the gut degrade the indigestible carbohydrates (food fiber) in brussels sprouts and produce gas that some people find distressing.

Food/Drug Interactions

Anticoagulants   Brussels sprouts are rich in vitamin K, the blood-clotting vitamin produced naturally by bacteria in the intestines. Consuming large quantities of this food may reduce the effectiveness of anticoagulants (blood thinners) such as warfarin (Coumadin). One cup of drained, boiled brussels sprouts contains 219 mcg vitamin K, nearly three times the RDA for a healthy adult.

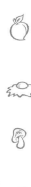

Butter

See also Vegetable oils.

Nutritional Profile

Energy value (calories per serving): *High*
Protein: *Low*
Fat: *High*
Saturated fat: *High*
Cholesterol: *High*
Carbohydrates: *Low*
Fiber: *None*
Sodium: *Low (unsalted butter)*
       High (salted butter)
Major vitamin contribution: *Vitamin A, vitamin D*
Major mineral contribution: *None*

About the Nutrients in This Food

Butterfat is 62 percent saturated fatty acids, 35 percent monounsaturated fatty acids, and 4 percent polyunsaturated fatty acids. One tablespoon of butter has 11 g of fat, 7.1 g of saturated fat, and 31 mg cholesterol, and 1,070 IU vitamin A (46 percent of the RDA for a woman, 36 percent of the RDA for a man). The vitamin A is derived from carotenoids in plants eaten by the milk-cow.

The Most Nutritious Way to Serve This Food

* * *

Diets That May Restrict or Exclude This Food

Low-cholesterol, controlled-fat diet
Sodium-restricted diet (salted butter)

Buying This Food

Look for: Fresh butter. Check the date on the package.

Storing This Food

Store butter in the refrigerator, tightly wrapped to protect it from air and prevent it from picking up the odors of other food. Even refrigerated butter will eventually turn rancid as its fat molecules combine with oxygen to produce hydroperoxides that, in turn, break down into chemicals with an unpleasant flavor and aroma. This reaction is slowed (but not stopped) by cold. Because salt retards the combination of fats with oxygen, salted butter stays fresh longer than plain butter. (Lard, which is pork fat, must also be refrigerated. Lard has a higher proportion of unsaturated fats than the butter. Since unsaturated fats combine with oxygen more easily than saturated fats, lard becomes rancid more quickly than butter.)

Preparing This Food

To measure a half-cup of butter. Pour four ounces of water into an eight-ounce measuring cup, then add butter until the water rises to the eight-ounce mark. Scoop out the butter, use as directed in recipe.

What Happens When You Cook This Food

Fats are very useful in cooking. They keep foods from sticking to the pot or pan; add flavor; and, as they warm, transfer heat from the pan to the food. In doughs and batters, fats separate the flour's starch granules from each other. The more closely the fat mixes with the starch, the smoother the bread or cake will be.

Heat speeds the oxidation and decomposition of fats. When fats are heated, they can catch fire spontaneously without boiling first at what is called the smoke point. Butter will burn at 250°F.

How Other Kinds of Processing Affect This Food

Freezing. Freezing slows the oxidation of fats more effectively than plain refrigeration; frozen butter keeps for up to nine months.

Whipping. When butter is whipped, air is forced in among the fat molecules to produce a foam. As a result, the whipped butter has fewer calories per serving, though not per ounce.

Medical Uses and/or Benefits

* * *

Adverse Effects Associated with This Food

Increased risk of heart disease. Like other foods from animals, butter contains cholesterol and saturated fats. Eating butter increases the amount of cholesterol circulating in your blood and raise your risk of heart disease. To reduce the risk of heart disease, USDA/Health and Human Services Dietary Guidelines for Americans recommends limiting the amount of cholesterol in your diet to no more than 300 mg a day. The guidelines also recommend limiting the amount of fat you consume to no more than 30 percent of your total calories, while holding your consumption of saturated fats to no more than 10 percent of your total calories (the calories from saturated fats are counted as part of the total calories from fat).

Increased risk of acid reflux.   Consuming excessive amounts of fats and fatty foods loosens the lower esophageal sphincter (LES), a muscular valve between the esophagus and the stomach. When food is swallowed, the valve opens to let food into the stomach, then closes tightly to keep acidic stomach contents from refluxing (flowing backwards) into the esophagus. If the LES does not close efficiently, the stomach contents reflux to cause heartburn, a burning sensation. Repeated reflux is a risk factor for esophageal cancer.

Food/Drug Interactions

* * *

Cabbage

(Bok choy [Chinese cabbage], green cabbage, red cabbage, savoy cabbage)

See also Broccoli, Brussels sprouts, Cabbage, Cauliflower, Lettuce, Radishes, Spinach, Turnips.

Nutritional Profile

Energy value (calories per serving): *Low*
Protein: *Moderate*
Fat: *Low*
Saturated fat: *Low*
Cholesterol: *None*
Carbohydrates: *High*
Fiber: *Low*
Sodium: *Low*
Major vitamin contribution: *Vitamin A, folate, vitamin C*
Major mineral contribution: *Calcium (moderate)*

About the Nutrients in This Food

All cabbage has some dietary fiber food: insoluble cellulose and lignin in the ribs and structure of the leaves. Depending on the variety, it has a little vitamin A, moderate amounts of the B vitamin folate and vitamin C.

One-half cup shredded raw bok choy has 0.1 g dietary fiber, 1,041 IU vitamin A (45 percent of the RDA for a woman, 35 percent of the RDA for a man), and 15.5 mg vitamin C (21 percent of the RDA for a woman, 17 percent of the RDA for a man).

One-half cup shredded raw green cabbage has 0.5 g dietary fiber, 45 IU vitamin A (1.9 percent of the RDA for a woman, 1.5 percent of the RDA for a man), 15 mcg folate (4 percent of the RDA), and 11 mg vitamin C (15 percent of the RDA for a woman, 12 percent of the RDA for a man).

One-half cup chopped raw red cabbage has 0.5 g dietary fiber, 7 mcg folate (2 percent of the RDA), and 20 mg vitamin C (27 percent of the RDA for a woman, 22 percent of the RDA for a man).

One-half cup chopped raw savoy cabbage has one gram dietary fiber, 322 IU vitamin A (14 percent of the RDA for a woman, 11 percent of the RDA for a man), and 11 mg vitamin C (15 percent of the RDA for a woman, 12 percent of the RDA for a man).

Raw red cabbage contains an antinutrient enzyme that splits the thiamin molecule so that the vitamin is no longer nutritionally useful. This thiamin inhibitor is inactivated by cooking.

The Most Nutritious Way to Serve This Food

Raw or lightly steamed to protect the vitamin C.

Diets That May Restrict or Exclude This Food

Antiflatulence diet
Low-fiber diet

Buying This Food

Look for: Cabbages that feel heavy for their size. The leaves should be tightly closed and attached tightly at the stem end. The outer leaves on a savoy cabbage may curl back from the head, but the center leaves should still be relatively tightly closed.

Also look for green cabbages that still have their dark-green, vitamin-rich outer leaves.

Avoid: Green and savoy cabbage with yellow or wilted leaves. The yellow carotene pigments show through only when the cabbage has aged and its green chlorophyll pigments have faded. Wilted leaves mean a loss of moisture and vitamins.

Storing This Food

Handle cabbage gently; bruising tears cells and activates ascorbic acid oxidase, an enzyme in the leaves that hastens the destruction of vitamin C.

Store cabbage in a cool, dark place, preferably a refrigerator. In cold storage, cabbage can retain as much as 75 percent of its vitamin C for as long as six months. Cover the cabbage to keep it from drying out and losing vitamin A.

Preparing This Food

Do not slice the cabbage until you are ready to use it; slicing tears cabbage cells and releases the enzyme that hastens the oxidation and destruction of vitamin C.

If you plan to serve cooked green or red cabbage in wedges, don't cut out the inner core that hold the leaves together.

To separate the leaves for stuffing, immerse the entire head in boiling water for a few minutes, then lift it out and let it drain until it is cool enough to handle comfortably. The leaves should pull away easily. If not, put the cabbage back into the hot water for a few minutes.

What Happens When You Cook This Food

Cabbage contains mustard oils (isothiocyanates) that break down into a variety of smelly sulfur compounds (including hydrogen sulfide and ammonia) when the cabbage is heated, a reaction that occurs more strongly in aluminum pots. The longer you cook the cabbage, the more smelly the compounds will be. Adding a slice of bread to the cooking water may lessen the odor. Keeping a lid on the pot will stop the smelly molecules from floating off into the air, but it will also accelerate the chemical reaction that turns cooked green cabbage drab.

Chlorophyll, the pigment that makes green vegetables green, is sensitive to acids. When you heat green cabbage, the chlorophyll in its leaves reacts chemically with acids in the cabbage or in the cooking water to form pheophytin, which is brown. The pheophytin gives the cooked cabbage its olive color.

To keep cooked green cabbage green, you have to reduce the interaction between the chlorophyll and the acids. One way to do this is to cook the cabbage in a large quantity of water, so the acids will be diluted, but this increases the loss of vitamin C.[*] Another alternative is to leave the lid off the pot so that the volatile acids can float off into the air, but this allows the smelly sulfur compounds to escape too. The best way may be to steam the cabbage very quickly in very little water so that it keeps its vitamin C and cooks before there is time for the chlorophyll/acid reaction to occur.

Red cabbage is colored with red anthocyanins, pigments that turn redder in acids (lemon juice, vinegar) and blue purple in bases (alkaline chemicals such as baking soda). To keep the cabbage red, make sweet-and-sour cabbage. But be careful not to make it in an iron or aluminum pot, since vinegar (which contains tannins) will react with these metals to create dark pigments that discolor both the pot and the vegetable. Glass, stainless-steel, or enameled pots do not produce this reaction.

How Other Kinds of Processing Affect This Food

Pickling. Sauerkraut is a fermented and pickled produce made by immersing cabbage in a salt solution strong enough to kill off pathological bacteria but allow beneficial ones to survive, breaking down proteins in the cabbage and producing the acid that gives sauerkraut its distinctive flavor. Sauerkraut contains more than 37 times as much sodium as fresh cabbage (661 mg sodium/100 grams canned sauerkraut with liquid) but only one third the vitamin C and one-seventh the vitamin A.

---

[*] According to USDA, if you cook three cups of cabbage in one cup of water you will lose only 10 percent of the vitamin C; reverse the ratio to four times as much water as cabbage and you will lose about 50 percent of the vitamin C. Cabbage will lose as much as 25 percent of its vitamin C if you cook it in water that is cold when you start. As it boils, water releases oxygen that would otherwise destroy vitamin C, so you can cut the vitamin loss dramatically simply by letting the water boil for 60 seconds before adding the cabbage.

Medical Uses and/or Benefits

Protection against certain cancers.   Naturally occurring chemicals (indoles, isothiocyanates, glucosinolates, dithiolethiones, and phenols) in cabbage, brussels sprouts, broccoli, cauliflower, and other cruciferous vegetables appear to reduce the risk of some cancers, perhaps by preventing the formation of carcinogens in your body or by blocking cancer-causing substances from reaching or reacting with sensitive body tissues or by inhibiting the transformation of healthy cells to malignant ones.

All cruciferous vegetables contain sulforaphane, a member of a family of chemicals known as isothiocyanates. In experiments with laboratory rats, sulforaphane appears to increase the body's production of phase-2 enzymes, naturally occurring substances that inactivate and help eliminate carcinogens. At Johns Hopkins University in Baltimore, Maryland, 69 percent of the rats injected with a chemical known to cause mammary cancer developed tumors vs. only 26 percent of the rats given the carcinogenic chemical plus sulforaphane.

In 1997, Johns Hopkins researchers discovered that broccoli seeds and three-day-old broccoli sprouts contain a compound converted to sulforaphane when the seed and sprout cells are crushed. Five grams of three-day-old broccoli sprouts contain as much sulforaphane as 150 grams of mature broccoli. The sulforaphane levels in other cruciferous vegetables have not yet been calculated.

Vision protection.   In 2004, the Johns Hopkins researchers updated their findings on sulforaphane to suggest that it may also protect cells in the eyes from damage due to ultraviolet light, thus reducing the risk of macular degeneration, the most common cause of age-related vision loss.

Lower risk of some birth defects.   As many as two of every 1,000 babies born in the United States each year may have cleft palate or a neural tube (spinal cord) defect due to their mothers' not having gotten adequate amounts of folate during pregnancy. The current RDA for folate is 180 mcg for a woman and 200 mcg for a man, but the FDA now recommends 400 mcg for a woman who is or may become pregnant. Taking a folate supplement before becoming pregnant and through the first two months of pregnancy reduces the risk of cleft palate; taking folate through the entire pregnancy reduces the risk of neural tube defects.

Possible lower risk of heart attack.   In the spring of 1998, an analysis of data from the records for more than 80,000 women enrolled in the long-running Nurses' Health Study at Harvard School of Public Health/Brigham and Women's Hospital, in Boston, demonstrated that a diet providing more than 400 mcg folate and 3 mg vitamin B_6 daily, either from food or supplements, might reduce a woman's risk of heart attack by almost 50 percent. Although men were not included in the study, the results were assumed to apply to them as well.

However, data from a meta-analysis published in the *Journal of the American Medical Association* in December 2006 called this theory into question. Researchers at Tulane University examined the results of 12 controlled studies in which 16,958 patients with preexisting cardiovascular disease were given either folic acid supplements or placebos ("look-alike" pills with no folic acid) for at least six months. The scientists, who found no reduction in the risk of further heart disease or overall death rates among those taking folic acid, concluded that further studies will be required to verify whether taking folic acid supplements reduces the risk of cardiovascular disease.

Adverse Effects Associated with This Food

Enlarged thyroid gland (goiter).   Cruciferous vegetables, including cabbage, contain goitrin, thiocyanate, and isothiocyanate. These chemicals, known collectively as goitrogens, inhibit the formation of thyroid hormones and cause the thyroid to enlarge in an attempt to produce more. Goitrogens are not hazardous for healthy people who eat moderate amounts of cruciferous vegetables, but they may pose problems for people who have a thyroid condition or are taking thyroid medication.

Intestinal gas.   Bacteria that live naturally in the gut degrade the indigestible carbohydrates (food fiber) in cabbage, producing gas that some people find distressing.

Food/Drug Interactions

Anticoagulants   Cabbage contains vitamin K, the blood-clotting vitamin produced naturally by bacteria in the intestines. Consuming large quantities of this food may reduce the effectiveness of anticoagulants (blood thinners) such as warfarin (Coumadin). One cup of shredded common green cabbage contains 163 mcg vitamin K, nearly three times the RDA for a healthy adult; one cup of drained boiled common green cabbage contains 73 mcg vitamin K, slightly more than the RDA for a healthy adult.

Monoamine oxidase (MAO) inhibitors.   Monoamine oxidase inhibitors are drugs used to treat depression. They inactivate naturally occurring enzymes in your body that metabolize tyramine, a substance found in many fermented or aged foods. Tyramine constricts blood vessels and increases blood pressure. If you eat a food such as sauerkraut which is high in tyramine while you are taking an MAO inhibitor, you cannot effectively eliminate the tyramine from your body. The result may be a hypertensive crisis.

Carob

Nutritional Profile

Energy value (calories per serving): *Moderate*
Protein: *Moderate*
Fat: *Low*
Saturated fat: *Low*
Cholesterol: *None*
Carbohydrates: *High*
Fiber: *High*
Sodium: *Low*
Major vitamin contribution: *Niacin*
Major mineral contribution: *Calcium*

About the Nutrients in This Food

Carob flour, which is milled from the dried pod of a Mediterranean evergreen tree, *Ceratonia siliqua,* looks like cocoa but has a starchy, beanlike
flavor. It can be mixed with sweeteners to make a cocoalike powder or
combined with fats and sweeteners to produce a candy that looks like and
has the same rich mouthfeel as milk chocolate but tastes more like honey.

Ounce for ounce, carob, which is also known as locust bean gum,
has more fiber and calcium but fewer calories than cocoa. Its carbohydrates
include the sugars sucrose, D-mannose, and D-galactose. (D-galactose is a
simple sugar that links up with other sugars to form the complex indigestible sugars raffinose and stachyose.) Carob also contains gums and pectins,
the indigestible food fibers commonly found in seeds.

The Most Nutritious Way to Serve This Food

As a substitute for cocoa or chocolate for people who are sensitive to
chocolate.

Diets That May Restrict or Exclude This Food

Low-carbohydrate diet

Buying This Food

Look for: Tightly sealed containers that will protect the flour from moisture and insects.

Storing This Food

Store carob flour in a cool, dark place in a container that protects it from air, moisture, and insects. Keep carob candy cool and dry.

Preparing This Food

Measure out carob flour by filling a cup or tablespoon and leveling it off with a knife. To substitute carob for regular flour, use ¼ cup carob flour plus ¾ cup regular flour for each cup ordinary flour. To substitute for chocolate, use three tablespoons of carob flour plus two tablespoons of water for each ounce of unsweetened chocolate. Carob flour is sweeter than unsweetened chocolate.

What Happens When You Cook This Food

Unlike cocoa powder, carob flour contains virtually no fat. It will burn, not melt, if you heat it in a saucepan. When the flour is heated with water, its starch granules absorb moisture and rupture, releasing a gum that can be used as a stabilizer, thickener, or binder in processed foods and cosmetics. In cake batters, it performs just like other flours (see FLOUR).

How Other Kinds of Processing Affect This Food

* * *

Medical uses and/or Benefits

Adsorbent and demulcent. Medically, carob flour has been used as a soothing skin powder.

As a chocolate substitute. People who are sensitive to chocolate can usually use carob instead. Like cocoa beans, carob is free of cholesterol. Unlike cocoa, which contains the central-nervous-system stimulant caffeine and the muscle stimulant theobromine, carob does not contain any stimulating methylxanthines.

Lower cholesterol levels. In 2001, a team of German nutrition researchers from the Institute for Nutritional Science at the University of Potsdam, the German Institute of Human Nutrition, Center for Conventional Medicine and Alternative Therapies (Berlin) Nutrinova Nutrition Specialties and Food Ingredients GmbH, and PhytoPharm Consulting, Institute for

Phytopharmaceuticals GmbH conducted a study to evaluate carob's effectiveness in lowering cholesterol. For a period of eight weeks, 47 volunteers with moderately high cholesterol levels (232–302 mg/dL) were fed 15 g of carob per day in breakfast cereal, fruit grain bars, and a drink made from powdered carob pulp as supplements to their normal diet. After four weeks, the volunteers' total cholesterol levels fell an average of 7 percent and their LDL (low density lipoprotein—"bad" cholesterol) levels fell an average 10.6 percent. At six weeks, the numbers were 7.8 percent and 10.6 percent. There was no effect on HDLs (high density lipoproteins, a.k.a. "good" cholesterol).

Adverse Effects Associated with This Food

* * *

Food/Drug Interactions

* * *

Carrots

Nutritional Profile

Energy value (calories per serving): *Low*
Protein: *Moderate*
Fat: *Low*
Saturated fat: *Low*
Cholesterol: *None*
Carbohydrates: *High*
Fiber: *High*
Sodium: *Moderate*
Major vitamin contribution: *Vitamin A*
Major mineral contribution: *Potassium*

About the Nutrients in This Food

Carrots are high-fiber food, roots whose crispness comes from cell walls stiffened with the insoluble dietary fibers cellulose and lignin. Carrots also contain soluble pectins, plus appreciable amounts of sugar (mostly sucrose) and a little starch. They are an extraordinary source of vitamin A derived from deep yellow carotenoids (including beta-carotene).

One raw carrot, about seven inches long, has two grams of dietary fiber and 20,250 IU vitamin A (nine times the RDA for a woman, seven times the RDA for a man).

The Most Nutritious Way to Serve This Food

Cooked, so that the cellulose- and hemicellulose-stiffened cell walls of the carrot have partially dissolved and the nutrients inside are more readily available.

Diets That May Restrict or Exclude This Food

Disaccharide-intolerance diet (for people who are sucrase- and/or invertase-deficient)
Low-fiber diet
Low-sodium diet (fresh and canned carrots)

Buying This Food

Look for: Firm, bright orange yellow carrots with fresh, crisp green tops.

Avoid: Wilted or shriveled carrots, pale carrots, or carrots with brown spots on the skin.

Storing This Food

Trim off the green tops before you store carrots. The leafy tops will wilt and rot long before the sturdy root.

Keep carrots cool. They will actually gain vitamin A during their first five months in storage. Protected from heat and light, they can hold to their vitamins at least another two and a half months.

Store carrots in perforated plastic bags or containers. Circulating air prevents the formation of the terpenoids that make the carrots taste bitter. Do not store carrots near apples or other fruits that manufacture ethylene gas as they continue to ripen; this gas encourages the development of terpenoids.

Store peeled carrots in ice water in the refrigerator to keep them crisp for as long as 48 hours.

Preparing This Food

Scrape the carrots. Very young, tender carrots can be cleaned by scrubbing with a vegetable brush.

Soak carrots that are slightly limp in ice water to firm them up. Don't discard slightly wilted intact carrots; use them in soups or stews where texture doesn't matter.

What Happens When You Cook This Food

Since carotenes do not dissolve in water and are not affected by the normal heat of cooking, carrots stay yellow and retain their vitamin A when you heat them. But cooking will dissolve some of the hemicellulose in the carrot's stiff cell walls, changing the vegetable's texture and making it easier for digestive juices to penetrate the cells and reach the nutrients inside.

How Other Kinds of Processing Affect This Food

Freezing. The characteristic crunchy texture of fresh carrots depends on the integrity of its cellulose- and hemicellulose-stiffened cell walls. Freezing cooked carrots creates ice crystals that rupture these membranes so that the carrots usually seem mushy when defrosted. If possible, remove the carrots before freezing a soup or stew and add fresh or canned carrots when you defrost the dish.

Medical Uses and/or Benefits

A reduced risk of some kinds of cancer. According to the American Cancer Society, carrots and other foods rich in beta-carotene, a deep yellow pigment that your body converts to a form of vitamin A, may lower the risk of cancers of the larynx, esophagus and lungs. There is no such benefit from beta-carotene supplements; indeed, one controversial study actually showed a higher rate of lung cancer among smokers taking the supplement.

Protection against vitamin A-deficiency blindness. In the body, the vitamin A from carrots becomes 11-cis retinol, the essential element in rhodopsin, a protein found in the rods (the cells inside your eyes that let you see in dim light). Rhodopsin absorbs light, triggering the chain of chemical reactions known as vision. One raw carrot a day provides more than enough vitamin A to maintain vision in a normal healthy adult.

Adverse Effects Associated with This Food

Oddly pigmented skin. The carotenoids in carrots are fat-soluble. If you eat large amounts of carrots day after day, these carotenoids will be stored in your fatty tissues, including the fat just under your skin, and eventually your skin will look yellow. If you eat large amounts of carrots *and* large amounts of tomatoes (which contain the red pigment lycopene), your skin may be tinted orange. This effect has been seen in people who ate two cups of carrots and two tomatoes a day for several months; when the excessive amounts of these vegetables were eliminated from the diet, skin color returned to normal.

False-positive test for occult blood in the stool. The active ingredient in the guaiac slide test for hidden blood in feces is alphaguaiaconic acid, a chemical that turns blue in the presence of blood. Carrots contain peroxidase, a natural chemical that also turns alphaguaiaconic acid blue and may produce a positive test in people who do not actually have blood in the stool.

Food/Drug Interactions

* * *

Cauliflower

Nutritional Profile

Energy value (calories per serving): *Low*
Protein: *High*
Fat: *Low*
Saturated fat: *Low*
Cholesterol: *None*
Carbohydrates: *High*
Fiber: *High*
Sodium: *Low*
Major vitamin contribution: *B vitamins, vitamin C*
Major mineral contribution: *Potassium*

About the Nutrients in This Food

Cauliflower is an excellent source of vitamin C and a moderately good source of folate, a member of the B vitamin family.

One-half cup cooked fresh cauliflower florets (the top of the plant) has one gram dietary fiber, 13.5 mcg folate (3 percent of the RDA), and 35 mg vitamin C (50 percent of the RDA for a woman, 39 percent of the RDA for a man).

The Most Nutritious Way to Serve This Food

Raw or lightly steamed to protect the vitamin C. Cooked or frozen cauliflower may have up to 50 percent less vitamin C than raw cauliflower.

Diets That May Restrict or Exclude This Food

Antiflatulence diet
Low-fiber diet

Buying This Food

Look for: Creamy white heads with tight, compact florets and fresh green leaves. The size of the cauliflower has no bearing on its nutritional value or its taste.

Avoid: Cauliflower with brown spots or patches.

Storing This Food

Keep cauliflower in a cool, humid place to safeguard its vitamin C content.

Preparing This Food

Pull off and discard any green leaves still attached to the cauliflower and slice off the woody stem and core. Then plunge the cauliflower, head down, into a bowl of salted ice water to flush out any insects hiding in the head. To keep the cauliflower crisp when cooked, add a teaspoon of vinegar to the water. You can steam or bake the cauliflower head whole or break it up into florets for faster cooking.

What Happens When You Cook This Food

Cauliflower contains mustard oils (isothiocyanates), natural chemicals that give the vegetable its taste but break down into a variety of smelly sulfur compounds (including hydrogen sulfide and ammonia) when the cauliflower is heated. The longer you cook the cauliflower, the better it will taste but the worse it will smell. Adding a slice of bread to the cooking water may lessen the odor; keeping a lid on the pot will stop the smelly molecules from floating off into the air.

Cooking cauliflower in an aluminum pot will intensify its odor and turn its creamy white anthoxanthin pigments yellow; iron pots will turn anthoxanthins blue green or brown. Like red and blue anthocyanin pigments (see BEETS, BLACKBERRIES, BLUEBERRIES), anthoxanthins hold their color best in acids. To keep cauliflower white, add a tablespoon of lemon juice, lime juice, vinegar, or milk to the cooking water.

Steaming or stir-frying cauliflower preserves the vitamin C that would be lost if the vegetable were cooked for a long time or in a lot of water.

How Other Kinds of Processing Affect This Food

Freezing. Before it is frozen, cauliflower must be blanched to inactivate catalase and peroxidase, enzymes that would otherwise continue to ripen and eventually deteriorate the vegetable. According to researchers at Cornell University, cauliflower will lose less vitamin C if it is blanched in very little water (two cups cauliflower in two tbsp. water) in a microwave-safe plastic bag in a microwave oven for four minutes at 600–700 watts. Leave the bag open an inch at the top so steam can escape and the bag does not explode.

Medical Uses and/or Benefits

Protection against certain cancers. Naturally occurring chemicals (indoles, isothiocyanates, glucosinolates, dithiolethiones, and phenols) in cauliflower, Brussels sprouts, broccoli, cabbage, and other cruciferous vegetables appear to reduce the risk of some cancers, perhaps by preventing the formation of carcinogens in your body or by blocking cancer-causing substances from reaching or reacting with sensitive body tissues or by inhibiting the transformation of healthy cells to malignant ones.

All cruciferous vegetables contain sulforaphane, a member of a family of chemicals known as isothiocyanates. In experiments with laboratory rats, sulforaphane appears to increase the body's production of phase-2 enzymes, naturally occurring substances that inactivate and help eliminate carcinogens. At the Johns Hopkins University in Baltimore, Maryland, 69 percent of the rats injected with a chemical known to cause mammary cancer developed tumors vs. only 26 percent of the rats given the carcinogenic chemical plus sulforaphane.

In 1997, Johns Hopkins researchers discovered that broccoli seeds and three-day-old broccoli sprouts contain a compound converted to sulforaphane when the seed and sprout cells are crushed. Five grams of three-day-old broccoli sprouts contain as much sulforaphane as 150 grams of mature broccoli. The sulforaphane levels in other cruciferous vegetables have not yet been calculated.

Vision protection. In 2004, the Johns Hopkins researchers updated their findings on sulforaphane to suggest that it may also protect cells in the eyes from damage due to UV (ultraviolet) light, thus reducing the risk of macular degeneration, the most common cause of age-related vision loss.

Adverse Effects Associated with This Food

Enlarged thyroid gland (goiter). Cruciferous vegetables, including cauliflower, contain goitrin, thiocyanate, and isothiocyanate. These chemicals, known collectively as goitrogens, inhibit the formation of thyroid hormones and cause the thyroid to enlarge in an attempt to produce more. Goitrogens are not hazardous for healthy people who eat moderate amounts of cruciferous vegetables, but they may pose problems for people who have a thyroid condition or are taking thyroid medication.

Intestinal gas. Bacteria that live naturally in the gut degrade the indigestible carbohydrates (food fiber) in cauliflower, producing intestinal gas that some people find distressing.

Food/Drug Interactions

Anticoagulants (blood thinners). All cruciferous vegetables (broccoli, brussels sprouts, cabbages, cauliflower, greens, radishes, and turnips) are high in vitamin K, a nutrient that decreases the anticoagulant effect of medicine such as warfarin (Coumadin). Multiple servings of this vegetable, i.e., several days a week, may interfere with the anticoagulant effect of the drug.

False-positive test for occult blood in the stool. The active ingredient in the guaiac slide test for hidden blood in feces is alphaguaiaconic acid, a chemical that turns blue in the presence of blood. Cauliflower contains peroxidase, a natural chemical that also turns alphaguaiaconic acid blue and may produce a positive test in people who do not actually have blood in the stool.

Caviar

Nutritional Profile

Energy value (calories per serving): *High*

Protein: *High*

Fat: *High*

Saturated fat: *Low*

Cholesterol: *High*

Carbohydrates: *Low*

Fiber: *None*

Sodium: *High*

Major vitamin contribution: *B vitamins*

Major mineral contribution: *Calcium, iron, phosphorus*

About the Nutrients in This Food

Caviar is a high-fat, high-cholesterol, high-protein, low-carbohydrate food. It is extremely high in sodium (650 mg/oz.) and, ounce for ounce, contains twice as much calcium as milk.

The Most Nutritious Way to Serve This Food

* * *

Diets That May Restrict or Exclude This Food

Low-cholesterol, controlled-fat diet

Low-salt/low-sodium diet

Buying This Food

Look for: Shiny, translucent, large-grained gray fresh caviar (sturgeon roe) with a clean aroma.

Look for: Tightly sealed tins and jars of less expensive roe. Lumpfish roe is small-grained and usually black. Cod, salmon, carp, pike, and tuna roe are large-grained and orangey red or pinkish.

Storing This Food

Store fresh caviar in the coldest part of the refrigerator; it will spoil within hours at temperatures above 39°F.

Store jars of caviar in a cool, dark place.

Preparing This Food

Always serve caviar in a dish (or jar) nestled in ice to keep it safe at room temperature. The roe contains so much salt that it will not freeze.

When making canapés, add the caviar last so that the oil does not spread and discolor the other ingredients.

What Happens When You Cook This Food

* * *

How Other Kinds of Processing Affect This Food

Pressing.   Pressed caviar is caviar with 10 percent of its moisture removed. As a result it contains more nutrients per ounce than regular caviar and is even higher in sodium.

Medical Uses and/or Benefits

Omega-3 fish oils.   Caviar contains the same protective oils found in other fish (see FISH).

Adverse Effects Associated with This Food

* * *

Food/Drug Interactions

MAO inhibitors.   Monoamine oxidase (MAO) inhibitors are drugs used as antidepressants or antihypertensives. They inhibit the action of enzymes that break down tyramine, a natural by-product of protein metabolism. Tyramine is a pressor amine, a chemical that constricts blood vessels and raises blood pressure. If you eat a food that contains tyramine while you are taking an MAO inhibitor, the pressor amine cannot be eliminated from your body and the result could be a hypertensive crisis (sustained elevated blood pressure). Caviar contains small amounts of tyramine.

Celeriac

Nutritional Profile

Energy value (calories per serving): *Low*
Protein: *Moderate*
Fat: *Low*
Saturated fat: *Low*
Cholesterol: *None*
Carbohydrates: *High*
Fiber: *Moderate*
Sodium: *Moderate*
Major vitamin contribution: *Vitamin C*
Major mineral contribution: *Potassium, phosphorus*

About the Nutrients in This Food

Celeriac is the starchy root of a variety of celery with moderate amounts of dietary fiber and vitamin C. One-half cup cooked celeriac has one gram dietary fiber and 4 mg vitamin C (5 percent of the RDA for a woman, 4 percent of the RDA for a man), and 134 mg potassium—about 40 percent as much potassium as one medium orange.

The Most Nutritious Way to Serve This Food

Fresh sliced in salads to protect the vitamin C.

Diets That May Restrict or Exclude This Food

Low-fiber diet
Low-sodium diet

Buying This Food

Look for: firm, small-to-medium, sprout-free celeriac roots

Avoid: large roots. Larger celeriac roots contain more cellulose and lignin, which gives them a "woody" texture.

Storing This Food

Do remove green tops from celeriac before storing the root.

Do refrigerate celeriac in plastic bags or in the vegetable crisper; it will keep fresh for about a week.

Preparing This Food

Scrub celeriac under cold running water. Cut off leaves, and extra root buds. Peel the root, slice it and either use it raw in salads or boil it to serve as a vegetable side dish.

When you cut into the celeriac, you tear its cell walls, releasing polyphenoloxidase, an enzyme that will turn the vegetable brown. You can slow the reaction (but not stop it completely) by dipping peeled, sliced raw celeriac in an acid such as lemon juice or a solution of vinegar and water.

What Happens When You Cook This Food

When celeriac is heated, the soluble fibers in its cell walls dissolves; the cooked vegetable is softer.

How Other Kinds of Processing Affect This Food

* * *

Medical Uses and/or Benefits

Lower risk of stroke. Potassium lowers blood pressure. According to new data from the Harvard University Health Professionals Study, a long-running survey of male doctors, a diet rich in high-potassium foods such as bananas may also reduce the risk of stroke. The men who ate the most potassium-rich foods (an average nine servings a day) had 38 percent fewer strokes than men who ate the least (less than four servings a day).

Adverse Effects Associated with This Food

* * *

Celery

Nutritional Profile

Energy value (calories per serving): *Low*
Protein: *Moderate*
Fat: *Low*
Saturated fat: *Low*
Cholesterol: *None*
Carbohydrates: *High*
Fiber: *Moderate*
Sodium: *High*
Major vitamin contribution: *Folate*
Major mineral contribution: *Potassium, phosphorus*

About the Nutrients in This Food

Celery has moderate amounts of dietary fiber and small amounts of the B vitamin folate.

One-half cup diced raw celery has one gram dietary fiber and 17 mcg folate (4 percent of the RDA).

The Most Nutritious Way to Serve This Food

Fresh, filled with cheese to add protein.

Diets That May Restrict or Exclude This Food

Low-fiber diet
Low-sodium diet

Buying This Food

Look for: Crisp, medium-size pale green celery with fresh leaves. Darker stalks have more vitamin A but are likely to be stringy.

Avoid: Wilted or yellowed stalks. Wilted stalks have lost moisture and are low in vitamins A and C. Yellowed stalks are no longer fresh; their chlorophyll pigments have faded enough to let the yellow carotenes show through.

Avoid bruised or rotten celery. Celery cells contain chemicals called furocoumarins (psoralens) that may turn carcinogenic when the cell membranes are damaged and the furocoumarins are exposed to light. Bruised or rotting celery may contain up to a hundred times the psoralens in fresh celery.

Storing This Food

Handle celery carefully to avoid damaging the stalks and releasing furocoumarins.

Refrigerate celery in plastic bags or in the vegetable crisper to keep them moist and crisp. They will stay fresh for about a week.

Preparing This Food

Rinse celery under cold running water to remove all sand and dirt. Cut off the leaves, blanch them, dry them thoroughly, and rub them through a sieve or food mill. The dry powder can be used to season salt or frozen for later use in soups or stews.

What Happens When You Cook This Food

When you cook celery the green flesh will soften as the pectin inside its cells dissolves in water, but the virtually indestructible cellulose and lignin "strings" on the ribs will stay stiff. If you don't like the strings, pull them off before you cook the celery.

Cooking also changes the color of celery. Chlorophyll, the pigment that makes green vegetables green, is very sensitive to acids. When you heat celery, the chlorophyll in its stalks reacts chemically with acids in the celery or in the cooking water to form pheophytin, which is brown. The pheophytin will turn the celery olive-drab or, if the stalks have a lot of yellow carotene, bronze.

You can prevent this natural chemical reaction and keep the celery green by cooking it so quickly that there is no time for the chlorophyll to react with the acids, or by cooking it in lots of water (which will dilute the acids), or by cooking it with the lid off the pot so that the volatile acids can float off into the air.

How Other Kinds of Processing Affect This Food

* * *

Medical Uses and/or Benefits

* * *

Adverse Effects Associated with This Food

Contact dermatitis. Celery contains limonene, an essential oil known to cause contact dermatitis in sensitive individuals. (Limonene is also found in dill, caraway seeds, and the peel of lemon and limes.)

Photosensitivity. The furocoumarins (psoralens) released by damaged or moldy celery are photosensitizers as well as potential mutagens and carcinogens. Constant contact with these chemicals can make skin very sensitive to light, a problem most common among food workers who handle large amounts of celery without wearing gloves.

Nitrate/nitrite poisoning. Like beets, eggplant, lettuce, radish, spinach, and collard and turnip greens, celery contains nitrates that convert naturally into nitrites in your stomach and then react with the amino acids in proteins to form nitrosamines. Although some nitrosamines are known or suspected carcinogens, this natural chemical conversion presents no known problems for a healthy adult. However, when these nitrate-rich vegetables are cooked and left to stand at room temperature, bacterial enzyme action (and perhaps some enzymes in the plants) convert the nitrates to nitrites at a much faster rate than normal. These higher-nitrite foods may be hazardous for infants; several cases of "spinach poisoning" have been reported among children who ate cooked spinach that had been left standing at room temperature.

Food/Drug Interactions

* * *

Cheese

Nutritional Profile

Energy value (calories per serving): *Moderate to high*
Protein: *Moderate to high*
Fat: *Low to high*
Saturated fat: *High*
Cholesterol: *Low to high*
Carbohydrates: *Low*
Fiber: *None*
Sodium: *High*
Major vitamin contribution: *Vitamin A, vitamin D, B vitamins*
Major mineral contribution: *Calcium*

About the Nutrients in This Food

Cheese making begins when *Lactobacilli* and/or *Streptococci* bacteria are added to milk. The bacteria digest lactose (milk sugar) and release lactic acid, which coagulates casein (milk protein) into curds. Rennet (gastric enzymes extracted from the stomach of calves) is added, and the mixture is put aside to set. The longer the curds are left to set, the firmer the cheese will be. When the curds are properly firm, they are pressed to squeeze out the whey (liquid) and cooked. Cooking evaporates even more liquid and makes the cheese even firmer.[*]

At this point, the product is "fresh" or "green" cheese: cottage cheese, cream cheese, farmer cheese. Making "ripe" cheese requires the addition of salt to pull out more moisture and specific organisms, such as *Penicillium roquefort* for Roquefort cheese, blue cheese, and Stilton, or *Penicillium cambembert* for Camembert and Brie.

The nutritional value of cheese is similar to the milk from which it is made. All cheese is a good source of high quality proteins with sufficient amounts of all the essential amino acids. Cheese is low to high in fat, moderate to high in cholesterol.

---

[*] *Natural cheese* is cheese made directly from milk. *Processed cheese* is natural cheese melted and combined with emulsifiers. *Pasteurized process cheese foods* contain ingredients that allow them to spread smoothly; they are lower in fat and higher in moisture than processed cheese.

Cholesterol and Saturated Fat Content of Selected Cheeses

Cheese	Serving	Cholesterol (mg)	Saturated fat (g)
American	oz.	25	5.3
Blue/Roquefort	oz.	21	5.3
Camembert	wedge	27	5.8
Cheddar	oz.	30	6.0
Cottage cheese			
creamed	cup	25–34	6.0–6.4
uncreamed	cup	10	0.4
Mozzarella			
part skim	oz.	15	3.1
whole milk	oz.	22	3.7
Muenster	oz.	27	5.4
Swiss	oz.	26	5.0

Source: USDA, *Nutritive Value of Foods,* Home and Garden Bulletin No. 72 (USDA, 1989).

All cheeses, except cottage cheese, are good sources of vitamin A. Orange and yellow cheeses are colored with carotenoid pigments, including bixin (the carotenoid pigment in annatto) and synthetic beta-carotene.

Hard cheeses are an excellent source of calcium; softer cheeses are a good source; cream cheese and cottage cheese are poor sources. The RDA for calcium is 1,000 mg for a woman, 1,200 mg for a man, and 1,500 mg for an older woman who is not on hormone-replacement therapy. All cheese, unless otherwise labeled, is high in sodium.

Calcium Content of Cheese

Cheese	Serving	Calcium (mg)
Blue	oz.	150
Camembert	wedge	147
Cheddar	oz.	204
Cottage cheese		
creamed	cup	135
uncreamed	cup	46
Muenster	oz.	203
Pasteurized processed American	oz.	174
Parmesan grated	tbsp.	69
Provolone	oz.	214
Swiss	oz.	272

Source: *Nutritive Value of Foods,* Home and Gardens Bulletin No. 72 (USDA, 1989).

The Most Nutritious Way to Serve This Food

With grains, bread, noodles, beans, nuts, or vegetables to add the essential amino acids missing from these foods, "complete" their proteins, and make them more nutritionally valuable.

Diets That May Restrict or Exclude This Food

Antiflatulence diet
Controlled-fat, low-cholesterol diet
Lactose- and galactose-free diet (lactose, a disaccharide [double sugar] is composed of one unit of galactose and one unit of glucose)
Low-calcium diet (for patients with kidney disease)
Sucrose-free diet (processed cheese)

Buying This Food

Look for: Cheese stored in a refrigerated case. Check the date on the package.

Avoid: Any cheese with mold that is not an integral part of the food.

Storing This Food

Refrigerate all cheese except unopened canned cheeses (such as Camembert in tins) or grated cheeses treated with preservatives and labeled to show that they can be kept outside the refrigerator. Some sealed packages of processed cheeses can be stored at room temperature but must be refrigerated once the package is opened.

Wrap cheeses tightly to protect them from contamination by other microorganisms in the air and to keep them from drying out. Well-wrapped, refrigerated hard cheeses that have not been cut or sliced will keep for up to six months; sliced hard cheeses will keep for about two weeks. Soft cheeses (cottage cheese, ricotta, cream cheese, and Neufchatel) should be used within five to seven days. Use all packaged or processed cheeses by the date stamped on the package.

Throw out moldy cheese (unless the mold is an integral part of the cheese, as with blue cheese or Stilton).

Preparing This Food

To grate cheese, chill the cheese so it won't stick to the grater.

The molecules that give cheese its taste and aroma are largely immobilized when the cheese is cold. When serving cheese with fruit or crackers, bring it to room temperature to activate these molecules.

What Happens When You Cook This Food

Heat changes the structure of proteins. The molecules are denatured, which means that they may be broken into smaller fragments or change shape or clump together. All of these changes may force moisture out of the protein tissue, which is why overcooked cheese is often stringy. Whey proteins, which do not clump or string at low temperatures, contain the sulfur atoms that give hot or burned cheese an unpleasant "cooked" odor. To avoid both strings and an unpleasant odor, add cheese to sauces at the last minute and cook just long enough to melt the cheese.

How Other Kinds of Processing Affect This Food

Freezing. All cheese loses moisture when frozen, so semisoft cheeses will freeze and thaw better than hard cheeses, which may be crumbly when defrosted.

Drying. The less moisture cheese contains, the less able it is to support the growth of organisms like mold. Dried cheeses keep significantly longer than ordinary cheeses.

Medical Uses and/or Benefits

To strengthen bones and reduce age-related loss of bone density. High-calcium foods protect bone density. The current recommended dietary allowance (RDA) for calcium is still 800 mg for adults 25 and older, but a 1984 National Institutes of Health (NIH) Conference advisory stated that lifelong protection for bones requires an RDA of 1,000 mg for healthy men and women age 25 to 50; 1,000 mg for older women using hormone replacement therapy; and 1,500 mg for older women who are not using hormones, and these recommendations have been confirmed in a 1994 NIH Consensus Statement on optimal calcium intake. A diet with adequate amounts of calcium-rich foods helps protect bone density. Low-fat and no-fat cheeses provide calcium without excess fat and cholesterol.

Protection against tooth decay. Studies at the University of Iowa (Iowa City) Dental School confirm that a wide variety of cheeses, including aged cheddar, Edam, Gouda, Monterey Jack, Muenster, mozzarella, Port Salut, Roquefort, Romano, Stilton, Swiss, and Tilsit—limit the tooth decay ordinarily expected when sugar becomes trapped in plaque, the sticky film on tooth surfaces where cavity-causing bacteria flourish. In a related experiment using only cheddar cheese, people who ate cheddar four times a day over a two-week period showed a 20 percent buildup of strengthening minerals on the surface of synthetic toothlike material attached to the root surfaces of natural teeth.

Protection against periodontal disease. A report in the January 2008 issue of the *Journal of Periodontology* suggests that consuming adequate amounts of dairy products may reduce the risk of developing periodontal disease. Examining the dental health of 942 subjects ages 40 to 79, researchers at Kyushu University, in Japan, discovered that those whose diets regularly included two ounces (55 g) of foods containing lactic acid (milk, cheese, and yogurt) were significantly less likely to have deep "pockets" (loss of attachment of tooth to gum) than those who consumed fewer dairy products.

Adverse Effects Associated with This Food

Increased risk of heart disease. Like other foods from animals, cheese is a source of cholesterol and saturated fats, which increase the amount of cholesterol circulating in your blood and raise your risk of heart disease. To reduce the risk of heart disease, the USDA/Health and Human Services Dietary Guidelines for Americans recommends limiting the amount of cholesterol in your diet to no more than 300 mg a day. The guidelines also recommend limiting the amount of fat you consume to no more than 30 percent of your total calories, while holding your consumption of saturated fats to more than 10 percent of your total calories (the calories from saturated fats are counted as part of the total calories from fat).

Food poisoning. Cheese made from raw (unpasteurized) milk may contain hazardous microorganisms, including *Salmonella* and *Listeria. Salmonella* causes serious gastric upset; *Listeria,* a flulike infection, encephalitis, or blood infection. Both may be life-threatening to the very young, the very old, pregnant women, and those whose immune systems are weakened either by illness (such as AIDS) or drugs (such as cancer chemotherapy). In 1998, the Federal Centers for Disease Control (CDC) released data identifying *Listeria* as the cause of nearly half the reported deaths from food poisoning.

Allergy to milk proteins. Milk is one of the foods most frequently implicated as a cause of allergic reactions, particularly upset stomach. However, in many cases the reaction is not a true allergy but the result of lactose intolerance (see below).

Lactose intolerance. Lactose intolerance—the inability to digest the sugar in milk—is an inherited metabolic deficiency that affects two thirds of all adults, including 90 to 95 percent of all Orientals, 70 to 75 percent of all blacks, and 6 to 8 percent of Caucasians. These people do not have sufficient amounts of lactase, the enzyme that breaks the disaccharide lactose into its easily digested components, galactose and glucose. When they drink milk, the undigested sugar is fermented by bacteria in the gut, causing bloating, diarrhea, flatulence, and intestinal discomfort. Some milk is now sold with added lactase to digest the lactose and make the milk usable for lactase-deficient people. In making cheese, most of the lactose in milk is broken down into glucose and galactose. There is very little lactose in cheeses other than the fresh ones—cottage cheese, cream cheese, and farmer cheese.

Galactosemia. Galactosemia is an inherited metabolic disorder in which the body lacks the enzymes needed to metabolize galactose, a component of lactose. Galactosemia is a recessive trait; you must receive the gene from both parents to develop the condition. Babies born with galactosemia will fail to thrive and may develop brain damage or cataracts if they are given milk. To prevent this, children with galactosemia are usually kept on a protective milk-free diet for several years, until their bodies have developed alternative pathways by which to metabolize galactose. Pregnant women who are known carriers of galactosemia may be advised to give up milk and milk products while pregnant lest the unmetabolized galactose in their bodies cause brain damage to the fetus (damage not detectable by amniocentesis). Genetic counseling is available to identify galactosemia carriers and assess their chances of producing a baby with the disorder.

Penicillin sensitivity. People who experience a sensitivity reaction the first time they take penicillin may have been sensitized by exposure to the *Penicillium* molds in the environment, including the *Penicillium* molds used to make brie, blue, camembert, roquefort, Stilton, and other "blue" cheeses.

Food/Drug Interactions

Tetracycline. The calcium ions in milk products, including cheese, bind tetracyclines into insoluble compounds. If you take tetracyclines with cheese, your body may not be able to absorb and use the drug efficiently.

Monoamine oxidase (MAO) inhibitors. Monoamine oxidase inhibitors are drugs used to treat depression. They inactivate naturally occurring enzymes in your body that metabolize tyramine, a substance found in many fermented or aged foods. Tyramine constricts blood vessels and increases blood pressure. If you eat a food such as aged or fermented cheese which is high in tyramine while you are taking an MAO inhibitor, your body may not be able to eliminate the tyramine. The result may be a hypertensive crisis.

Tyramine Content of Cheeses

High
Boursault, Camembert, Cheddar, Emmenthaler, Stilton
Medium to high
Blue, brick, Brie, Gruyère, mozzarella, Parmesan, Romano, Roquefort
Low
Processed American cheese
Very little or none
Cottage and cream cheese

Sources: *The Medical Letter Handbook of Adverse Drug Interactions* (1985); *Handbook of Clinical Dietetics* (The American Dietetic Association, 1981).

False-positive test for pheochromocytoma. Pheochromocytomas (tumors of the adrenal glands) secrete adrenalin that is converted by the body to vanillyl-mandelic acid (VMA) and excreted in the urine. Tests for this tumor measure the level of VMA in the urine. Since cheese contains VMA, taking the test after eating cheese may result in a false-positive result. Ordinarily, cheese is prohibited for at least 72 hours before this diagnostic test.

Cherries

Nutritional Profile

Energy value (calories per serving): *Low*
Protein: *Moderate*
Fat: *Low*
Saturated fat: *Low*
Cholesterol: *None*
Carbohydrates: *High*
Fiber: *Moderate*
Sodium: *Low**
Major vitamin contribution: *Vitamin A (sour cherries), vitamin C*
Major mineral contribution: *Potassium*

About the Nutrients in This Food

Cherries have moderate amounts of fiber, insoluble cellulose and lignin in the skin and soluble pectins in the flesh, plus vitamin C.

One cup fresh red sweet cherries (two ounces, without pits) has 3.2 g dietary fiber, 64 IU vitamin A (.2 percent of the RDA) and 10.8 mg vitamin C (14 percent of the RDA for a woman, 12 percent of the RDA for a man). One-half cup canned water-packed sour/tart cherries has 0.5 g dietary fiber and 1.5 mg vitamin C, and 377 IU vitamin A (16 percent of the RDA for a woman, 13 percent of the RDA for a man).

Like apple seeds and apricot, peach, or plum pits, cherry pits contain amygdalin, a naturally occurring cyanide/sugar compound that breaks down into hydrogen cyanide in the stomach. While accidentally swallowing a cherry pit once in a while is not a serious hazard, cases of human poisoning after eating apple seeds have been reported (see APPLES). NOTE: Some wild cherries are poisonous.

The Most Nutritious Way to Serve This Food

Sweet cherries can be eaten raw to protect their vitamin C; sour ("cooking") cherries are more palatable when cooked.

---

*   Except for maraschino cherries, which are high in sodium.

Diets That May Restrict or Exclude This Food

Low-sodium diet (maraschino cherries)

Buying This Food

Look for: Plump, firm, brightly colored cherries with glossy skin whose color may range from pale golden yellow to deep red to almost black, depending on the variety. The stems should be green and fresh, bending easily and snapping back when released.

Avoid: Sticky cherries (they've been damaged and are leaking), red cherries with very pale skin (they're not fully ripe), and bruised cherries whose flesh will be discolored under the bruise.

Storing This Food

Store cherries in the refrigerator to keep them cold and humid, conserving their nutrient and flavor. Cherries are highly perishable; use them as quickly as possible.

Preparing This Food

Handle cherries with care. When you bruise, peel, or slice a cherry you tear its cell walls, releasing polyphenoloxidase—an enzyme that converts phenols in the cherry into brown compounds that darken the fruit. You can slow this reaction (but not stop it completely) by dipping raw sliced or peeled cherries into an acid solution (lemon juice and water or vinegar and water) or by mixing them with citrus fruits in a fruit salad. Polyphenoloxidase also works more slowly in the cold, but storing sliced or peeled cherries in the refrigerator is much less effective than bathing them in an acid solution.

What Happens When You Cook This Food

Depending on the variety, cherries get their color from either red anthocyanin pigments or yellow to orange to red carotenoids. The anthocyanins dissolve in water, turn redder in acids and bluish in bases (alkalis). The carotenoids are not affected by heat and do not dissolve in water, which is why cherries do not lose vitamin A when you cook them. Vitamin C, however, is vulnerable to heat.

How Other Kinds of Processing Affect This Food

Canning and freezing. Canned and frozen cherries contain less vitamin C and vitamin A than fresh cherries. Sweetened canned or frozen cherries contain more sugar than fresh cherries.

Candying. Candied cherries are much higher in calories and sugar than fresh cherries. Maraschino cherries contain about twice as many calories per serving as fresh cherries and are high in sodium.

Medical Uses and/or Benefits

Anti-inflammatory effects. In a series of laboratory studies conducted from 1998 through 2001, researchers at the Bioactive Natural Products Laboratory in the Department of Horticulture and National Food Safety and Toxicology Center at Michigan State University discovered that the anthocyanins (red pigments) in tart cherries effectively block the activity of two enzymes, COX-1 and COX-2, essential for the production of prostaglandins, which are natural chemicals involved in the inflammatory response (which includes redness, heat, swelling, and pain). In other words, the anthocyanins appeared to behave like aspirin and other traditional nonsteroidal anti-inflammatory drugs, such as ibuprofen and naproxen. In 2004, scientists at the USDA Human Nutrition Research Center in Davis, California, released data from a study showing that women who ate 45 bing (sweet) cherries at breakfast each morning had markedly lower blood levels of uric acid, a by-product of protein metabolism linked to pain and inflammation, during an acute episode of gout (a form of arthritis). The women in the study also had lower blood levels of C-reactive protein and nitric acid, two other chemicals linked to inflammation. These effects are yet to be proven in larger studies with a more diverse group of subjects.

Adverse Effects Associated with This Food

* * *

Food/Drug Interactions

* * *

Chocolate

(Cocoa, milk chocolate, sweet chocolate)

Nutritional Profile[*]

Energy value (calories per serving): *Moderate*

Protein: *Low (cocoa powder)*
　　　　　High (chocolate)

Fat: *Moderate*

Saturated fat: *High*

Cholesterol: *None*

Carbohydrates: *Low (chocolate)*
　　　　　　　High (cocoa powder)

Fiber: *Moderate (chocolate)*
　　　High (cocoa powder)

Sodium: *Moderate*

Major vitamin contribution: *B vitamins*

Major mineral contribution: *Calcium, iron, copper*

About the Nutrients in This Food

Cocoa beans are high-carbohydrate, high-protein food, with less dietary fiber and more fat than all other beans, excepting SOY BEANS.

The cocoa bean's dietary fiber includes pectins and gums. Its proteins are limited in the essential amino acids lysine and isoleucine. Cocoa butter, the fat in cocoa beans, is the second most highly saturated vegetable fat (coconut oil is number one), but it has two redeeming nutritional qualities. First, it rarely turns rancid. Second, it melts at 95°F, the temperature of the human tongue. Cocoa butter has no cholesterol; neither does plain cocoa powder or plain dark chocolate.

Cocoa beans have B vitamins (thiamine, riboflavin, niacin) plus minerals (iron, magnesium, potassium, phosphorus, and copper).

All chocolate candy is made from chocolate liquor, a thick paste produce by roasting and grinding cocoa beans. Dark (sweet) chocolate is made of chocolate liquor, cocoa butter, and sugar. Milk chocolate is made of chocolate liquor, cocoa butter, sugar, milk or milk powder, and vanilla. White

---

* These values apply to plain cocoa powder and plain unsweetened chocolate. Adding other foods, such as milk or sugar, changes these values. For example, there is no cholesterol in plain bitter chocolate, but there is cholesterol in milk chocolate.

chocolate is made of cocoa butter, sugar, and milk powder. Baking chocolate is unsweetened dark chocolate. The most prominent nutrient in chocolate is its fat.

Fat Content in One Ounce of Chocolate

	Saturated fat (g)	Monounsaturated fat (g)	Polyunsaturated fat (g)	Cholesterol (mg)
Dark (sweet) chocolate	5.6	3.2	0.3	0
Milk chocolate	5.9	4.5	0.4	6.6
Baking chocolate	9	5.6	0.3	0
White chocolate	5.5	2.6	0.3	0

Source: USDA Nutrient Data Laboratory. National Nutrient Database for Standard Reference. Available online. URL: http://www.nal.usda.gov/fnic/foodcomp/search/.

Because chocolate is made from a bean, it also contains dietary fiber and measurable amounts of certain minerals. For example, one ounce of dark chocolate, the most nutritious "eating" chocolate, has 1.6 g dietary fiber, 0.78 mg iron (4 percent of the RDA for a woman, 10 percent of the RDA for a man), 32 mg magnesium (11 percent of the RDA for a woman, 8 percent of the RDA for a man), and .43 mg zinc (5 percent of the RDA for a woman, 4 percent of the RDA for a man).

Cocoa beans, cocoa, and chocolate contain caffeine, the muscle stimulant theobromine, and the mood-altering chemicals phenylethylalanine and anandamide (see below).

The Most Nutritious Way to Serve This Food

With low-fat milk to complete the proteins without adding saturated fat and cholesterol. NOTE: Both cocoa and chocolate contain oxalic acid, which binds with calcium to form calcium oxalate, an insoluble compound, but milk has so much calcium that the small amount bound to cocoa and chocolate hardly matters. Chocolate skim milk is a source of calcium.

Diets That May Restrict or Exclude This Food

Antiflatulence diet
Low-calcium and low-oxalate diet (to prevent the formation of calcium oxalate kidney stones)
Low-calorie diet
Low-carbohydrate diet
Low-fat diet
Low-fat, controlled-cholesterol diet (milk chocolates)
Low-fiber diet
Potassium-regulated (low-potassium) diet

Buying This Food

Look for: Tightly sealed boxes or bars. When you open a box of chocolates or unwrap a candy bar, the chocolate should be glossy and shiny. Chocolate that looks dull may be stale, or it may be inexpensively made candy without enough cocoa butter to make it gleam and give it the rich creamy mouthfeel we associate with the best chocolate. (Fine chocolate melts evenly on the tongue.) Chocolate should also smell fresh, not dry and powdery, and when you break a bar or piece of chocolate it should break cleanly, not crumble. One exception: If you have stored a bar of chocolate in the refrigerator, it may splinter if you break it without bringing it to room temperature first.

Storing This Food

Store chocolate at a constant temperature, preferably below 78°F. At higher temperatures, the fat in the chocolate will rise to the surface and, when the chocolate is cooled, the fat will solidify into a whitish powdery *bloom*. Bloom is unsightly but doesn't change the chocolate's taste or nutritional value. To get rid of bloom, melt the chocolate. The chocolate will turn dark, rich brown again when its fat recombines with the other ingredients. Chocolate with bloom makes a perfectly satisfactory chocolate sauce.

   Dark chocolate (bitter chocolate, semisweet chocolate) ages for at least six months after it is made, as its flavor becomes deeper and more intense. Wrapped tightly and stored in a cool, dry cabinet, it can stay fresh for a year or more. Milk chocolate ages only for about a month after it is made and holds its peak flavor for about three to six months, depending on how carefully it is stored. Plain cocoa, with no added milk powder or sugar, will stay fresh for up to a year if you keep it tightly sealed and cool.

Preparing This Food

* * *

What Happens When You Cook This Food

Chocolate burns easily. To melt it without mishap, stir the chocolate in a bowl over a pot of hot water or in the top of a double boiler or put the chocolate in a covered dish and melt it in the microwave (which does not get as hot as a pot on the store).

   Simple chemistry dictates that chocolate cakes be leavened with baking soda rather than baking powder. Chocolate is so acidic that it will upset the delicate balance of acid (cream of tartar) and base (alkali = sodium bicarbonate = baking soda) in baking powder. But it is not acidic enough to balance plain sodium bicarbonate. That's why we add an acidic sour-milk product such as buttermilk or sour cream or yogurt to a chocolate cake. Without the sour milk, the batter would be so basic that the chocolate would look red, not brown, and taste very bitter.

How Other Kinds of Processing Affect This Food

Freezing. Chocolate freezes and thaws well. Pack it in a moistureproof container and defrost it in the same package to let it reabsorb moisture it gave off while frozen.

Medical Uses and/or Benefits

Mood elevator. Chocolate's reputation for making people feel good is based not only on its caffeine content—19 mg caffeine per ounce of dark (sweet) chocolate, which is one-third the amount of caffeine in a five-ounce cup of brewed coffee—but also on its naturally occurring mood altering chemicals phenylethylalanine and anandamide. Phenylethylalanine is found in the blood of people in love. Anandamide stimulates areas of your brain also affected by the active ingredients in marijuana. (NOTE: As noted by the researchers at the Neurosciences Institute in San Diego who identified anandamide in chocolate in 1996, to get even the faintest hint of marijuana-like effects from chocolate you would have to eat more than 25 pounds of the candy all at once.)

Possible heart health benefits. Chocolate is rich in catechins, the antioxidant chemicals that give tea its reputation as a heart-protective anticancer beverage (see TEA). In addition, a series of studies beginning with those at the USDA Agricultural Research Center in Peoria, Illinois, suggest that consuming foods rich in stearic acid like chocolate may reduce rather than raise the risk of a blood clot leading to a heart attack.

Possible slowing of the aging process. Chocolate is a relatively good source of copper, a mineral that may play a role in slowing the aging process by decreasing the incidence of "protein glycation," a reaction in which sugar molecules (*gly = sugar*) hook up with protein molecules in the bloodstream, twisting the protein molecules out of shape and rendering them unusable. This can lead to bone loss, rising cholesterol, cardiac abnormalities, and a slew of other unpleasantries. In people with diabetes, excess protein glycation may be one factor involved in complications such as loss of vision. Ordinarily, increased protein glycation is age-related. But at the USDA Grand Forks Human Nutrition Research Center in North Dakota, agricultural research scientist Jack T. Saari has found that rats on copper-deficient diets experience more protein glycation at any age than other rats. A recent USDA survey of American eating patterns says that most of us get about 1.2 mg copper a day, considerably less than the Estimated Safe and Adequate Daily Dietary Intake (ESADDI) or 1.5 mg to 3 mg a day. Vegetarians are less likely to be copper deficient because, as Saari notes, the foods highest in copper are whole grains, nuts, seeds, and beans, including the cocoa bean. One ounce of dark chocolate has .25 mg copper (8–17 percent of the ESADDI).

Adverse Effects Associated with This Food

Possible loss of bone density. In 2008, a team of Australian researchers at Royal Perth Hospital, and Sir Charles Gairdner Hospital published a report in the *American Journal of Clinical Nutrition* suggesting that women who consume chocolate daily had 3.1 percent lower bone density than women who consume chocolate no more than once a week. No explanation for the reaction was proposed; the finding remains to be confirmed.

Possible increase in the risk of heart disease. Cocoa beans, cocoa powder, and plain dark chocolate are high in saturated fats. Milk chocolate is high in saturated fats and cholesterol. Eating foods high in saturated fats and cholesterol increases the amount of cholesterol in your blood and raises your risk of heart disease.

NOTE: Plain cocoa powder and plain dark chocolate may be exceptions to this rule. In studies at the USDA Agricultural Research Center in Peoria, Illinois, volunteers who consumed foods high in stearic acid, the saturated fat in cocoa beans, cocoa powder, and chocolate, had a lower risk of blood clots. In addition, chocolate is high in flavonoids, the antioxidant chemicals that give red wine its heart-healthy reputation.

Mild jitters. There is less caffeine in chocolate than in an equal size serving of coffee: A five-ounce cup of drip-brewed coffee has 110 to 150 mg caffeine; a five-ounce cup of cocoa made with a tablespoon of plain cocoa powder ($1/3$ oz.) has about 18 mg caffeine. Nonetheless, people who are very sensitive to caffeine may find even these small amounts problematic.

Allergic reaction. According to the *Merck Manual,* chocolate is one of the 12 foods most likely to trigger the classic food allergy symptoms: hives, swelling of the lips and eyes, and upset stomach.* The others are berries (blackberries, blueberries, raspberries, strawberries), corn, eggs, fish, legumes (green peas, lima beans, peanuts, soybeans), milk, nuts, peaches, pork, shellfish, and wheat (see WHEAT CEREALS).

Food/Drug Interactions

Monoamine oxidase (MAO) inhibitors. Monoamine oxidase inhibitors are drugs used to treat depression. They inactivate naturally occurring enzymes in your body that metabolize tyramine, a substance found in many fermented or aged foods. Tyramine constricts blood vessels and increases blood pressure. Caffeine is a substance similar to tyramine. If you consume excessive amounts of a caffeinated food, such as cocoa or chocolate, while you are taking an MAO inhibitor, the result may be a hypertensive crisis.

False-positive test for pheochromocytoma. Pheochromocytoma, a tumor of the adrenal gland, secretes adrenalin, which the body converts to VMA (vanillylmandelic acid). VMA is excreted in urine, and, until recently, the test for this tumor measured the level of VMA in the urine. In the past, chocolate and cocoa, both of which contain VMA, were eliminated from the patient's diet prior to the test lest they elevate the level of VMA in the urine and produce a false-positive result. Today, more finely drawn tests usually make this unnecessary.

---

* The evidence linking chocolate to allergic or migraine headaches is inconsistent. In some people, phenylethylamine (PEA) seems to cause headaches similar to those induced by tyramine, another pressor amine. The PEA-induced headache is unusual in that it is a delayed reaction that usually occurs 12 or more hours after the chocolate is eaten.

Coconut

See also Nuts.

Nutritional Profile

Energy value (calories per serving): *High*
Protein: *Low*
Fat: *High*
Saturated fat: *High*
Cholesterol: *None*
Carbohydrates: *Low*
Fiber: *High*
Sodium: *Low*
Major vitamin contribution: *B vitamins, vitamin C*
Major mineral contribution: *Iron, potassium, phosphorus*

About the Nutrients in This Food

Coconut is high in fiber, but its most plentiful nutrient is fat, the oil that accounts for 85 percent of the calories in coconut meat. Coconut oil, which is 89 percent saturated fatty acids, is the most highly saturated dietary fat (see BUTTER, VEGETABLE OILS).

One piece of fresh coconut, 2" × 2"× 1/2", has four grams dietary fiber and 15 g fat (13 g saturated fat, 0.6 g monounsaturated fat, 0.2 g polyunsaturated fat). Like other nuts and seeds, coconut is a good source of some minerals, including 1.1 mg iron (6 percent of the RDA for a woman, 14 percent of the RDA for a man), 0.5 mg zinc (6 percent of the RDA for a woman, 5 percent of the RDA for a man), and 4.5 mg selenium (8 percent of the RDA).

The Most Nutritious Way to Serve This Food

In small servings, as a condiment.

Diets That May Restrict or Exclude This Food

Low-fat diet
Low-fiber, low-residue diet

Buying This Food

Look for: Coconuts that are heavy for their size. You should be able to hear the liquid sloshing around inside when you shake a coconut; if you don't, the coconut has dried out. Avoid nuts with a wet "eye" (the dark spots at the top of the nut) or with mold anywhere on the shell.

Storing This Food

Store whole fresh coconuts in the refrigerator and use them within a week.

Shredded fresh coconut should be refrigerated in a covered container and used in a day or so while it is still fresh and moist.

Refrigerate dried, shredded coconut in an air- and moistureproof container once you have opened the can or bag.

Preparing This Food

Puncture one of the "eyes" of the coconut with a sharp, pointed tool. Pour out the liquid. Then crack the coconut by hitting it with a hammer in the middle, where the shell is widest. Continue around the nut until you have cracked the shell in a circle around the middle and can separate the two halves. Pry the meat out of the shell.

To shred coconut meat, break the shell into small pieces, peel off the hard shell and the brown papery inner covering, then rub the meat against a regular food grater.

What Happens When You Cook This Food

Toasting caramelizes sugars on the surface of the coconut meat and turns it golden. Toasting also reduces the moisture content of the coconut meat, concentrating the nutrients.

How Other Kinds of Processing Affect This Food

Drying.   Drying concentrates all the nutrients in coconut. *Unsweetened* dried shredded coconut has about twice as much protein, fat, carbohydrate, iron, and potassium as an equal amount of fresh coconut. (*Sweetened* dried shredded coconut has six times as much sugar.)

Coconut milk and cream.   Coconut cream is the liquid wrung out of fresh coconut meat; coconut milk is the liquid wrung from fresh coconut meat that has been soaked in water; coconut water is the liquid in the center of the whole coconut. Coconut milk and cream are high in fat, coconut water is not. All coconut liquids should be refrigerated if not used immediately.

Medical Uses and/or Benefits

* * *

Adverse Effects Associated with This Food

Increased risk of cardiovascular disease. Foods high in saturated fats increase the risk of heart attack from clogged arteries.

Allergic reaction. According to the *Merck Manual,* nuts are one of the 12 foods most likely to trigger the classic food allergy symptoms: hives, swelling of the lips and eyes, and upset stomach. The others are berries (blackberries, blueberries, raspberries, strawberries), chocolate, corn, eggs fish, legumes (green peas, lima beans, peanuts, soybeans), milk, peaches, pork, shellfish, and wheat (see WHEAT CEREALS).

Food/Drug Interactions

* * *

Coffee

Nutritional Profile

Energy value (calories per serving): *Low*

Protein: *Trace*

Fat: *Trace*

Saturated fat: *None*

Cholesterol: *None*

Carbohydrates: *Trace*

Fiber: *Trace*

Sodium: *Low*

Major vitamin contribution: *None*

Major mineral contribution: *None*

About the Nutrients in This Food

Coffee beans are roasted seeds from the fruit of the evergreen coffee tree. Like other nuts and seeds, they are high in proteins (11 percent), sucrose and other sugars (8 percent), oils (10 to 15 percent), assorted organic acids (6 percent), B vitamins, iron, and the central nervous system stimulant caffeine (1 to 2 percent). With the exceptions of caffeine, none of these nutrients is found in coffee.

Like spinach, rhubarb, and tea, coffee contains oxalic acid (which binds calcium ions into insoluble compounds your body cannot absorb), but this is of no nutritional consequence as long as your diet contains adequate amounts of calcium-rich foods.

Coffee's best known constituent is the methylxanthine central nervous system stimulant caffeine. How much caffeine you get in a cup of coffee depends on how the coffee was processed and brewed. Caffeine is

Caffeine Content/Coffee Servings

Brewed coffee	60 mg/five-ounce cup
Brewed/decaffeinated	5 mg/five-ounce cup
Espresso	64 mg/one-ounce serving
Instant	47 mg/rounded teaspoon

Source: USDA Nutrient Data Laboratory. National Nutrient Database for Standard Reference. Available online. URL: http://www.nal.usda.gov/fnic/foodcomp/search/.

water-soluble. *Instant, freeze-dried,* and *decaffeinated* coffees all have less caffeine than plain ground roasted coffee.

The Most Nutritious Way to Serve This Food

In moderation, with high-calcium foods. Like spinach, rhubarb, and tea, coffee has oxalic acid, which binds calcium into insoluble compounds. This will have no important effect as long as you keep your consumption moderate (two to four cups of coffee a day) and your calcium consumption high.

Diets That May Restrict or Exclude This Food

Bland diet
Gout diet
Diet for people with heart disease (regular coffee)

Buying This Food

Look for: Ground coffee and coffee beans in tightly sealed, air- and moisture-proof containers.

Avoid: Bulk coffees or coffee beans stored in open bins. When coffee is exposed to air, the volatile molecules that give it its distinctive flavor and richness escape, leaving the coffee flavorless and/or bitter.

Storing This Food

Store unopened vacuum-packed cans of ground coffee or coffee beans in a cool, dark cabinet—where they will stay fresh for six months to a year. They will lose some flavor in storage, though, because it is impossible to can coffee without trapping some flavor-destroying air inside the can.

Once the can or paper sack has been opened, the coffee or beans should be sealed as tight as possible and stored in the refrigerator. Tightly wrapped, refrigerated ground coffee will hold its freshness and flavor for about a week, whole beans for about three weeks. For longer storage, freeze the coffee or beans in an air- and moistureproof container. (You can brew coffee directly from frozen ground coffee and you can grind frozen beans without thawing them.)

Preparing This Food

If you make your coffee with tap water, let the water run for a while to add oxygen. Soft water makes "cleaner"-tasting coffee than mineral-rich hard water. Coffee made with chlorinated water will taste better if you refrigerate the water overnight in a glass (not plastic) bottle so that the chlorine evaporates.

Never make coffee with hot tap water or water that has been boiled. Both lack oxygen, which means that your coffee will taste flat.

Always brew coffee in a scrupulously clean pot. Each time you make coffee, oils are left on the inside of the pot. If you don't scrub them off, they will turn rancid and the next pot of coffee you brew will taste bitter. To clean a coffee pot, wash it with detergent, rinse it with water in which you have dissolved a few teaspoons of baking soda, then rinse one more time with boiling water.

What Happens When You Cook This Food

In making coffee, your aim is to extract flavorful solids (including coffee oils and sucrose and other sugars) from the ground beans without pulling bitter, astringent tannins along with them. How long you brew the coffee determines how much solid material you extract and how the coffee tastes. The longer the brewing time, the greater the amount of solids extracted. If you brew the coffee long enough to extract more than 30 percent of its solids, you will get bitter compounds along with the flavorful ones. (These will also develop by letting coffee sit for a long time after brewing it.)

Ordinarily, drip coffee tastes less bitter than percolator coffee because the water in a drip coffeemaker goes through the coffee only once, while the water in the percolator pot is circulated through the coffee several times. To make strong but not bitter coffee, increase the amount of coffee—not the brewing time.

How Other Kinds of Processing Affect This Food

Drying. Soluble coffees (freeze-dried, instant) are made by dehydrating concentrated brewed coffee. These coffees are often lower in caffeine than regular ground coffees because caffeine, which dissolves in water, is lost when the coffee is dehydrated.

Decaffeinating. Decaffeinated coffee is made with beans from which the caffeine has been extracted, either with an organic solvent (methylene chloride) or with water. How the coffee is decaffeinated has no effect on its taste, but many people prefer water-processed decaffeinated coffee because it is not a chemically treated food. (Methylene chloride is an animal carcinogen, but the amounts that remain in coffees decaffeinated with methylene chloride are so small that the FDA does not consider them hazardous. The carcinogenic organic solvent trichloroethylene [TCE], a chemical that causes liver cancer in laboratory animals, is no longer used to decaffeinate coffee.)

Medical Uses and/or Benefits

As a stimulant and mood elevator. Caffeine is a stimulant. It increases alertness and concentration, intensifies muscle responses, quickens heartbeat, and elevates mood. Its effects derive from the fact that its molecular structure is similar to that of adenosine, a natural chemical by-product of normal cell activity. Adenosine is a regular chemical that keeps nerve cell activity within safe limits. When caffeine molecules hook up to sites in the brain when adenosine molecules normally dock, nerve cells continue to fire indiscriminately, producing the jangly feeling sometimes associated with drinking coffee, tea, and other caffeine products.

As a rule, it takes five to six hours to metabolize and excrete caffeine from the body. During that time, its effects may vary widely from person to person. Some find its stimulation pleasant, even relaxing; others experience restlessness, nervousness, hyperactivity, insomnia, flushing, and upset stomach after as little as one cup a day. It is possible to develop a tolerance for caffeine, so people who drink coffee every day are likely to find it less immediately stimulating than those who drink it only once in a while.

Changes in blood vessels.   Caffeine's effects on blood vessels depend on site: It dilates coronary and gastrointestinal vessels but constricts blood vessels in your head and may relieve headache, such as migraine, which symptoms include swollen cranial blood vessels. It may also increase pain-free exercise time in patients with angina. However, because it speeds up heartbeat, doctors often advise patients with heart disease to avoid caffeinated beverages entirely.

As a diuretic.   Caffeine is a mild diuretic sometimes included in over-the-counter remedies for premenstrual tension or menstrual discomfort.

Adverse Effects Associated with This Food

Stimulation of acid secretion in the stomach.   Both regular and decaffeinated coffees increase the secretion of stomach acid, which suggests that the culprit is the oil in coffee, not its caffeine.

Elevated blood levels of cholesterol and homocysteine.   In the mid-1990s, several studies in the Netherlands and Norway suggested that drinking even moderate amounts of coffee (five cups a day or less) might raise blood levels of cholesterol and homocysteine (by-product of protein metabolism considered an independent risk factor for heart disease), thus increasing the risk of cardiovascular disease. Follow-up studies, however, showed the risk limited to drinking unfiltered coffees such as coffee made in a coffee press, or boiled coffees such as Greek, Turkish, or espresso coffee. The unfiltered coffees contain problematic amounts of cafestol and kahweol, two members of a chemical family called diterpenes, which are believed to affect cholesterol and homocysteine levels. Diterpenes are removed by filtering coffee, as in a drip-brew pot.

Possible increased risk of miscarriage.   Two studies released in 2008 arrived at different conclusions regarding a link between coffee consumption and an increased risk of miscarriage. The first, at Kaiser Permanente (California), found a higher risk of miscarriage among women consuming even two eight-ounce cups of coffee a day. The second, at Mt. Sinai School of Medicine (New York), found no such link. However, although the authors of the Kaiser Permanente study described it as a "prospective study" (a study in which the researchers report results that occur after the study begins), in fact nearly two-thirds of the women who suffered a miscarriage miscarried before the study began, thus confusing the results.

Increased risk of heartburn/acid reflux. The natural oils in both regular and decaffeinated coffees loosen the lower esophageal sphincter (LES), a muscular valve between the esophagus and the stomach. When food is swallowed, the valve opens to let food into the stomach, then closes tightly to keep acidic stomach contents from refluxing (flowing backwards) into the esophagus. If the LES does not close efficiently, the stomach contents reflux and cause heartburn, a burning sensation. Repeated reflux is a risk factor for esophageal cancer.

Masking of sleep disorders. Sleep deprivation is a serious problem associated not only with automobile accidents but also with health conditions such as depression and high blood pressure. People who rely on the caffeine in a morning cup of coffee to compensate for lack of sleep may put themselves at risk for these disorders.

Withdrawal symptoms. Caffeine is a drug for which you develop a tolerance; the more often you use it, the more likely you are to require a larger dose to produce the same effects and the more likely you are to experience withdrawal symptoms (headache, irritation) if you stop using it. The symptoms of coffee-withdrawal can be relieved immediately by drinking a cup of coffee.

Food/Drug Interactions

Drugs that make it harder to metabolize caffeine. Some medical drugs slow the body's metabolism of caffeine, thus increasing its stimulating effect. The list of such drugs includes cimetidine (Tagamet), disulfiram (Antabuse), estrogens, fluoroquinolone antibiotics (e.g., ciprofloxacin, enoxacin, norfloxacin), fluconazole (Diflucan), fluvoxamine (Luvox), mexiletine (Mexitil), riluzole (Rilutek), terbinafine (Lamisil), and verapamil (Calan). If you are taking one of these medicines, check with your doctor regarding your consumption of caffeinated beverages.

Drugs whose adverse effects increase due to consumption of large amounts of caffeine.
This list includes such drugs as metaproterenol (Alupent), clozapine (Clozaril), ephedrine, epinephrine, monoamine oxidase inhibitors, phenylpropanolamine, and theophylline. In addition, suddenly decreasing your caffeine intake may increase blood levels of lithium, a drug used to control mood swings. If you are taking one of these medicines, check with your doctor regarding your consumption of caffeinated beverages.

Allopurinol. Coffee and other beverages containing methylxanthine stimulants (caffeine, theophylline, and theobromine) reduce the effectiveness of the antigout drug allopurinol, which is designed to inhibit xanthines.

Analgesics. Caffeine strengthens over-the-counter painkillers (acetaminophen, aspirin, and other nonsteroidal anti-inflammatories [NSAIDS] such as ibuprofen and naproxen). But it also makes it more likely that NSAIDS will irritate your stomach lining.

Antibiotics. Coffee increases stomach acidity, which reduces the rate at which ampicillin, erythromycin, griseofulvin, penicillin, and tetracyclines are absorbed when they are taken by mouth. (There is no effect when the drugs are administered by injection.)

Antiulcer medication.   Coffee increases stomach acidity and reduces the effectiveness of normal doses of cimetidine and other antiulcer medication.

False-positive test for pheochromocytoma.   Pheochromocytoma, a tumor of the adrenal glands, secretes adrenalin, which is converted to VMA (vanillylmandelic acid) by the body and excreted in the urine. Until recently, the test for this tumor measured the levels of VMA in the patient's urine and coffee, which contains VMA, was eliminated from patients' diets lest it elevate the level of VMA in the urine, producing a false-positive test result. Today, more finely drawn tests make this unnecessary.

Iron supplements.   Caffeine binds with iron to form insoluble compounds your body cannot absorb. Ideally, iron supplements and coffee should be taken at least two hours apart.

Birth control pills.   Using oral contraceptives appears to double the time it takes to eliminate caffeine from the body. Instead of five to six hours, the stimulation of one cup of coffee may last as long as 12 hours.

Monoamine oxidase (MAO) inhibitors.   Monoamine oxidase inhibitors are drugs used to treat depression. They inactivate naturally occurring enzymes in your body that metabolize tyramine, a substance found in many fermented or aged foods. Tyramine constricts blood vessels and increases blood pressure. Caffeine is a substance similar to tyramine. If you consume excessive amounts of a caffeinated beverage such as coffee while you are taking an MAO inhibitor, the result may be a hypertensive crisis.

Nonprescription drugs containing caffeine.   The caffeine in coffee may add to the stimulant effects of the caffeine in over-the-counter cold remedies, diuretics, pain relievers, stimulants, and weight-control products containing caffeine. Some cold pills contain 30 mg caffeine, some pain relievers 130 mg, and some weight-control products as much as 280 mg caffeine. There are 110–150 mg caffeine in a five-ounce cup of drip-brewed coffee.

Sedatives.   The caffeine in coffee may counteract the drowsiness caused by sedative drugs; this may be a boon to people who get sleepy when they take antihistamines. Coffee will not, however, "sober up" people who are experiencing the inebriating effects of alcoholic beverages.

Theophylline.   Caffeine relaxes the smooth muscle of the bronchi and may intensify the effects (and/or increase the risk of side effects) of this antiasthmatic drug.

Corn

(Hominy)

See also Flour, Vegetable oils, Wheat cereals.

Nutritional Profile

Energy value (calories per serving): *Moderate*
Protein: *Moderate*
Fat: *Low*
Saturated fat: *Low*
Cholesterol: *None*
Carbohydrates: *High*
Fiber: *High*
Sodium: *Low*
Major vitamin contribution: *Vitamin A (in yellow corn), B vitamins, vitamin C*
Major mineral contribution: *Potassium*

About the Nutrients in This Food

Like other grains, corn is a high-carbohydrate, high-fiber food. Eighty-one percent of the solid material in the corn kernel consists of sugars, starch, and dietary fiber, including insoluble cellulose and noncarbohydrate lignin in the seed covering and soluble pectins and gums in the kernel.[*] Corn has small amounts of vitamin A, the B vitamin folate, and vitamin C.

Corn is a moderately good source of plant proteins, but zein (its major protein) is deficient in the essential amino acids lysine, cystine, and tryptophan. Corn is low in fat and its oils are composed primarily of unsaturated fatty acids.

Yellow corn, which gets its color from the xanthophyll pigments lutein and zeaxanthin plus the vitamin A-active pigments carotene and cryptoxanthin, contains a little vitamin A; white corn has very little.

One fresh ear of yellow corn, 5.5–6.5 inches long, has three grams dietary fiber, one gram fat (0.1 g saturated fat, 0.3 g monounsaturated fat, 0.4 mg polyunsaturated fat), 137 IU vitamin A (6 percent of the RDA for a woman, 5 percent of the RDA for a man), 34 mcg folate (9 percent of the RDA), and 5 mg vitamin C (7 percent of the RDA for a woman, 6 percent of the RDA for a man).

---

[*] The most plentiful sugar in sweet corn is glucose; hydrolysis (chemical splitting) of corn starch is the principal industrial source of glucose. Since glucose is less sweet than sucrose, sucrose and fructose are added to commercial corn syrup to make it sweeter.

The Most Nutritious Way to Serve This Food

With beans (which are rich in lysine) or milk (which is rich in lysine and tryptophan), to complement the proteins in corn.

With meat or a food rich in vitamin C, to make the iron in corn more useful.

Diets That May Restrict or Exclude This Food

Low-fiber diet

Buying This Food

Look for: Cobs that feel cool or are stored in a refrigerated bin. Keeping corn cool helps retain its vitamin C and slows the natural conversion of the corn's sugars to starch.

Choose fresh corn with medium-sized kernels that yield slightly when you press them with your fingertip. Very small kernels are immature; very large ones are older and will taste starchy rather than sweet. Both yellow and white kernels may be equally tasty, but the husk of the corn should always be moist and green. A dry yellowish husk means that the corn is old enough for the chlorophyll pigments in the husk to have faded, letting the carotenes underneath show through.

Storing This Food

Refrigerate fresh corn. At room temperature, fresh-picked sweet corn will convert nearly half its sugar to starch within 24 hours and lose half its vitamin C in four days. In the refrigerator, it may keep all its vitamin C for up to a week and may retain its sweet taste for as long as ten days.

Preparing This Food

Strip off the husks and silk, and brush with a vegetable brush to get rid of clinging silky threads. Rinse the corn briefly under running water, and plunge into boiling water for four to six minutes, depending on the size of the corn.

What Happens When You Cook This Food

Heat denatures (breaks apart) the long-chain protein molecules in the liquid inside the corn kernel, allowing them to form a network of protein molecules that will squeeze out moisture and turn rubbery if you cook the corn too long. Heat also allows the starch granules inside the kernel to absorb water so that they swell and eventually rupture, releasing the nutrients inside. When you cook corn, the trick is to cook it just long enough to rupture its starch granules while keeping its protein molecules from turning tough and chewy.

Cooking fresh corn for several minutes in boiling water may destroy at least half of its vitamin C. At Cornell University, food scientists found that cooking fresh corn in the microwave oven (two ears/without water if very fresh/4 minutes/600–700 watts) preserves most of the vitamin C.

How Other Kinds of Processing Affect This Food

Canning and freezing. Canned corn and frozen corn both have less vitamin C than fresh-cooked corn. The vitamin is lost when the corn is heated during canning or blanched before freezing to destroy the natural enzymes that would otherwise continue to ripen it. Blanching in a microwave oven rather than in boiling water can preserve the vitamin C in frozen corn (see above).

Milling. Milling removes the hull and germ from the corn kernel, leaving what is called *hominy*. Hominy, which is sometimes soaked in wood ash (lye) to increase its calcium content, can be dried and used as a cereal (grits) or ground into corn flour. Coarsely ground corn flour is called *cornmeal*.

Processed corn cereals. All processed, ready-to-eat corn cereals are much higher in sodium and sugar than fresh corn.

Added calcium carbonate. Pellagra is a niacin-deficiency disease that occurs most commonly among people for whom corn is the staple food in a diet lacking protein foods with the essential amino acid tryptophan, which can be converted to niacin in the human body. Pellagra is not an inevitable result of a diet high in corn, however, since the niacin in corn can be made more useful by soaking the corn in a solution of calcium carbonate (lime) and water. In Mexico, for example, the corn used to make tortillas is boiled in a dilute solution of calcium carbonate (from shells or limestone) and water, then washed, drained, and ground. The alkaline bath appears to release the bound niacin in corn so that it can be absorbed by the body.

Medical Uses and/or Benefits

As a wheat substitute in baking. People who are allergic to wheat or cannot tolerate the gluten in wheat flour or wheat cereals can often use corn flour or hominy instead.

Bath powder. Corn starch, a fine powder refined from the endosperm (inner part) of the corn kernel, can be used as an inexpensive, unperfumed body or face powder. Because it absorbs oils, it is also used as an ingredient in dry shampoos.

Adverse Effects Associated with This Food

Allergic reaction. According to the *Merck Manual,* corn is one of the 12 foods most likely to trigger the classic food allergy symptoms: hives, swelling of the lips and eyes, and upset stomach. The others are berries (blackberries, blueberries, raspberries, strawberries), chocolate, eggs, fish, legumes (green peas, lima beans, peanuts, soybeans), milk, nuts, peaches, pork, shellfish, and wheat (see WHEAT CEREALS).

Food/Drug Interactions

* * *

Cranberries

Nutritional Profile

Energy value (calories per serving): *Low*
Protein: *Low*
Fat: *Low*
Saturated fat: *Low*
Cholesterol: *None*
Carbohydrates: *High*
Fiber: *Low*
Sodium: *Moderate*
Major vitamin contribution: *Vitamin C*
Major mineral contribution: *Iron, potassium*

About the Nutrients in This Food

Cranberries are nearly 90 percent water. The rest is sugars and dietary fiber, including insoluble cellulose in the skin and soluble gums and pectins in the flesh. Pectin dissolves as the fruit ripens; the older and riper the cranberries, the less pectin they contain.

Cranberries also have a bit of protein and a trace of fat, plus moderate amounts of vitamin C.

One-half cup cranberries has 1.6 g dietary fiber and 6.5 mg vitamin C (9 percent of the RDA for a woman, 7 percent of the RDA for a man). One-half cup cranberry sauce has 1.5 g dietary fiber and 3 mg vitamin C (4 percent of the RDA for a woman, 3 percent of the RDA for a man).

The Most Nutritious Way to Serve This Food

Relish made of fresh, uncooked berries (to preserve the vitamin C, which is destroyed by heat) plus oranges.

Diets That May Restrict or Exclude This Food

Low-fiber diet

Buying This Food

Look for: Firm, round, plump, bright red berries that feel cool and dry to the touch.

Avoid: Shriveled, damp, or moldy cranberries. Moldy cranberries may be contaminated with fusarium molds, which produce toxins that can irritate skin and damage tissues by inhibiting the synthesis of DNA and protein.

Storing This Food

Store packaged cranberries, unwashed, in the refrigerator, or freeze unwashed berries in sealed plastic bags for up to one year.

Preparing This Food

Wash the berries under running water, drain them, and pick them over carefully to remove shriveled, damaged, or moldy berries.

Rinse frozen berries. It is not necessary to thaw before cooking.

What Happens When You Cook This Food

First, the heat will make the water inside the cranberry swell, so that if you cook it long enough the berry will burst. Next, the anthocyanin pigments that make cranberries red will dissolve and make the cooking water red. Anthocyanins stay bright red in acid solutions and turn bluish if the liquid is basic (alkaline). Cooking cranberries in lemon juice and sugar preserves the color as well as brightens the taste. Finally, the heat of cooking will destroy some of the vitamin C in cranberries. Cranberry sauce has about one-third the vitamin C of an equal amount of fresh cranberries.

How Other Kinds of Processing Affect This Food

* * *

Medical Uses and/or Benefits

Urinary antiseptic. Cranberry juice is a long-honored folk remedy for urinary infections. In 1985, researchers at Youngstown (Ohio) State University found a "special factor" in cranberries that appeared to keep disease-causing bacteria from adhering to the surface of cells in the bladder and urinary tract. In 1999, scientists at study at Rutgers University (in New

Jersey) identified specific tannins in cranberries as the effective agents. In 2004, researchers at Beth Israel Medical Center (New York) published a review of 19 recent studies of cranberries. The report, in the journal *American Family Physician,* suggested that a regimen of eight ounces of unsweetened cranberry juice or one 300–400 mg cranberry extract tablet twice a day for up to 12 months safely reduced the risk of urinary tract infections. In 2008, a similar review by scientists at the University of Stirling (Scotland) of 10 studies showed similar results.

Adverse Effects Associated with This Food

Increased risk of kidney stones. Long-term use of cranberry products may increase the risk of stone formation among patients known to form oxalate stones (stones composed of calcium and/or other minerals).

Food/Drug Interactions

Anticoagulants Anticoagulants (blood thinners) are drugs used to prevent blood clots. They are most commonly prescribed for patients with atrial fibrillation, an irregular heartbeat that allows blood to pool in the heart and possibly clot before being pumped out into the body. In 2006 researchers at the College of Pharmacy and the Antithrombosis Center at the University of Illinois (Chicago) reported that consuming cranberry juice while using the anticoagulant warafin (Coumadin) might cause fluctuations in blood levels of the anticoagulant, thus reducing the drug's ability to prevent blood clots.

Cucumbers

(Pickles)

Nutritional Profile

Energy value (calories per serving): *Low*
Protein: *Moderate*
Fat: *Low*
Saturated fat: *Low*
Cholesterol: *None*
Carbohydrates: *High*
Fiber: *Low*
Sodium: *Low*
Major vitamin contribution: *Vitamin C*
Major mineral contribution: *Iron, potassium*

About the Nutrients in This Food

Cucumbers are mostly (96 percent) water. Their dietary fiber is unique in that it can hold up to 30 times its weight in water compared to the fiber in wheat bran, which holds only four to six times its weight in water. But cucumbers have so much water that there is little room for anything else. Two ounces of fresh cucumber slices has less than one gram dietary fiber—and no significant amounts of vitamins or minerals.

The Most Nutritious Way to Serve This Food

Raw, fresh-sliced, with the unwaxed skin.

Diets That May Restrict or Exclude This Food

Antiflatulence diet
Low-fiber diet

Buying This Food

Look for: Firm cucumbers with a green, unwaxed skin. In the natural state, the skin of the cucumber is neither shiny nor deep green, characteristics it picks up when the cucumber is waxed to keep it from losing moisture during shipping and storage. The wax is edible, but some people prefer not to eat it, which means missing out on fiber. To get your cucumbers without wax, ask for pickling cucumbers, and note the difference in color and texture.

Choose cucumbers with a clean break at the stem end; a torn, uneven stem end means that the cucumber was pulled off the vine before it was ready. Technically, all the cucumbers we buy are immature; truly ripe cucumbers have very large, hard seeds that make the vegetable unpalatable.

Avoid: Cucumbers with yellowing skin; the vegetable is so old that its chlorophyll pigments have faded and the carotenes underneath are showing through. Puffy, soft cucumbers are also past their prime.

Storing This Food

Store cucumbers in the refrigerator and use them as soon as possible. The cucumber has no starch to convert to sugar as it ages, so it won't get sweeter off the vine, but it will get softer as the pectins in its cell wall absorb water. You can make a soft cucumber crisp again by slicing it and soaking the slices in salted water. By osmotic action, the unsalted, lower-density water in the cucumber's cells will flow out across the cell walls out into the higher-density salted water and the cucumber will feel snappier.

Preparing This Food

Rinse the cucumber under cold, running water. Check to see if the cucumber has been waxed by scraping the skin gently with the tip of your fingernail and then looking for waxy residue under the nail. If the skin is waxed, you can peel it off—but not until you are ready to use it, since slicing the cucumber tears its cell walls, releasing an enzyme that oxidizes and destroys vitamin C.

What Happens When You Cook This Food

* * *

How Other Kinds of Processing Affect This Food

Pickling. Cucumbers are not a good source of iron, but pickles may be. If processed in iron vats, the pickles have picked up iron and will give you about 1 mg per pickle. Pickles made in stainless steel vats have no iron, nor do pickles made at home in glass or earthenware.

Medical Uses and/or Benefits

* * *

Adverse Effects Associated with This Food

Intestinal gas.   Some sensitive people find cucumbers "gassy." Pickling, marinating, and heating, which inactivate enzymes in the cucumber, may reduce this gassiness for certain people—although others find pickles even more upsetting than fresh cucumbers.

Food/Drug Interactions

False-positive test for occult blood in the stool.   The active ingredient in the guaiac slide test for hidden blood in feces is alphaguaiaconic acid, a chemical that turns blue in the presence of blood. Alphaguaiaconic acid also turns blue in the presence of peroxidase, a chemical that occurs naturally in cucumbers. Eating cucumbers in the 72 hours before taking the guaiac test may produce a false-positive result in people who not actually have any blood in their stool.

Monoamine oxidase (MAO) inhibitors.   Monoamine oxidase inhibitors are drugs used to treat depression. They inactivate naturally occurring enzymes in your body that metabolize tyramine, a substance found in many fermented or aged foods. Tyramine constricts blood vessels and increases blood pressure. If you eat a food, such as pickles, containing tyramine while you are taking an MAO inhibitor, you cannot effectively eliminate the tyramine from your body. The result may be a hypertensive crisis.

Currants

(Gooseberries)

See also Raisins.

Nutritional Profile

Energy value (calories per serving): *Low*
Protein: *Moderate*
Fat: *Low*
Saturated fat: *Low*
Cholesterol: *None*
Carbohydrates: *High*
Fiber: *Moderate*
Sodium: *Low*
Major vitamin contribution: *Vitamin C*
Major mineral contribution: *Potassium*

About the Nutrients in This Food

Fresh currants have moderate amounts of dietary fiber and are an excellent source of vitamin C. Black currants, the berries used to make crème de cassis, are more nutritious than red currants. NOTE: Dried "currants" are grapes, not currants.

One-half cup fresh black currant has 1.3 g dietary fiber and 101 mg vitamin C (135 percent of the RDA for a woman, 112 percent of the RDA for a man). One-half cup fresh red currants have 1.9 g dietary fiber and 23 mg vitamin C (31 percent of the RDA for a woman, 26 percent of the RDA for a man). One-half cup gooseberries has 1.4 g dietary fiber and 11 mg vitamin C (28 percent of the RDA for a woman, 23 percent of the RDA for a man).

The Most Nutritious Way to Serve This Food

Fresh.

Diets That May Restrict or Exclude This Food

* * *

Buying This Food

Look for: Plump, firm, well-colored currants. Gooseberries, which are members of the same species as currants, should have a slight golden blush.

Avoid: Sticky packages of currants or berries, moldy fruit, or fruit with lots of stems and leaves.

Storing This Food

Refrigerate ripe currants or gooseberries and use them within a day or so. Dried currants can be stored at room temperature in an air- and moisture-proof package.

Preparing This Food

Wash fresh currants or gooseberries under cold running water, pull off stems and leaves, and drain the berries.

What Happens When You Cook This Food

When fresh currants and gooseberries are heated, the water under the skin expands; if you cook them long enough, the berries will eventually burst.

How Other Kinds of Processing Affect This Food

Canning.   The heat of canning destroys vitamin C; canned gooseberries have only about one-third the vitamin C of fresh gooseberries.

Medical Uses and/or Benefits

* * *

Adverse Effects Associated with This Food

* * *

Food/Drug Interactions

* * *

Dates

Nutritional Profile

Energy value (calories per serving): *High*
Protein: *Low*
Fat: *Low*
Saturated fat: *Low*
Cholesterol: *None*
Carbohydrates: *High*
Fiber: *Very high*
Sodium: *Low (fresh or dried fruit)*
        High (dried fruit treated with sodium sulfur compounds)
Major vitamin contribution: *B vitamins*
Major mineral contribution: *Iron, potassium*

About the Nutrients in This Food

Dates are a high-carbohydrate food, rich in fiber and packed with sugar (as much as 70 percent of the total weight of the fruit). Dates are also a good source of nonheme iron, the inorganic iron found in plant foods, plus potassium, niacin, thiamin, and riboflavin, but they are an unusual fruit because they have no vitamin C at all.

A serving of 10 whole pitted Medjool dates has 16 g dietary fiber and 2.2 mg iron (12 percent of the RDA for a woman, 27 percent of the RDA for a man).

The Most Nutritious Way to Serve This Food

With meat or with a vitamin C- rich food. Both enhance your body's ability to use the nonheme iron in plants (which is ordinarily much less useful than heme iron, the organic iron in foods of animal origin).

Diets That May Restrict or Exclude This Food

Low-carbohydrate diet
Low-fiber/low-residue diet
Low-potassium diet
Low-sodium diet (dried dates, if treated with sodium sulfite)

Buying This Food

Look for: Soft, shiny brown dates in tightly sealed packages.

Storing This Food

Store opened packages of dates in the refrigerator, tightly wrapped to keep the fruit from drying out. (The dates sold in American markets are partly dried; they retain sufficient moisture to keep them soft and tasty.) Properly stored dates will stay fresh for several weeks.

Preparing This Food

To slice dates neatly, chill them in the refrigerator or freezer for an hour. The colder they are, the easier it will be to slice them.

If you're adding dates to a cake or bread batter, coat them first with flour to keep them from dropping through the batter.

What Happens When You Cook This Food

The dates will absorb moisture from a cake or bread batter and soften.

How Other Kinds of Processing Affect This Food

* * *

Medical Uses and/or Benefits

Potassium benefits. Because potassium is excreted in urine, potassium-rich foods are often recommended for people taking diuretics. In addition, a diet rich in potassium (from food) is associated with a lower risk of stroke. A 1998 Harvard School of Public Health analysis of data from the long-running Health Professionals Study shows 38 percent fewer strokes among men who ate nine servings of high potassium foods a day vs. those who ate less than four servings. Among men with high blood pressure, taking a daily 1,000 mg potassium supplement—about the amount of potassium in ¾ cup pitted dates—reduced the incidence of stroke 60 percent.

Adverse Effects Associated with This Food

Sulfite sensitivity. Dates contain polyphenoloxidase, an enzyme that oxidizes phenols in the fruit to brown compounds that turn its flesh dark in the presence of air. To keep dates from darkening when they are dried, they may be treated with sulfur compounds called sulfites (sulfur dioxide, sodium bisulfite, or sodium metabisulfite). Treated dates may trigger serious allergic reactions, including potentially fatal anaphylactic shock, in people sensitive to sulfites.

Food/Drug Interactions

* * *

Distilled Spirits

(Brandy, gin, rum, tequila, whiskey, vodka)

Nutritional Profile

Energy value (calories per serving): *Moderate to high*

Protein: *None*

Fat: *None*

Saturated fat: *None*

Cholesterol: *None*

Carbohydrates: *None* (except for cordials which contain added sugar)

Fiber: *None*

Sodium: *Low*

Major vitamin contribution: *None*

Major mineral contribution: *Phosphorus*

About the Nutrients in This Food

Spirits are the clear liquids produced by distilling the fermented sugars of grains, fruit, or vegetables. The yeasts that metabolize these sugars and convert them into alcohol stop growing when the concentration of alcohol rises above 12–15 percent. In the United States, the proof of an alcoholic beverage is defined as twice its alcohol content by volume: a beverage with 20 percent alcohol by volume is 40 proof.

This is high enough for most wines, but not high enough for most whiskies, gins, vodkas, rums, brandies, and tequilas. To reach the concentration of alcohol required in these beverages, the fermented sugars are heated and distilled. Ethyl alcohol (the alcohol in beer, wine, and spirits) boils at a lower temperature than water. When the fermented sugars are heated, the ethyl alcohol escapes from the distillation vat and condenses in tubes leading from the vat to a collection vessel. The clear liquid that collects in this vessel is called *distilled spirits* or, more technically, *grain neutral spirits.*

Gins, whiskies, cordials, and many vodkas are made with spirits distilled from grains. *American whiskeys* (which include bourbon, rye, and blended whiskeys) and *Canadian, Irish,* and *Scotch whiskies* are all made from spirits aged in wood barrels. They get their flavor from the grains and their color from the barrels. (Some whiskies are also colored with caramel.)

Vodka is made from spirits distilled and filtered to remove all flavor. By law, vodkas made in America must be made with spirits distilled from grains. Imported vodkas may be made with spirits distilled either from grains or potatoes and may contain additional flavoring agents such as citric acid or pepper. *Aquavit,* for example, is essentially vodka flavored with caraway seeds. *Gin* is a clear spirit flavored with an infusion of juniper berries and other herbs (botanicals). *Cordials* (also called liqueurs) and *schnapps* are flavored spirits; most are sweetened with added sugar. Some cordials contain cream.

Rum is made with spirits distilled from sugar cane (molasses). *Tequila* is made with spirits distilled from the blue agave plant. *Brandies* are made with spirits distilled from fruit. (Armagnac and *cognac* are distilled from fermented grapes, *calvados* and *applejack* from fermented apples, *kirsch* from fermented cherries, *slivovitz* from fermented plums.)

Unless they contain added sugar or cream, spirits have no nutrients other than alcohol. Unlike food, which has to be metabolized before your body can use it for energy, alcohol can be absorbed into the blood-stream directly from the gastrointestinal tract. Ethyl alcohol provides 7 calories per gram.

The Most Nutritious Way to Serve This Food

The USDA/Health and Human Services Dietary Guidelines for Americans defines one drink as 12 ounces of beer, five ounces of wine, or 1.25 ounces of distilled spirits, and "moderate drinking" as two drinks a day for a man, one drink a day for a woman.

Diets That May Restrict or Exclude This Food

Bland diet
Lactose-free diet (cream cordials made with cream or milk)
Low-purine (antigout) diet

Buying This Food

Look for: Tightly sealed bottles stored out of direct sunlight, whose energy might disrupt the structure of molecules in the beverage and alter its flavor.

Choose spirits sold only by licensed dealers. Products sold in these stores are manufactured under the strict supervision of the federal government.

Storing This Food

Store sealed or opened bottles of spirits in a cool, dark cabinet.

Preparing This Food

All spirits except unflavored vodkas contain volatile molecules that give the beverage its characteristic taste and smell. Warming the liquid excites these molecules and intensifies the flavor and aroma, which is the reason we serve brandy in a round glass with a narrower top that captures the aromatic molecules as they rise toward the air when we warm the glass by holding it in our hands. Whiskies, too, though traditionally served with ice in America, will have a more intense flavor and aroma if served at room temperature.

What Happens When You Cook This Food

The heat of cooking evaporates the alcohol in spirits but leaves the flavoring intact. Like other alcoholic beverages, spirits should be added to a recipe near the end of the cooking time to preserve the flavor while cooking away any alcohol bite.

Alcohol is an acid. If you cook it in an aluminum or iron pot, it will combine with metal ions to form dark compounds that discolor the pot and the food you are cooking. Any recipe made with spirits should be prepared in an enameled, glass, or stainless-steel pot.

How Other Kinds of Processing Affect This Food

* * *

Medical Uses and/or Benefits

Reduced risk of heart attack.   Data from the American Cancer Society's Cancer Prevention Study 1, a 12-year survey of more than 1 million Americans in 25 states, shows that men who take one drink a day have a 21 percent lower risk of heart attack and a 22 percent lower risk of stroke than men who do not drink at all. Women who have up to one drink a day also reduce their risk of heart attack. Numerous later studies have confirmed these findings.

Lower cholesterol levels.   Beverage alcohol decreases the body's production and storage of low density lipoproteins (LDLs), the protein and fat particles that carry cholesterol into your arteries. As a result, people who drink moderately tend to have lower cholesterol levels and higher levels of high density lipoproteins (HDLs), the fat and protein particles that carry cholesterol out of the body. Numerous later studies have confirmed these findings.

Lower risk of stroke.   In January 1999, the results of a 677-person study published by researchers at New York Presbyterian Hospital-Columbia University showed that moderate alcohol consumption reduces the risk of stroke due to a blood clot in the brain among older people (average age: 70). How alcohol prevents stroke is still unknown, but it is clear that moderate use is a key. Heavy drinkers (those who consume more than seven drinks a day) have a higher risk of stroke. People who once drank heavily, but cut their consumption to moderate levels, reduce their risk of stroke.

Stimulating the appetite. Alcoholic beverages stimulate the production of saliva and the gastric acids that cause the stomach contractions we call hunger pangs. Moderate amounts of alcoholic beverages, which may help stimulate appetite, are often prescribed for geriatric patients, convalescents, and people who do not have ulcers or other chronic gastric problems that might be exacerbated by the alcohol.

Dilation of blood vessels. Alcoholic beverages dilate the tiny blood vessels just under the skin, bringing blood up to the surface. That's why moderate amounts of alcoholic beverages (0.2–1 gram per kilogram of body weight, or two ounces of whiskey for a 150-pound adult) temporarily warm the drinker. But the warm blood that flows up to the surface of the skin will cool down there, making you even colder when it circulates back into the center of your body. Then an alcohol flush will make you perspire, so you lose more heat. Excessive amounts of beverage alcohol may depress the mechanism that regulates body temperature.

Adverse Effects Associated with This Food

Alcoholism. Alcoholism is an addiction disease, the inability to control one's alcohol consumption. It is a potentially life-threatening condition, with a higher risk of death by accident, suicide, malnutrition, or acute alcohol poisoning, a toxic reaction that kills by paralyzing body organs, including the heart.

Fetal alcohol syndrome. Fetal alcohol syndrome is a specific pattern of birth defects—low birth weight, heart defects, facial malformations, learning disabilities, and mental retardation—first recognized in a study of babies born to alcoholic women who consumed more than six drinks a day while pregnant. Subsequent research has found a consistent pattern of milder defects in babies born to women who drink three to four drinks a day or five drinks on any one occasion while pregnant. To date there is no evidence of a consistent pattern of birth defects in babies born to women who consume less than one drink a day while pregnant, but two studies at Columbia University have suggested that as few as two drinks a week while pregnant may raise a woman's risk of miscarriage. (One drink is 12 ounces of beer, five ounces of wine, or 1.25 ounces of distilled spirits.)

Increased risk of breast cancer. In 2008, scientists at the National Cancer Institute released data from a seven-year survey of more than 100,000 postmenopausal women showing that even moderate drinking (one to two drinks a day) may increase by 32 percent a woman's risk of developing estrogen-receptor positive (ER+) and progesterone-receptor positive (PR+) breast cancer, tumors whose growth is stimulated by hormones. No such link was found between consuming alcohol and the risk of developing ER-/PR- tumors (not fueled by hormones). The finding applies to all types of alcohol: beer, wine, and distilled spirits.

Increased risk of oral cancer (cancer of the mouth and throat). Numerous studies confirm the American Cancer Society's warning that men and women who consume more than two drinks a day are at higher risk of oral cancer than are nondrinkers or people who drink less.

Increased risk of cancer of the colon and rectum.   In the mid-1990s, studies at the University of Oklahoma suggested that men who drink more than five beers a day are at increased risk of rectal cancer. Later studies suggested that men and women who are heavy beer or spirits drinkers (but not those who are heavy wine drinkers) have a higher risk of colorectal cancers. Further studies are required to confirm these findings.

Malnutrition.   While moderate alcohol consumption stimulates appetite, alcohol abuses depresses it. In addition, an alcoholic may drink instead of eating. When an alcoholic does eat, excess alcohol in his/her body prevents absorption of nutrients and reduces the ability to synthesize new tissue.

Hangover.   Alcohol is absorbed from the stomach and small intestine and carried by the bloodstream to the liver, where it is oxidized to acetaldehyde by alcohol dehydrogenase (ADH), the enzyme our bodies use every day to metabolize the alcohol we produce when we digest carbohydrates. The acetaldehyde is converted to acetyl coenzyme A and either eliminated from the body or used in the synthesis of cholesterol, fatty acids, and body tissues. Although individuals vary widely in their capacity to metabolize alcohol, an adult of average size can metabolize the alcohol in four ounces (120 ml) whiskey in approximately five to six hours. If he or she drinks more than that, the amount of alcohol in the body will exceed the available supply of ADH. The surplus, unmetabolized alcohol will pile up in the bloodstream, interfering with the liver's metabolic functions. Since alcohol decreases the reabsorption of water from the kidneys and may inhibit the secretion of an antidiuretic hormone, the drinker will begin to urinate copiously, losing magnesium, calcium, and zinc but retaining uric acid, which is irritating. The level of lactic acid in the body will increase, making him or her feel tired and out of sorts; the acid-base balance will be out of kilter; the blood vessels in the head will swell and throb; and the stomach, its lining irritated by the alcohol, will ache. The ultimate result is a hangover whose symptoms will disappear only when enough time has passed to allow the body to marshal the ADH needed to metabolize the extra alcohol in the person's blood.

Changes in body temperature.   Alcohol dilates capillaries, tiny blood vessels just under the skin, producing a "flush" that temporarily warms the drinker. But drinking is not an effective way to stay warm in cold weather. Warm blood flowing up from the body core to the surface capillaries is quickly chilled, making you even colder when it circulates back into your organs. In addition, an alcohol flush triggers perspiration, further cooling your skin. Finally, very large amounts of alcohol may actually depress the mechanism that regulates body temperature.

Impotence.   Excessive drinking decreases libido (sexual desire) and interferes with the ability to achieve or sustain an erection.

Migraine headache.   Some alcoholic beverages contain chemicals that inhibit PST, an enzyme that breaks down certain alcohols in spirits so that they can be eliminated from the body. If they are not broken down by PST, these alcohols will build up in the bloodstream and may trigger a migraine headache. Gin and vodka appear to be the distilled spirits least likely to trigger headaches, brandy the most likely.

Food/Drug Interactions

Acetaminophen (Tylenol, etc.). FDA recommends that people who regularly have three or more drinks a day consult a doctor before using acetaminophen. The alcohol/acetaminophen combination may cause liver failure.

Anti-alcohol abuse drugs (disulfiram [Antabuse]). Taken concurrently with alcohol, the anti-alcoholism drug disulfiram can cause flushing, nausea, a drop in blood pressure, breathing difficulty, and confusion. The severity of the symptoms, which may vary among individuals, generally depends on the amount of alcohol consumed and the amount of disulfiram in the body.

Anticoagulants. Alcohol slows the body's metabolism of anticoagulants (blood thinners), intensifying the effect of the drugs and increasing the risk of side effects such as spontaneous nosebleeds.

Antidepressants. Alcohol may strengthen the sedative effects of antidepressants.

Aspirin, ibuprofen, ketoprofen, naproxen and nonsteroidal anti-inflammatory drugs. Like alcohol, these analgesics irritate the lining of the stomach and may cause gastric bleeding. Combining the two intensifies the effect.

Insulin and oral hypoglycemics. Alcohol lowers blood sugar and interferes with the metabolism of oral antidiabetics; the combination may cause severe hypoglycemia.

Sedatives and other central nervous system depressants (tranquilizers, sleeping pills, antidepressants, sinus and cold remedies, analgesics, and medication for motion sickness). Alcohol intensifies the sedative effects of these medications and, depending on the dose, may cause drowsiness, sedation, respiratory depression, coma, or death.

MAO inhibitors. Monoamine oxidase (MAO) inhibitors are drugs used as antidepressants or antihypertensives. They inhibit the action of natural enzymes that break down tyramine, a substance formed naturally when proteins are metabolized. Tyramine is a pressor amine, a chemical that constricts blood vessel and raises blood pressure. If you eat a food that contains tyramine while you are taking an MAO inhibitor, the pressor amine cannot be eliminated from your body and the result may be a hypertensive crisis (sustained elevated blood pressure). Brandy, a distilled spirit made from wine (which is fermented) contains tyramine. All other distilled spirits may be excluded from your diet when you are taking an MAO inhibitor because the spirits and the drug, which are both sedatives, may be hazardous in combination.

Eggplant

Nutritional Profile

Energy value (calories per serving): *Low*

Protein: *Moderate*

Fat: *Low*

Saturated fat: *Low*

Cholesterol: *None*

Carbohydrates: *High*

Fiber: *High*

Sodium: *Low*

Major vitamin contribution: *Vitamin C (low)*

Major mineral contribution: *Potassium (low)*

About the Nutrients in This Food

Eggplant is a high-fiber food with only minimum amounts of vitamins and minerals. One cup (100 g/3.5 ounces) boiled eggplant has 2.5 mg dietary fiber and 1.3 mg vitamin C (2 percent of the RDA for a woman, 1 percent of the RDA for a man).

In 1992, food scientists at the Autonomous University of Madrid studying the chemistry of the eggplant discovered that the vegetable's sugar content rises through the end of the sixth week of growth and then falls dramatically over the next 10 days. The same thing happens with other flavor chemicals in the vegetable and with vitamin C, so the researchers concluded that eggplants taste best and are most nutritious after 42 days of growth. NOTE: Eggplants are members of the nightshade family, Solanacea. Other members of this family are potatoes, tomatoes, and red and green peppers. These plants produce natural neurotoxins (nerve poisons) called glycoalkaloids. It is estimated that an adult would have to eat 4.5 pounds of eggplant at one sitting to get a toxic amount of solanine, the glycoalkaloid in eggplant.

The Most Nutritious Way to Serve This Food

The eggplant's two culinary virtues are its meaty texture and its ability to assume the flavor of sauces in which it is cooked. As a result, it is often used as a vegetarian, no-cholesterol substitute for veal or chicken in Italian cuisine, specifically dishes *ala parmigiana* and spaghetti sauces. However, in cooking, the eggplant absorbs very large amounts of oil. To keep eggplant *parmigiana* low in fat, use non-fat cheese and ration the olive oil.

Diets That May Restrict or Exclude This Food

* * *

Buying This Food

Look for: Firm, purple to purple-black or umblemished white eggplants that are heavy for their size.

Avoid: Withered, soft, bruised, or damaged eggplants. Withered eggplants will be bitter; damaged ones will be dark inside.

Storing This Food

Handle eggplants carefully. If you bruise an eggplant, its damaged cells will release polyphenoloxidase, an enzyme that hastens the oxidation of phenols in the eggplant's flesh, producing brown compounds that darken the vegetable.

Refrigerate fresh eggplant to keep it from losing moisture and wilting.

Preparing This Food

Do not slice or peel an eggplant until you are ready to use it, since the polyphenoloxidase in the eggplant will begin to convert phenols to brown compounds as soon as you tear the vegetable's cells. You can slow this chemical reaction (but not stop it completely) by soaking sliced eggplant in ice water—which will reduce the eggplant's already slim supply of water-soluble vitamin C and B vitamins—or by painting the slices with a solution of lemon juice or vinegar.

To remove the liquid that can make a cooked eggplant taste bitter, slice the eggplant, salt the slices, pile them on a plate, and put a second plate on top to weight the slices down. Discard the liquid that results.

What Happens When You Cook This Food

A fresh eggplant's cells are full of air that escapes when you heat the vegetable. If you cook an eggplant with oil, the empty cells will soak it up. Eventually, however, the cell walls will collapse and the oil will leak out, which is why eggplant parmigiana often seems to be served in a pool of olive oil.

Eggplant should never be cooked in an aluminum pot, which will discolor the eggplant. If you cook the eggplant in its skin, adding lemon juice or vinegar to the dish will turn the skin, which is colored with red anthocyanin pigments, a deeper red-purple. Red anthocyanin pigments get redder in acids and turn bluish in basic (alkaline) solutions.

Cooking reduces the eggplant's supply of water-soluble vitamins, but you can save the Bs if you serve the eggplant with its juices.

How Other Kinds of Processing Affect This Food

* * *

Medical Uses and/or Benefits of This Food

* * *

Adverse Effects Associated with This Food

Nitrate/nitrite reactions.   Eggplant—like beets, celery, lettuce, radish, spinach, and collard and turnip greens—contains nitrates that convert naturally into nitrites in your stomach, and then react with the amino acids in proteins to form nitrosamines. Although some nitrosamines are known or suspected carcinogens, this natural chemical conversion presents no known problems for a healthy adult. However, when these nitrate-rich vegetables are cooked and left to stand at room temperature, bacterial enzyme action (and perhaps some enzymes in the plants) convert the nitrates to nitrites at a much faster rate than normal. These higer-nitrite foods may be hazardous for infants; several cases of "spinach poisoning" have been reported among children who ate cooked spinach that had been left standing at room temperature.

Food/Drug Interactions

MAO inhibitors.   Monoamine oxidase (MAO) inhibitors are drugs used as antidepressants or antihypertensives. They inhibit the action of enzymes that break down tyramine, a natural by-product of protein metabolism, so that it can be eliminated from the body. Tyramine is a pressor amine, a chemical that constricts blood vessels and raises blood pressure. If you eat a food rich in tyramine while you are taking an MAO inhibitor, the pressor amine cannot be eliminated from your body, and the result may be a hypertensive crisis (sustained elevated blood pressure). Eggplants contain small amounts of tyramine.

False-positive urine test for carcinoid tumors.   Carcinoid tumors (tumors that may arise in tissues of the endocrine and gastrointestinal systems) secrete serotonin, which is excreted in urine. The test for these tumors measures the level of serotonin in your urine. Eating eggplant, which is rich in serotonin, in the 72 hours before a test for a carcinoid tumor might raise the serotonin levels in your urine high enough to cause a false-positive test result. (Other fruits and vegetables rich in serotonin are bananas, tomatoes, plums, pineapple, avocados, and walnuts.)

Eggs

Nutritional Profile*

Energy value (calories per serving): *Moderate*
Protein: *High*
Fat: *High*
Saturated fat: *Moderate*
Cholesterol: *High*
Carbohydrates: *Low*
Fiber: *None*
Sodium: *Moderate to high*
Major vitamin contribution: *Vitamin A, riboflavin, vitamin D*
Major mineral contribution: *Iron, calcium*

About the Nutrients in This Food

An egg is really three separate foods, the whole egg, the white, and the yolk, each with its own distinct nutritional profile.

A whole egg is a high-fat, high-cholesterol, high-quality protein food packaged in a high-calcium shell that can be ground and added to any recipe. The proteins in eggs, with sufficient amounts of all the essential amino acids, are 99 percent digestible, the standard by which all other proteins are judged.

The egg white is a high-protein, low-fat food with virtually no cholesterol. Its only important vitamin is riboflavin (vitamin B$_2$), a visible vitamin that gives egg white a slightly greenish cast. Raw egg whites contain avidin, an antinutrient that binds biotin a B complex vitamin formerly known as vitamin H, into an insoluble compound. Cooking the egg inactivates avidin.

An egg yolk is a high-fat, high-cholesterol, high-protein food, a good source of vitamin A derived from carotenes eaten by the laying hen, plus vitamin D, B vitamins, and heme iron, the form of iron most easily absorbed by your body.

One large whole egg (50 g/1.8 ounce) has five grams fat (1.5 g saturated fat, 1.9 g monounsaturated fat, 0.7 g polyunsaturated fat), 212 mg cholesterol, 244 IU vitamin A (11 percent of the RDA for a woman, 9 percent

---

* Values are for a whole egg.

of the RDA for a man), 0.9 mg iron (5 percent of the RDA for a woman, 11 percent of the RDA for a man) and seven grams protein. The fat in the egg is all in the yolk. The protein is divided: four grams in the white, three grams in the yolk.

The Most Nutritious Way to Serve This Food

With extra whites and fewer yolks to lower the fat and cholesterol per serving.

Diets That May Restrict or Exclude This Food

Controlled-fat, low-cholesterol diet
Low-protein diet

Buying This Food

Look for: Eggs stored in the refrigerated dairy case. Check the date for freshness. NOTE: In 1998, the FDA and USDA Food Safety and Inspection Service (FSIS) proposed new rules that would require distributors to keep eggs refrigerated on the way to the store and require stores to keep eggs in a refrigerated case. The egg package must have a "refrigeration required" label plus safe-handling instructions on eggs that have not been treated to kill *Salmonella.*

Look for: Eggs that fit your needs. Eggs are graded by the size of the yolk and the thickness of the white, qualities that affect appearance but not nutritional values. The higher the grade, the thicker the yolk and the thicker the white will be when you cook the egg. A Grade AA egg fried sunny side up will look much more attractive than a Grade B egg prepared the same way, but both will be equally nutritions. Egg sizes (Jumbo, Extra large, Large, Medium, Small) are determined by how much the eggs weigh per dozen. The color of the egg's shell depends on the breed of the hen that laid the egg and has nothing to do with the egg's food value.

Storing This Food

Store fresh eggs with the small end down so that the yolk is completely submerged in the egg white (which contains antibacterial properties, nature's protection for the yolk—or a developing chick embryo in a fertilized egg). *Never* wash eggs before storing them: The water will make the egg shell more porous, allowing harmful microorganisms to enter.

Store separated leftover yolks and whites in small, tightly covered containers in the refrigerator, where they may stay fresh for up to a week. Raw eggs are very susceptible to *Salmonella* and other bacterial contamination; discard *any* egg that looks or smells the least bit unusual.

Refrigerate hard-cooked eggs, including decorated Easter eggs. They, too, are suscep-tible to *Salmonella* contamination and should *never* be left at room temperature.

Preparing This Food

First, find out how fresh the eggs really are. The freshest ones are the eggs that sink and lie flat on their sides when submerged in cool water. These eggs can be used for any dish. By the time the egg is a week old, the air pocket inside, near the broad end, has expanded so that the broad end tilts up as the egg is submerged in cool water. The yolk and the white inside have begun to separate; these eggs are easier to peel when hard-cooked. A week or two later, the egg's air pocket has expanded enough to cause the broad end of the egg to point straight up when you put the egg in water. By now the egg is runny and should be used in sauces where it doesn't matter if it isn't picture-perfect. After four weeks, the egg will float. Throw it away.

Eggs are easily contaminated with *Salmonella* microorganisms that can slip through an intact shell. *NEVER EAT OR SERVE A DISH OR BEVERAGE CONTAINING RAW FRESH EGGS. SALMONELLA IS DESTROYED BY COOKING EGGS TO AN INTERNAL TEMPERATURE OF 145°F; EGG-MILK DISHES SUCH AS CUSTARDS MUST BE COOKED TO AN INTERNAL TEMPERATURE OF 160°F.*

If you separate fresh eggs by hand, wash your hands thoroughly before touching other food, dishes, or cooking tools. When you have finished preparing raw eggs, wash your hands and all utensils thoroughly with soap and hot water. *NEVER STIR COOKED EGGS WITH A UTENSIL USED ON RAW EGGS.*

When you whip an egg white, you change the structure of its protein molecules which unfold, breaking bonds between atoms on the same molecule and forming new bonds to atoms on adjacent molecules. The result is a network of protein molecules that hardens around air trapped in bubbles in the net. If you beat the whites too long, the foam will turn stiff enough to hold its shape even if you don't cook it, but it will be too stiff to expand natu-rally if you heat it, as in a soufflé. When you do cook properly whipped egg white foam, the hot air inside the bubbles will expand. Ovalbumin, an elastic protein in the white, allows the bubble walls to bulge outward until they are cooked firm and the network is stabilized as a puffy soufflé.

The bowl in which you whip the whites should be absolutely free of fat or grease, since the fat molecules will surround the protein molecules in the egg white and keep them from linking up together to form a puffy white foam. Eggs whites will react with metal ions from the surface of an aluminum bowl to form dark particles that discolor the egg-white foam. You can whip eggs successfully in an enamel or glass bowl, but they will do best in a copper bowl because copper ions bind to the egg and stabilize the foam.

What Happens When You Cook This Food

When you heat a whole egg, its protein molecules behave exactly as they do when you whip an egg white. They unfold, form new bonds, and create a protein network, this time with molecules of water caught in the net. As the egg cooks, the protein network tightens, squeezing out moisture, and the egg becomes opaque. The longer you cook the egg, the tighter the network will be. If you cook the egg too long, the protein network will contract strongly enough to force out all the moisture. That is why overcooked egg custards run and why overcooked eggs are rubbery.

If you mix eggs with milk or water before you cook them, the molecules of liquid will surround and separate the egg's protein molecules so that it takes more energy (higher heat) to make the protein molecules coagulate. Scrambled eggs made with milk are softer than plain scrambled eggs cooked at the same temperature.

When you boil an egg in its shell, the air inside expands and begins to escape through the shell as tiny bubbles. Sometimes, however, the force of the air is enough to crack the shell. Since there's no way for you to tell in advance whether any particular egg is strong enough to resist the pressure of the bubbling air, the best solution is to create a safety vent by sticking a pin through the broad end of the egg before you start to boil it. Or you can slow the rate at which the air inside the shell expands by starting the egg in cold water and letting it warm up naturally as the water warms rather than plunging it cold into boiling water—which makes the air expand so quickly that the shell is virtually certain to crack.

As the egg heats, a little bit of the protein in its white will decompose, releasing sulfur that links up with hydrogen in the egg, forming hydrogen sulfide, the gas that gives rotten eggs their distinctive smell. The hydrogen sulfide collects near the coolest part of the egg—the yolk. The yolk contains iron, which now displaces the hydrogen in the hydrogen sulfide to form a green iron-sulfide ring around the hard-cooked yolk.

How Other Kinds of Processing Affect This Food

Egg substitutes.   Fat-free, cholesterol-free egg substitutes are made of pasteurized egg whites, plus artificial or natural colors, flavors, and texturizers (food gums) to make the product look and taste like eggs, plus vitamins and minerals to produce the nutritional equivalent of a full egg. Pasteurized egg substitutes may be used without additional cooking, that is, in salad dressings and eggnog.

Drying.   Dried eggs have virtually the same nutritive value as fresh eggs. Always refrigerate dried eggs in an air- and moistureproof container. At room temperature, they will lose about a third of their vitamin A in six months.

Medical Uses and/or Benefits

Protein source.   The protein in eggs, like protein from all animal foods, is complete. That is, protein from animal foods provides all the essential amino acids required by human beings. In fact, the protein from eggs is so well absorbed and utilized by the human body that it is considered the standard by which all other dietary protein is measured. On a scale known as biological value, eggs rank 100; milk, 93; beef and fish, 75; and poultry, 72.

Vision protection. The egg yolk is a rich source of the yellow-orange carotenoid pigments lutein and zeaxanthin. Both appear to play a role in protecting the eyes from damaging ultraviolet light, thus reducing the risk of cataracts and age-related macular degeneration, a leading cause of vision of loss in one-third of all Americans older than 75. Just 1.3 egg yolks a day appear to increase blood levels of lutein and zeaxanthin by up to 128 percent. Perhaps as a result, data released by the National Eye Institute's 6,000-person Beaver Dam (Wisconsin) Eye Study in 2003 indicated that egg consumption was inversely associated with cataract risk in study participants who were younger than 65 years of age when the study started. The relative risk of cataracts was 0.4 for people in the highest category of egg consumption, compared to a risk of 1.0 for those in the lowest category.

External cosmetic effects. Beaten egg whites can be used as a facial mask to make your skin look smoother temporarily. The mask works because the egg proteins constrict as they dry on your face, pulling at the dried layer of cells on top of your skin. When you wash off the egg white, you also wash off some of these loose cells. Used in a rinse or shampoo, the protein in a beaten raw egg can make your hair look smoother and shinier temporarily by filling in chinks and notches on the hair shaft.

Adverse Effects Associated with This Food

Increased risk of cardiovascular disease. Although egg yolks are high in cholesterol, data from several recent studies suggest that eating eggs may not increase the risk of heart disease. In 2003, a report from a 14-year, 177,000-plus person study at the Harvard School of Public Health showed that people who eat one egg a day have exactly the same risk of heart disease as those who eat one egg or fewer per week. A similar report from the Multiple Risk Factor Intervention Trial showed an inverse relationship between egg consumption and cholesterol levels—that is, people who ate more eggs had lower cholesterol levels.

Nonetheless, in 2006 the National Heart, Lung, and Blood Institute still recommends no more than four egg yolks a week (including the yolk in baked goods) for a heart-healthy diet. The American Heart Association says consumers can have one whole egg a day if they limit cholesterol from other sources to the amount suggested by the National Cholesterol Education Project following the Step I and Step II diets. (Both groups permit an unlimited number of egg whites.)

The Step I diet provides no more than 30 percent of total daily calories from fat, no more than 10 percent of total daily calories from saturated fat, and no more than 300 mg of cholesterol per day. It is designed for healthy people whose cholesterol is in the range of 200–239 mg/dL.

The Step II diet provides 25–35 percent of total calories from fat, less than 7 percent of total calories from saturated fat, up to 10 percent of total calories from polyunsaturated fat, up to 20 percent of total calories from monounsaturated fat, and less than 300 mg cholesterol per day. This stricter regimen is designed for people who have one or more of the following conditions:

- Existing cardiovascular disease
- High levels of low-density lipoproteins (LDLs, or "bad" cholesterol) or low levels of high-density lipoproteins (HDLs, or "good" cholesterol)
- Obesity
- Type 1 diabetes (insulin-dependent diabetes, or diabetes mellitus)
- Metabolic syndrome, a.k.a. insulin resistance syndrome, a cluster of risk factors that includes type 2 diabetes (non-insulin-dependent diabetes)

Food poisoning.   Raw eggs (see above) and egg-rich foods such as custards and cream pies are excellent media for microorganisms, including the ones that cause food poisoning. To protect yourself against egg-related poisoning, always cook eggs thoroughly: poach them five minutes over boiling water or boil at least seven minutes or fry two to three minutes on each side (no runny center) or scramble until firm. Bread with egg coating, such as French toast, should be cooked crisp. Custards should be firm and, once cooked, served very hot or refrigerated and served very cold.

Allergic reaction.   According to the *Merck Manual,* eggs are one of the 12 foods most likely to trigger the classic food allergy symptoms: hives, swelling of the lips and eyes, and upset stomach. The others are berries (blackberries, blueberries, raspberries, strawberries), chocolate, corn, fish, legumes (green peas, lima beans, peanuts, soybeans), milk, nuts, peaches, pork, shellfish, and wheat (see WHEAT CEREALS).

Food/Drug Interactions

Sensitivity to vaccines.   Live-virus measles vaccine, live-virus mumps vaccine, and the vaccines for influenza are grown in either chick embryo or egg culture. They may all contain minute residual amounts of egg proteins that may provoke a hypersensitivity reaction in people with a history of anaphylactic reactions to eggs (hives, swelling of the mouth and throat, difficulty breathing, a drop in blood pressure, or shock).

Figs

Nutritional Profile

Energy value (calories per serving): *Moderate (fresh figs)*
High (dried figs)
Protein: *Low*
Fat: *Low*
Saturated fat: *Low*
Cholesterol: *None*
Carbohydrates: *High*
Fiber: *Very high*
Sodium: *Low (fresh or dried fruit)*
       High (dried fruit treated with sodium sulfur compounds)
Major vitamin contribution: *B vitamins*
Major mineral contribution: *Iron (dried figs)*

About the Nutrients in This Food

Figs, whether fresh or dried, are high-carbohydrate food, an extraordinarily good source of dietary fiber, natural sugars, iron, calcium, and potassium.

Ninety-two percent of the carbohydrates in dried figs are sugars (42 percent glucose, 31 percent fructose, 0.1 percent sucrose). The rest is dietary fiber, insoluble cellulose in the skin, soluble pectins in fruit. The most important mineral in dried figs is iron. Gram for gram, figs have about 50 percent as much iron as beef liver (0.8 mg/gram vs. 1.9 mg/gram).

One medium fresh fig has 1.4 g dietary fiber, six grams sugars, and 0.18 mg iron (1 percent of the RDA for a woman, 2 percent of the RDA for a man). A similar size dried, uncooked fig has 0.8 g fiber, four grams sugars and the same amount of iron as a fresh fig.

The Most Nutritious Way to Serve This Food

Dried (but see *How other kinds of processing affect this food,* below).

Diets That May Restrict or Exclude This Food

Low-fiber, low-residue diets
Low-sodium (dried figs treated with sulfites)

Buying This Food

Look for: Plump, soft fresh figs whose skin may be green, brown, or purple, depending on the variety. As figs ripen, the pectin in their cell walls dissolves and the figs grow softer to the touch. The largest, best-tasting figs are generally the ones harvested and shipped in late spring and early summer, during June and July.

Choose dried figs in tightly sealed airtight packages.

Avoid: Fresh figs that smell sour. The odor indicates that the sugars in the fig have fermented; such fruit is spoiled.

Storing This Food

Refrigerate fresh figs. Dried figs can be stored in the refrigerator or at room temperature; either way, wrap them tightly in an air- and moistureproof container to keep them from losing moisture and becoming hard. Dried figs may keep for several months.

Preparing This Food

Wash fresh figs under cool water; use dried figs right out of the package. If you want to slice the dried figs, chill them first in the refrigerator or freezer: cold figs slice clean.

What Happens When You Cook This Food

Fresh figs contain ficin, a proteolytic (protein-breaking) enzyme similar to papain in papayas and bromelin in fresh pineapple. Proteolytic enzymes split long-chain protein molecules into smaller units, which is why they help tenderize meat. Ficin is most effective at about 140–160°F, the temperature at which stews simmer, and it will continue to work after you take the stew off the stove until the food cools down. Temperatures higher than 160°F inactivate ficin; canned figs—which have been exposed to very high heat in processing—will not tenderize meat.

Both fresh and dried figs contain pectin, which dissolves when you cook the figs, making them softer. Dried figs also absorb water and swell.

How Other Kinds of Processing Affect This Food

Drying. Figs contain polyphenoloxidase, an enzyme that hastens the oxidation of phenols in the fig, creating brownish compounds that darken its flesh. To prevent this reaction, figs may be treated with a sulfur compound such as sulfur dioxide or sodium sulfite. People who are sensitive to sulfites may suffer serious allergic reactions, including potentially fatal anaphylactic shock, if they eat figs that have been treated with one of these compounds.

Canning. Canned figs contain slightly less vitamin C, thiamin, riboflavin, and niacin than fresh figs, and no active ficin.

Medical Uses and/or Benefits

Iron supplementation. Dried figs are an excellent source of iron.

As a laxative. Figs are a good source of the indigestible food fiber lignin. Cells whose walls are highly lignified retain water and, since they are impossible to digest, help bulk up the stool. In addition, ficin has some laxative effects. Together, the lignin and the ficin make figs (particularly dried figs) an efficient laxative food.

Lower risk of stroke. Potassium lowers blood pressure. According to new data from the Harvard University Health Professionals Study, a long-running survey of male doctors, a diet rich in high-potassium foods such as bananas may also reduce the risk of stroke. The men who ate the most potassium-rich foods (an average nine servings a day) had 38 percent fewer strokes than men who ate the least (less than four servings a day).

Adverse Effects Associated with This Food

Sulfite allergies. See *How other kinds of processing affect this food.*

Food/Drug Interactions

MAO inhibitors. Monoamine oxidase (MAO) inhibitors are drugs used as antidepressants or antihypertensives. They inhibit the action of natural enzymes that break down tyramine, a nitrogen compound formed when proteins are metabolized, so it can be eliminated from the body. Tyramine is a pressor amine, a chemical that constricts blood vessels and raises blood pressure. If you eat a food rich in one of these chemicals while you are taking an MAO inhibitor, the pressor amines cannot be eliminated from your body, and the result may be a hypertensive crisis (sustained elevated blood pressure). There has been one report of such a reaction in a patient who ate canned figs while taking an MAO inhibitor.

Fish

See also Shellfish, Squid.

Nutritional Profile

Energy value (calories per serving): *Moderate*

Protein: *High*

Fat: *Low to moderate*

Saturated fat: *Low to moderate*

Cholesterol: *Moderate*

Carbohydrates: *Low*

Fiber: *None*

Sodium: *Low (fresh fish)*

      High (some canned or salted fish)

Major vitamin contribution: *Vitamin A, vitamin D*

Major mineral contribution: *Iodine, selenium, phosphorus, potassium, iron, calcium*

About the Nutrients in This Food

Like meat, poultry, milk, and eggs, fish are an excellent source of high-quality proteins with sufficient amount of all the essential amino acids.

While some fish have as much or more fat per serving than some meats, the fat content of fish is always lower in saturated fat and higher in unsaturated fats. For example, 100 g/3.5 ounce cooked pink salmon (a fatty fish) has 4.4 g total fat, but only 0.7 g saturated fat, 1.2 g monounsaturated fat, and 1.7 g polyunsaturated fat; 100 g/3.5 ounce lean top sirloin has four grams fat but twice as much saturated fat (1.5 g), plus 1.6 g monounsaturated fat and only 0.2 g polyunsaturated fat.

Omega-3 Fatty Acid Content of Various Fish

Fish	Grams/ounce
Atlantic mackerel	0.61
Chinook salmon (fresh)	0.60
Pink salmon	0.55
Coho salmon, canned	0.45
Sockeye salmon	0.45
Sardines	0.32

Omega-3 Fatty Acid Content of Various Fish *(Continued)*

Fish	Grams/ounce
Rainbow trout	0.30
Lake whitefish	0.25

Source: "Food for the Heart," *American Health,* April 1985.

Fish oils are one of the few natural food sources of vitamin D. Salmon also has vitamin A derived from carotenoid pigments in the plants eaten by the fish. The soft bones in some canned salmon and sardines are an excellent source of calcium. CAUTION: *DO NOT EAT THE BONES IN RAW OR COOKED FISH. THE ONLY BONES CONSIDERED EDIBLE ARE THOSE IN THE CANNED PRODUCTS.*

The Most Nutritious Way to Serve This Food

Cooked, to kill parasites and potentially pathological microorganisms living in raw fish.

Broiled, to liquify fat and eliminate the fat-soluble environmental contaminants found in some freshwater fish.

With the soft, mashed, calcium-rich bones (in canned salmon and canned sardines).

Diets That May Restrict or Exclude This Food

Low-purine (antigout) diet
Low-sodium diet (canned, salted, or smoked fish)

Buying This Food

Look for: Fresh-smelling whole fish with shiny skin; reddish pink, moist gills; and clear, bulging eyes. The flesh should spring back when you press it lightly.

Choose fish fillets that look moist, not dry.

Choose tightly sealed, solidly frozen packages of frozen fish.

In 1998, the FDA/National Center for Toxicological Research released for testing an inexpensive indicator called "Fresh Tag." The indicator, to be packed with seafood, changes color if the product spoils.

Avoid: Fresh whole fish whose eyes have sunk into the head (a clear sign of aging); fillets that look dry; and packages of frozen fish that are stained (whatever leaked on the package may have seeped through onto the fish) or are coated with ice crystals (the package may have defrosted and been refrozen).

Storing This Food

Remove fish from plastic wrap as soon as you get it home. Plastic keeps out air, encouraging the growth of bacteria that make the fish smell bad. If the fish smells bad when you open the package, throw it out.

Refrigerate all fresh and smoked fish immediately. Fish spoils quickly because it has a high proportion of polyunsaturated fatty acids (which pick up oxygen much more easily than saturated or monounsaturated fatty acids). Refrigeration also slows the action of microorganisms on the surface of the fish that convert proteins and other substances to mucopolysaccharides, leaving a slimy film on the fish.

Keep fish frozen until you are ready to use it.

Store canned fish in a cool cabinet or in a refrigerator (but not the freezer). The cooler the temperature, the longer the shelf life.

Preparing This Food

Fresh fish. Rub the fish with lemon juice, then rinse it under cold running water. The lemon juice (an acid) will convert the nitrogen compounds that make fish smell "fishy" to compounds that break apart easily and can be rinsed off the fish with cool running water. Rinsing your hands in lemon juice and water will get rid of the fishy smell after you have been preparing fresh fish.

Frozen fish. Defrost plain frozen fish in the refrigerator or under cold running water. Prepared frozen fish dishes should not be thawed before you cook them since defrosting will make the sauce or coating soggy.

Salted dried fish. Salted dried fish should be soaked to remove the salt. How long you have to soak the fish depends on how much salt was added in processing. A reasonable average for salt cod, mackerel, haddock (finnan haddie), or herring is three to six hours, with two or three changes of water.

When you are done, clean all utensils thoroughly with hot soap and hot water. Wash your cutting board, wood or plastic, with hot water, soap, and a bleach-and-water solution. For ultimate safety in preventing the transfer of microorganisms from the raw fish to other foods, keep one cutting board exclusively for raw fish, meats, and poultry, and a second one for everything else. Finally, don't forget to wash your hands.

What Happens When You Cook This Food

Heat changes the structure of proteins. It denatures the protein molecules so that they break apart into smaller fragments or change shape or clump together. These changes force moisture out of the tissues so that the fish turns opaque. The longer you cook fish, the more moisture it will lose. Cooked fish flakes because the connective tissue in fish "melts" at a relatively low temperature.

Heating fish thoroughly destroys parasites and microorganisms that live in raw fish, making the fish safer to eat.

How Other Kinds of Processing Affect This Food

Marinating.   Like heat, acids coagulate the proteins in fish, squeezing out moisture. Fish marinated in citrus juices and other acids such as vinegar or wine has a firm texture and looks cooked, but the acid bath may not inactivate parasites in the fish.

Canning.   Fish is naturally low in sodium, but canned fish often contains enough added salt to make it a high-sodium food. A 3.5-ounce serving of baked, fresh red salmon, for example, has 55 mg sodium, while an equal serving of regular canned salmon has 443 mg. If the fish is canned in oil it is also much higher in calories than fresh fish.

Freezing.   When fish is frozen, ice crystals form in the flesh and tear its cells so that moisture leaks out when the fish is defrosted. Commercial flash-freezing offers some protection by freezing the fish so fast that the ice crystals stay small and do less damage, but all defrosted fish tastes drier and less palatable than fresh fish. Freezing slows but does not stop the oxidation of fats that causes fish to deteriorate.

Curing.   Fish can be cured (preserved) by smoking, drying, salting, or pickling, all of which coagulate the muscle tissue and prevent microorganisms from growing. Each method has its own particular drawbacks. Smoking adds potentially carcinogenic chemicals. Drying reduces the water content, concentrates the solids and nutrients, increases the calories per ounce, and raises the amount of sodium.

Medical Uses and/or Benefits

Protection against cardiovascular disease.   The most important fats in fish are the polyunsaturated acids known as omega-3s. These fatty acids appear to work their way into heart cells where they seem to help stabilize the heart muscle and prevent potentially fatal arrhythmia (irregular heartbeat). Among 85,000 women in the long-running Nurses' Health Study, those who ate fatty fish at least five times a week were nearly 50 percent less likely to die from heart disease than those who ate fish less frequently. Similar results appeared in men in the equally long-running Physicians' Health Study. Some studies suggest that people may get similar benefits from omega-3 capsules. Researchers at the Consorzio Mario Negri Sud in Santa Maria Imbaro (Italy) say that men given a one-gram fish oil capsule once a day have a risk of sudden death 42 percent lower than men given placebos ("look-alike" pills with no fish oil). However, most nutrition scientists recommend food over supplements.

Omega-3 Content of Various Food Fish

Fish* (3 oz.)	Omega-3 (grams)
Salmon, Atlantic	1.8
Anchovy, canned*	1.7
Mackerel, Pacific	1.6
Salmon, pink, canned*	1.4
Sardine, Pacific, canned*	1.4
Trout, rainbow	1.0
Tuna, white, canned*	0.7
Mussels	0.7

* cooked, without sauce
* drained

Source: National Fisheries Institute; USDA Nutrient Data Laboratory. National Nutrient Database for Standard Reference. Available online. URL: http://www.nal.usda.gov/fnic/foodcomp/search/.

Adverse Effects Associated with This Food

Allergic reaction. According to the *Merck Manual,* fish is one of the 12 foods most likely to trigger classic food allergy symptoms: hives, swelling of the lips and eyes, and upset stomach. The others are berries (blackberries, blueberries, raspberries, strawberries), chocolate, corn, eggs, legumes (green peas, lima beans, peanuts, soybeans), milk, nuts, peaches, pork, shellfish, and wheat (see WHEAT CEREALS). NOTE: Canned tuna products may contain sulfites in vegetable proteins used to enhance the tuna's flavor. People sensitive to sulfites may suffer serious allergic reactions, including potentially fatal anaphylactic shock, if they eat tuna containing sulfites. In 1997, tuna manufacturers agreed to put warning labels on products with sulfites.

Environmental contaminants. Some fish are contaminated with methylmercury, a compound produced by bacteria that chemically alters naturally occurring mercury (a metal found in rock and soil) or mercury released into water through industrial pollution. The methylmercury is absorbed by small fish, which are eaten by larger fish, which are then eaten by human beings. The larger the fish and the longer it lives the more methylmercury it absorbs. The measurement used to describe the amount of methylmercury in fish is ppm (parts per million). Newly-popular tilapia, a small fish, has an average 0.01 ppm, while shark, a big fish, may have up to 4.54 ppm, 450 times as much.

That is a relatively small amount of methylmercury; it will soon make its way harmlessly out of the body. But even small amounts may be hazardous during pregnancy because methylmercury targets the developing fetal nervous system. Repeated studies have shown that women who eat lots of high-mercury fish while pregnant are more likely to deliver babies with developmental problems. As a result, the FDA and the Environmental Protection Agency have now warned that women who may become pregnant, who are pregnant, or who are nursing should avoid shark, swordfish, king mackerel, and tilefish, the fish most likely to contain large amounts of methylmercury. The same prohibition applies to very young children; although there are no studies of newborns and babies, the young brain continues to develop after birth and the logic is that the prohibition during pregnancy should extend into early life.

That does not mean no fish at all should be eaten during pregnancy. In fact, a 2003 report in the *Journal of Epidemiology and Community Health* of data from an 11,585-woman study at the University of Bristol (England) shows that women who don't eat any fish while pregnant are nearly 40 percent more likely to deliver low birth-weight infants than are women who eat about an ounce of fish a day, the equivalent of 1/3 of a small can of tuna. One theory is that omega-3 fatty acids in the fish may increase the flow of nutrient-rich blood through the placenta to the fetus. University of Southern California researchers say that omega-3s may also protect some children from asthma. Their study found that children born to asthmatic mothers who ate oily fish such as salmon at least once a month while pregnant were less likely to develop asthma before age five than children whose asthmatic pregnant mothers never ate oily fish.

The following table lists the estimated levels of mercury in common food fish. For the complete list of mercury levels in fish, click onto www.cfsan.fda.gov/~frf/sea-mehg.html.

Mercury Levels in Common Food Fish

Low levels (0.01–0.12 ppm* average)
Anchovies, butterfish, catfish, clams, cod, crab (blue, king, snow), crawfish, croaker (Atlantic), flounder, haddock, hake, herring, lobster (spiny/Atlantic) mackerel, mullet, ocean perch, oysters, pollock, salmon (canned/fresh frozen), sardines, scallops, shad (American), shrimp, sole, squid, tilapia, trout (freshwater), tuna (canned, light), whitefish, whiting

Mid levels (0.14–0.54 ppm* average)
Bass (saltwater), bluefish, carp, croaker (Pacific), freshwater perch, grouper, halibut, lobster (Northern American), mackerel (Spanish), marlin, monkfish, orange roughy, skate, snapper, tilefish (Atlantic), tuna (canned albacore, fresh/frozen), weakfish/sea trout

High levels (0.73–1.45 ppm* average)
King mackerel, shark, swordfish, tilefish

* *ppm* = parts per million, i.e. parts of mercury to 1,000,000 parts fish

Source: U.S. Food and Drug Administration, Center for Food Safety and Applied Nutrition, "Mercury Levels in Commercial Fish and Shellfish." Available online. URL: www.cfsan.fda.gov/~frf/sea-mehg.html.

Parasitical, viral, and bacterial infections.   Like raw meat, raw fish may carry various pathogens, including fish tapeworm and flukes in freshwater fish and *Salmonella* or other microorganisms left on the fish by infected foodhandlers. Cooking the fish destroys these organisms.

Scombroid poisoning.   Bacterial decomposition that occurs after fish is caught produces a histaminelike toxin in the flesh of mackerel, tuna, bonito, and albacore. This toxin may trigger a number of symptoms, including a flushed face immediately after you eat it. The other signs of scombroid poisoning—nausea, vomiting, stomach pain, and hives—show up a few minutes later. The symptoms usually last 24 hours or less.

Food/Drug Interactions

Monoamine oxidase (MAO) inhibitors.   Monoamine oxidase inhibitors are drugs used to treat depression. They inactivate naturally occurring enzymes in your body that metabolize tyramine, a substance found in many fermented or aged foods. Tyramine constricts blood vessels and increases blood pressure. If you eat a food such as pickled herring, which is high in tyramine, while you are taking an MAO inhibitor, your body may not be able to eliminate the tyramine and the result may be a hypertensive crisis.

Flour

See also Bread, Corn, Oats, Pasta, Potatoes, Rice, Soybeans, Wheat cereals.

Nutritional Profile

Energy value (calories per serving): *High*

Protein: *Moderate*

Fat: *Low*

Saturated fat: *Low*

Cholesterol: *None*

Carbohydrates: *High*

Fiber: *Low to high*

Sodium: *Low (except self-rising flour)*

Major vitamin contribution: *B vitamins*

Major mineral contribution: *Iron*

About the Nutrients in This Food

Flour is the primary source of the carbohydrates (starch and fiber) in bread, pasta, and baked goods. All wheat and rye flours also provide some of the food fibers, including pectins, gums, and cellulose. Flour also contains significant amounts of protein but, like other plant foods, its proteins are "incomplete" because they are deficient in the essential amino acid lysine. The fat in the wheat germ is primarily polyunsaturated; flour contains no cholesterol. Flour is a good source of iron and the B vitamins. Iodine and iodophors used to clean the equipment in grain-processing plants may add iodine to the flour.

In 1998, the Food and Drug Administration ordered food manufacturers to add folates—which protect against birth defects of the spinal cord and against heart disease—to flour, rice, and other grain products. One year later, data from the Framingham Heart Study, which has followed heart health among residents of a Boston suburb for nearly half a century, showed a dramatic increase in blood levels of folic acid. Before the fortification of foods, 22 percent of the study participants had a folic acid deficiency; after, the number fell to 2 percent.

Whole grain flour, like other grain products, contains phytic acid, an antinutrient that binds calcium, iron, and zinc ions into insoluble compounds your body cannot absorb. This has no practical effect so long as your diet includes foods that provide these minerals.

Whole wheat flours.   Whole wheat flours use every part of the kernel: the fiber-rich bran with its B vitamins, the starch- and protein-rich endosperm with its iron and B vitamins, and the oily germ with its vitamin E.[*] Because they contain bran, whole-grain flours have much more fiber than refined white flours. However, some studies suggest that the size of the fiber particles may have some bearing on their ability to absorb moisture and "bulk up" stool and that the fiber particles found in fine-ground whole wheat flours may be too small to have a bulking effect.

Finely ground whole wheat flour is called *whole wheat cake flour;* coarsely ground whole wheat flour is called *graham flour. Cracked wheat* is a whole wheat flour that has been cut rather than ground; it has all the nutrients of whole wheat flour, but its processing makes it less likely to yield its starch in cooking. When dried and parboiled, cracked wheat is known as *bulgur,* a grain used primarily as a cereal, although it can be mixed with other flours and baked. *Gluten flour* is a low-starch, high-protein product made by drying and grinding hard-wheat flour from which the starch has been removed.

Refined ("white") flours.   Refined flours are paler than whole wheat flours because they do not contain the brown bran and germ. They have less fiber and fat and smaller amounts of vitamins and minerals than whole wheat flours, but *enriched refined flours* are fortified with B vitamins and iron. Refined flour has no phytic acid.

Some refined flours are bleached with chlorine dioxide to destroy the xanthophylls (carotenoid pigments) that give white flours a natural cream color. Unlike carotene, the carotenoid pigment that is converted to vitamin A in the body, xanthophylls have no vitamin A activity; bleaching does not lower the vitamin A levels in the flour, but it does destroy vitamin E.

There are several kinds of white flours. *All-purpose* white flour is a mixture of hard and soft wheats, high in protein and rich in gluten.[†] *Cake flour* is a finely milled soft-wheat flour; it has less protein than all-purpose flour. *Self-rising* flour is flour to which baking powder has been added and is very high in sodium. *Instant flour* is all-purpose flour that has been ground extra-fine so that it will combine quickly with water. *Semolina* is a pale high-protein, low-gluten flour made from durum wheat and used to make pasta.

Rye flours.   Rye flour has less gluten than wheat flour and is less elastic, which is why it makes a denser bread.[‡]

Like whole wheat flour, dark rye flour (the flour used for pumpernickel bread) contains the bran and the germ of the rye grain; light rye flour (the flour used for ordinary rye bread)

---

[*]   The bran is the kernel's hard, brown outer cover, an extraordinarily rich source of cellulose and lignin. The endosperm is the kernel's pale interior, where the vitamins abound. The germ, a small particle in the interior, is the part of the kernel that sprouts.

[†]   Hard wheat has less starch and more protein than soft wheat. It makes a heavier, denser dough.

[‡]   Gluten is the sticky substance formed when kneading the dough relaxes the long-chain molecules in the proteins gliadin and glutenin so that some of their intermolecular bonds (bonds between atoms in the same molecule) break and new intramolecular bonds (bonds between atoms on different molecules) are formed.

does not. Triticale flour is milled from triticale grain, a rye/wheat hybrid. It has more protein and less gluten than all-purpose wheat flour.

The Most Nutritious Way to Serve This Food

With beans or a "complete" protein food (meat, fish, poultry, eggs, milk, cheese) to provide the essential amino acid lysine, in which wheat and rye flours are deficient.

Diets That May Restrict or Exclude This Food

Low-calcium diet (whole grain and self-rising flours)
Low-fiber diet (whole wheat flours)
Low-gluten diet (all wheat and rye flour)
Sucrose-free diet

Buying This Food

Look for: Tightly sealed bags or boxes. Flours in torn packages or in open bins are exposed to air and to insect contamination.

Avoid: Stained packages—the liquid that stained the package may have seeped through into the flour.

Storing This Food

Store all flours in air- and moistureproof canisters. Whole wheat flours, which contain the germ and bran of the wheat and are higher in fat than white flours, may become rancid if exposed to air; they should be used within a week after you open the package. If you plan to hold the flour for longer than that, store it in the freezer, tightly wrapped to protect it against air and moisture. You do not have to thaw the flour when you are ready to use it; just measure it out and add it directly to the other ingredients.

Put a bay leaf in the flour canister to help protect against insect infections. Bay leaves are natural insect repellents.

Preparing This Food

* * *

What Happens When You Cook This Food

Protein reactions.   The wheat kernel contains several proteins, including gliadin and glutenin. When you mix flour with water, gliadin and glutenin clump together in a sticky mass.

Kneading the dough relaxes the long gliadin and glutenin molecules, breaking internal bonds between individual atoms in each gliadin and glutenin molecule and allowing the molecules to unfold and form new bonds between atoms in different molecules. The result is a network structure made of a new gliadin-glutenin compound called *gluten.*

Gluten is very elastic. The gluten network can stretch to accommodate the gas (carbon dioxide) formed when you add yeast to bread dough or heat a cake batter made with baking powder or baking soda (sodium bicarbonate), trapping the gas and making the bread dough or cake batter rise. When you bake the dough or batter, the gluten network hardens and the bread or cake assumes its finished shape.

Starch reactions. Starch consists of molecules of the complex carbohydrates amylose and amylopectin packed into a starch granule. When you heat flour in liquid, the starch granules absorb water molecules, swell, and soften. When the temperature of the liquid reaches approximately 140°F the amylose and amylopectin molecules inside the granules relax and unfold, breaking some of their internal bonds (bonds between atoms on the same molecule) and forming new bonds between atoms on different molecules. The result is a network that traps and holds water molecules. The starch granules then swell, thickening the liquid. If you continue to heat the liquid (or stir it too vigorously), the network will begin to break down, the liquid will leak out of the starch granules, and the sauce will separate.[*]

Combination reaction. Coating food with flour takes advantage of the starch reaction (absorbing liquids) and the protein reaction (baking a hard, crisp protein crust).

How Other Kinds of Processing Affect This Food

* * *

Medical Uses and/or Benefits

A lower risk of some kinds of cancer. In 1998, scientists at Wayne State University in Detroit conducted a meta-analysis of data from more than 30 well-designed animal studies measuring the anti-cancer effects of wheat bran, the part of grain with highest amount of the insoluble dietary fibers cellulose and lignin. They found a 32 percent reduction in the risk of colon cancer among animals fed wheat bran; now they plan to conduct a similar meta-analysis of human studies. Whole wheat flours are a good source of wheat bran. NOTE: The amount of fiber per serving listed on a food package label shows the total amount of fiber (insoluble and soluble).

Early in 1999, however, new data from the long-running Nurses Health Study at Brigham Women's Hospital/Harvard University School of Public Health showed that women who ate a high-fiber diet had a risk of colon cancer similar to that of women who ate a low-fiber diet.

---

[*] Amylose is a long, unbranched, spiral molecule; amylopectin is a short, compact, branched molecule. Amylose has more room for forming bonds to water. Wheat flours, which have a higher ratio of amylose to amylopectin, are superior thickeners.

Because this study contradicts literally hundreds of others conducted over the past 30 years, researchers are awaiting confirming evidence before changing dietary recommendations.

Adverse Effects Associated with This Food

Allergic reactions. According to the *Merck Manual,* wheat is one of the foods most commonly implicated as a cause of allergic upset stomach, hives, and angioedema (swollen lips and eyes). For more information, see under WHEAT CEREALS.

Gluten intolerance (celiac disease). Celiac disease is an intestinal allergic disorder that makes it impossible to digest gluten and gliadin (proteins found in wheat and some other grains). Corn flour, potato flour, rice flour, and soy flour are all gluten- and gliadin-free.

Ergot poisoning. Rye and some kinds of wheat will support ergot, a parasitic fungus related to lysergic acid (LSD). Because commercial flours are routinely checked for ergot contamination, there has not been a major outbreak of ergot poisoning from bread since a 1951 incident in France. Since baking does not destroy ergot toxins, the safest course is to avoid moldy flour altogether.

Food/Drug Interactions

* * *

Game Meat

(Bison, rabbit, venison)

Nutritional Profile

Energy value (calories per serving): *Moderate*
Protein: *High*
Fat: *Low*
Saturated fat: *High*
Cholesterol: *Moderate*
Carbohydrates: *None*
Fiber: *None*
Sodium: *Low*
Major vitamin contribution: *B vitamins*
Major mineral contribution: *Iron, zinc*

About the Nutrients in This Food

Like other animal foods, game meat has high-quality proteins with sufficient amounts of all the essential amino acids. Some game meat has less fat, saturated fat, and cholesterol than beef. All game meat is an excellent source of B vitamins, plus heme iron, the form of iron most easily absorbed by your body, and zinc. For example, one four-ounce serving of roast bison has 28 g protein, 2.7 g fat (1.04 g saturated fat), 93.7 mg cholesterol, 3.88 mg iron (25.8 percent of the RDA for a woman of childbearing age), and 4.1 mg zinc (27 percent of the RDA for a man).

The Nutrients in Roasted Game Meat (4-ounce serving)

Meat	Protein (g)	Fat (g)	Saturated fat (g)	Cholesterol (mg)	Iron (mg)	Zinc (mg)
Bison	28.44	2.7	1.04	93.7	3.88	4.1
Rabbit	33	9	2.7	93	2.57	2.59
Venison	34	4	1.4	127	5.07	3.12
Beef (lean)	33	6	2.3	90	3	8

Source: USDA Nutrient Database: www.nal.usda.gov/fnic/cgi-bin/nut_search. pl, *Nutritive Value of Foods,* Home and Garden Bulletin No. 72 (USDA, 1989).

The Most Nutritious Way to Serve This Food

With a food rich in vitamin C. Vitamin C increases the absorption of iron.

Diets That May Restrict or Exclude This Food

Low-protein diet (for kidney disease)

Buying This Food

In American markets, game meats are usually sold frozen. Choose a package with no leaks or stains to suggest previous defrosting.

Storing This Food

Keep frozen game meat well wrapped in the freezer until you are ready to use it. The packaging protects the meat from oxygen that can change its pigments from reddish to brown. Freezing prolongs the freshness of the meat by slowing the natural multiplication of bacteria that digest proteins and other substances on the surface, converting them to a slimy film. The bacteria also change the meat's sulfur-containing amino acids methionine and cystine into smelly chemicals called mercaptans. When the mercaptans combine with myoglobin, they produce the greenish pigment that gives spoiled meat its characteristic unpleasant appearance. Large cuts of game meat can be safely frozen, at 0°F, for six months to a year.

Preparing This Food

Defrost the meat in the refrigerator to protect it from spoilage. Trim the meat to dispose of all visible fat, thus reducing the amount of fat and cholesterol in each serving.

When you are done, clean all utensils thoroughly with hot soap and hot water. Wash your cutting board, wood or plastic, with hot water, soap, and a bleach-and-water solution. For ultimate safety in preventing the transfer of microorganisms from the raw meat to other foods, keep one cutting board exclusively for raw meats, fish, and poultry, and a second one for everything else. Finally, don't forget to wash your hands.

What Happens When You Cook This Food

Cooking changes the way meat looks and tastes, alters its nutritional value, makes it safer, and extends its shelf life.

Browning meat before you cook it does not "seal in the juices," but it does change the flavor by caramelizing proteins and sugars on the surface. Because meat's only sugars are the small amounts of glycogen in muscle tissue, we add sugars in marinades or basting liquids that may also contain acids (vinegar, lemon juice, wine) to break down muscle fibers and tenderize the meat. (NOTE: Browning has one minor nutritional drawback. It breaks amino acids on the surface of the meat into smaller compounds that are no longer useful proteins.)

When meat is heated, it loses water and shrinks. Its pigments, which combine with oxygen, are denatured (broken into fragments) by the heat. They turn brown, the natural color of well-done meat. At the same time, the fats in the meat are oxidized, a reaction that produces a characteristic warmed-over flavor when the cooked meat is refrigerated and then reheated. Cooking and storing the meat under a blanket of *antioxidants*—catsup or a gravy made of tomatoes, peppers and other vitamin-C rich vegetables—reduces fat oxidation and lessens the warmed-over flavor. Meat reheated in a microwave oven is also less likely to taste warmed-over.

How Other Kinds of Processing Affect This Food

Aging.   Hanging fresh meat exposed to air in a cold room evaporates moisture and shrinks the meat slightly. At the same time, bacterial action on the surface of the meat breaks down proteins, producing an "aged" flavor. (See below, *Food/drug interactions.*)

Curing.   Salt-curing preserves meat through osmosis, the physical reaction in which liquids flow across a membrane, such as the wall of a cell, from a less dense to a more dense solution. The salt or sugar used in curing dissolve in the liquid on the surface of the meat to make a solution that is more dense than the liquid inside the cells of the meat. Water flows out of the meat *and* out of the cells of any microorganisms living on the meat, killing the micro-organisms and protecting the meat from bacterial damage. Salt-cured meat is higher in sodium than fresh meat.

Smoking.   Hanging fresh meat over an open fire slowly dries the meat, kills microorganisms on its surface, and gives the meat a rich, smoky flavor. The flavor varies with the wood used in the fire. Meats smoked over an open fire are exposed to carcinogenic chemicals in the smoke, including *a*-benzopyrene. Artificial smoke flavoring is commercially treated to remove tar and *a*-benzopyrene.

Medical Uses and/or Benefits

Treating and/or preventing iron deficiency.   Without meat in the diet, it is virtually impossible for an adult woman to meet her iron requirement without supplements.

Adverse Effects Associated with This Food

Increased risk of cardiovascular disease.   Like all foods from animals, game meats are a source of cholesterol. To reduce the risk of heart disease, the National Cholesterol Education Project recommends following the Step I and Step II diets.

The Step I diet provides no more than 30 percent of total daily calories from fat, no more than 10 percent of total daily calories from saturated fat, and no more than 300 mg of cholesterol per day. It is designed for healthy people whose cholesterol is in the range of 200–239 mg/dL.

The Step II diet provides 25–35 percent of total calories from fat, less than 7 percent of total calories from saturated fat, up to 10 percent of total calories from polyunsaturated fat, up to 20 percent of total calories from monounsaturated fat, and less than 300 mg cholesterol per day. This stricter regimen is designed for people who have one or more of the following conditions:

◆ Existing cardiovascular disease
◆ High levels of low-density lipoproteins (LDLs, or "bad" cholesterol) or low levels of high-density lipoproteins (HDLs, or "good" cholesterol)
◆ Obesity
◆ Type 1 diabetes (insulin-dependent diabetes, or diabetes mellitus)
◆ Metabolic syndrome, a.k.a. insulin resistance syndrome, a cluster of risk factors that includes type 2 diabetes (non-insulin-dependent diabetes)

Food-borne illness. Improperly cooked meat contaminated with *E. coli* O157:H7 has been linked to a number of fatalities in several parts of the United States. In addition, meat contaminated with other bacteria, viruses, or parasites poses special problems for people with a weakened immune system: the very young, the very old, cancer chemotherapy patients, and people with HIV. Cooking meat to an internal temperature of 140°F should destroy *Salmonella* and *Campylobacter jejuni;* to 165°F, *E. coli,* and to 212°F, *Listeria monocytogenes.*

Decline in kidney function. Proteins are nitrogen compounds. When metabolized, they yield ammonia that is excreted through the kidneys. In laboratory animals, a sustained high-protein diet increases the flow of blood through the kidneys, accelerating the natural age-related decline in kidney function. Some experts suggest that this may also occur in human beings.

Food/Drug Interactions

Monoamine oxidase (MAO) inhibitors. Meat "tenderized" with papaya or a papain powder can interact with the class of antidepressant drugs known as monoamine oxidase inhibitors. Papain meat tenderizers work by breaking up the long chains of protein molecules. One by-product of this process is tyramine, a substance that constructs blood vessels and raises blood pressure. MAO inhibitors inactivate naturally occurring enzymes in your body that metabolize tyramine. If you eat a food such as papain-tenderized meat, which is high in tyramine, while you are taking an MAO inhibitor, you cannot effectively eliminate the tyramine from your body. The result may be a hypertensive crisis.

Garlic

See also Onions.

Nutritional Profile

Energy value (calories per serving): *Low*
Protein: *Moderate*
Fat: *Low*
Saturated fat: *Low*
Cholesterol: *None*
Carbohydrates: *High*
Fiber: *High*
Sodium: *Low*
Major vitamin contribution: *Vitamin C*
Major mineral contribution: *Iron, selenium*

About the Nutrients in This Food

Although raw garlic has some fiber and protein plus vitamins and minerals, we rarely eat enough garlic to get useful amounts of these nutrients.

Nutrient	Garlic cloves (2)	Garlic powder (1 tsp)
Carbohydrates (g)	2.98	2
Protein (g)	0.6	0.5
Dietary fiber (g)	0.2	0.3
Vitamin C (mg)	2.8	0.5
Iron (mg)	0.2	0.1
Selenium (mcg)	1.3	1.1

Source: USDA Nutrient Data Laboratory. National Nutrient Database for Standard Reference. Available online. URL: http://www.nal.usda.gov/fnic/foodcomp/search/.

Elephant garlic, a cross between an onion and garlic that may grow as large as a grapefruit, has a milder flavor than regular garlic.

Garlic contains alliin and allicin, two sulfur compounds with antibiotic activity. In a number of laboratory experiments, garlic juice appears to inhibit the growth of a broad variety of bacteria, yeast, and fungi growing in test tubes, but its effects on human beings have yet to be proven.

Diets That May Restrict or Exclude This Food

Antiflatulence diet
Bland diet

Buying This Food

Look for: Firm, solid cloves with tight clinging skin. If the skin is papery and pulling away from the cloves and the head feels light for its size, the garlic has withered or rotted away inside.

The Most Nutritious Way to Serve This Food

Fresh.

Storing This Food

Store garlic in a cool, dark, airy place to keep it from drying out or sprouting. (When garlic sprouts, diallyl disulfide—the sulfur compound that gives fresh garlic its distinctive taste and odor—goes into the new growth and the garlic itself becomes milder.) An unglazed ceramic "garlic keeper" will protect the garlic from moisture while allowing air to circulate freely around the head and cloves. Properly stored, garlic will keep for several months.

Do not refrigerate garlic unless you live in a very hot and humid climate.

Preparing This Food

To peel garlic easily, blanch the cloves in boiling water for about 30 seconds, then drain and cool. Slice off the root end, and the skin should come right off without sticking to your fingers. Or you can put a head of fresh, raw garlic on a flat surface and hit the flat end with the flat side of a knife. The head will come apart and the skin should come off easily.

To get the most "garlicky" taste from garlic cloves, chop or mash them or extract the oil with a garlic press. When you cut into a garlic clove, you tear its cell walls, releasing an enzyme that converts sulfur compounds in the garlic into ammonia, pyruvic acid, and diallyl disulfide.

What Happens When You Cook This Food

Heating garlic destroys its diallyl disulfide, which is why cooked garlic is so much milder tasting than raw garlic.

How Other Kinds of Processing Affect This Food

Drying. Drying removes moisture from garlic but leaves the oils intact. Powdered garlic and garlic salt should be stored in a cool, dry place to keep their oils from turning rancid. Garlic salt is much higher in sodium than either raw garlic, garlic powder, or dried garlic flakes.

Medical Uses and/or Benefits

Protection against some cancers. The organic sulfur compounds in garlic and onions appear to reduce the risk of some forms of cancer perhaps by preventing the formation of carcinogens in your body or by blocking carcinogens from reaching or reacting with sensitive body tissues or by inhibiting the transformation of healthy cells to malignant ones.

Protection against circulatory diseases. In a number of laboratory studies during the 1980s, adding garlic oil to animal feeds reduced levels of low-density lipoproteins (LDLs), the fat and protein particles that carry cholesterol into your arteries, and raised levels of high density lipoproteins (HDLs), the particles that carry cholesterol out of the body. However, current studies are contradictory. One year-long study at the Harbor-UCLA Medical Center showed that daily doses of aged garlic (brand name Kyolic) appeared to reduce the formation of cholesterol deposits in arteries while lowering blood levels of homocysteine, an amino acid the American Heart Association calls an independent risk factor for heart disease. But another study funded by the National Center for Complementary and Alternative Medicine (NCCAM), a division of the National Institutes of Health, to determine the safety and effectiveness of garlic showed that neither fresh garlic nor powdered garlic nor garlic tablets have any effect on cholesterol levels.

Adverse Effects Associated with This Food

Body odor, halitosis. Diallyl disulfide is excreted in perspiration and in the air you exhale, which is why eating garlic makes you smell garlicky.

Food/Drug Interactions

Anticoagulants (blood thinners). Garlic appears to reduce blood's ability to clot, thus increasing the effect of anticoagulants, including aspirin. NCCAM recommends using garlic with caution before surgery, including dental surgery. Patients who have a clotting disorder should consult their own doctors before using garlic.

Gelatin

Nutritional Profile*

Energy value (calories per serving): *Low*
Protein: *Low*
Fat: *Low*
Saturated fat: *Low*
Cholesterol: *Low*
Carbohydrates: *None*
Fiber: *None*
Sodium: *Low*
Major vitamin contribution: *None*
Major mineral contribution: *None*

About the Nutrients in This Food

Although gelatin is made from the collagen (connective tissue) of cattle hides and bones or pig skin, its proteins are limited in the essential acid tryptophan, which is destroyed when the bones and skin are treated with acid, and is deficient in several others, including lysine. In fact, gelatin's proteins are of such poor quality that, unlike other foods of animal origin (meat, milk), gelatin cannot sustain life. Laboratory rats fed a diet in which gelatin was the primary protein did not grow as they should; half died within 48 days, even though the gelatin was supplemented with some of the essential amino acids.

Plain gelatin has no carbohydrates and fiber. It is low in fat. Flavored gelatin desserts, however, are high in carbohydrates because of the added sugar.

The Most Nutritious Way to Serve This Food

With a protein food rich in complete proteins. Gelatin desserts whipped with milk fit the bill.

Diets That May Restrict or Exclude This Food

Low-carbohydrate diet (gelatin desserts prepared with sugar)
Low-sodium diet (commercial gelatin powders)
Sucrose-free diet (gelatin desserts prepared with sugar)

---

* Values are for prepared unsweetened gelatin.

Buying This Food

Look for: Tightly sealed, clean boxes.

Storing This Food

Store gelatin boxes in a cool, dry cabinet.

Preparing This Food

Commercial unflavored gelatin comes in premeasured 1-tablespoon packets. One tablespoon of gelatin will thicken about two cups of water. To combine the gelatin and water, first heat ¾ cup water to boiling. While it is heating, add the gelatin to ¼ cup cold liquid and let it absorb moisture until it is translucent. Then add the boiling water. (Flavored fruit gelatins can be dissolved directly in hot water.)

What Happens When You Cook This Food

When you mix gelatin with hot water, its protein molecules create a network that stiffens into a stable, solid gel as it squeezes out moisture. The longer the gel sits, the more intermolecular bonds it forms, the more moisture it loses and the firmer it becomes. A day-old gel is much firmer than one you've just made.

Gelatin is used as a thickener in prepared foods and can be used at home to thicken sauces. Flavored gelatin dessert powders have less stiffening power than plain gelatin because some of their protein has been replaced by sugar.

To build a layered gelatin mold, let each layer harden before you add the next.

How Other Kinds of Processing Affect This Food

* * *

Medical Uses and/or Benefits

* * *

Adverse Effects Associated with This Food

* * *

Food/Drug Interactions

* * *

Grapefruit

(Ugli fruit)

Nutritional Profile

Energy value (calories per serving): *Low*

Protein: *Low*

Fat: *Low*

Saturated fat: *Low*

Cholesterol: *None*

Carbohydrates: *High*

Fiber: *Moderate*

Sodium: *Low*

Major vitamin contribution: *Vitamin A, vitamin C*

Major mineral contribution: *Potassium*

About the Nutrients in This Food

Grapefruit and ugli fruit (a cross between the grapefruit and the tangerine) have moderate amounts of dietary fiber and, like all citrus fruits, are most prized for their vitamin C. Pink or red grapefruits have moderate amounts of vitamin A.

One-half medium (four-inch diameter) pink grapefruit has 1.4 g dietary fiber, 1,187 IU vitamin A (51 percent of the RDA for a woman, 40 percent of the RDA for a man), and 44 mg vitamin C (59 percent of the RDA for a woman, 49 percent of the RDA for a man). One half medium (3.75-inch diameter) white grapefruit has 1.3 g dietary fiber, 39 IU vitamin A (2 percent of the RDA for a woman, 1 percent of the RDA for a man), and 39 mg vitamin C (52 percent of the RDA for a woman, 43 percent of the RDA for a man).

Pink and red grapefruits also contain lycopene, a red carotenoid (plant pigment), a strong antioxidant that appears to lower the risk of cancer of the prostate. The richest source of lycopene is cooked TOMATOES.

The Most Nutritious Way to Serve This Food

Fresh fruit or fresh-squeezed juice.

Diets That May Restrict or Exclude This Food

* * *

Buying This Food

Look for: Firm fruit that is heavy for its size, which means that it will be juicy. The skin should be thin, smooth, and fine-grained. Most grapefruit have yellow skin that, depending on the variety, may be tinged with red or green. In fact, a slight greenish tint may mean that the grapefruit is high in sugar. Ugli fruit, which looks like misshapen, splotched grapefruit, is yellow with green patches and bumpy skin.

Avoid: Grapefruit or ugli fruit with puffy skin or those that feel light for their size; the flesh inside is probably dry and juiceless.

Storing This Food

Store grapefruit either at room temperature (for a few days) or in the refrigerator.

Refrigerate grapefruit juice in a tightly closed glass bottle with very little air space at the top. As you use up the juice, transfer it to a smaller bottle, again with very little air space at the top. The aim is to prevent the juice from coming into contact with oxygen, which destroys vitamin C. (Most plastic juice bottles are oxygen-permeable.) Properly stored and protected from oxygen, fresh grapefruit juice can hold its vitamin C for several weeks.

Preparing This Food

Grapefruit are most flavorful at room temperature, which liberates the aromatic molecules that give them their characteristic scent and taste.

Before cutting into the grapefruit, rinse it under cool running water to flush debris off the peel.

To section grapefruit, cut a slice from the top, then cut off the peel in strips—starting at the top and going down—or peel it in a spiral fashion. You can remove the bitter white membrane, but some of the vitamin C will go with it. Finally, slice the sections apart. Or you can simply cut the grapefruit in half and scoop out the sections with a curved, serrated grapefruit knife.

What Happens When You Cook This Food

Broiling a half grapefruit or poaching grapefruit sections reduces the fruit's supply of vitamin C, which is heat-sensitive.

How Other Kinds of Processing Affect This Food

Commercially prepared juices.   How well a commercially prepared juice retains its vitamin C depends on how it is prepared, stored, and packaged. Commercial flash-freezing preserves as much as 95 percent of the vitamin C in fresh grapefruit juices. Canned juice stored in the refrigerator may lose only 2 percent of its vitamin C in three months. Prepared, pasteurized "fresh" juices lose vitamin C because they are sold in plastic bottles or waxed-paper cartons that let oxygen in.

Commercially prepared juices are pasteurized to stop the natural enzyme action that would otherwise turn sugars to alcohols. Pasteurization also protects juices from potentially harmful bacterial and mold contamination. Following several deaths attributed to unpasteurized apple juices containing *E. coli* O157:H7, the FDA ruled that all fruit and vegetable juices must carry a warning label telling you whether the juice has been pasteurized. Around the year 2000, all juices must be processed to remove or inactivate harmful bacteria.

Medical Uses and/or Benefits

Antiscorbutic.   All citrus fruits are superb sources of vitamin C, the vitamin that prevents or cures scurvy, the vitamin C-deficiency disease.

Increased absorption of supplemental or dietary iron.   If you eat foods rich in vitamin C along with iron supplements or foods rich in iron, the vitamin C will enhance your body's ability to absorb the iron.

Wound healing.   Your body needs vitamin C in order to convert the amino acid proline into hydroxyproline, an essential ingredient in collagen, the protein needed to form skin, tendons, and bones. As a result people with scurvy do not heal quickly, a condition that can be remedied with vitamin C, which cures the scurvy and speeds healing. Whether taking extra vitamin C speeds healing in healthy people remains to be proved.

Possible inhibition of virus that causes chronic hepatitis C infection.   In January 2008, researchers at Massachusetts General Hospital Center for Engineering in Medicine (Boston) published a report in the medical journal *Hepatology* detailing the effect of naringenin, a compound in grapefruit, on the behavior of hepatitis viruses in liver cells. In laboratory studies, naringenin appeared to inhibit the ability of the virus to multiply and/or pass out from the liver cells. To date, there are no studies detailing the effect of naringenin in human beings with hepatitis C.

Adverse Effects Associated with This Food

Contact dermatitis.   The essential oils in the peel of citrus fruits may cause skin irritation in sensitive people.

Food/Drug Interactions

Aspirin and other nonsteroidal anti-inflammatory drugs (NSAIDs) such as ibuprofen, naproxen and others.   Taking aspirin or NSAIDs with acidic foods such as grapefruit may intensify the drug's ability to irritate your stomach and cause gastric bleeding.

Antihistamines, anticoagulants, benzodiazepines (tranquilizers or sleep medications), calcium channel blockers (blood pressure medication), cyclosporine (immunosuppressant drug used in organ transplants), theophylline (asthma drug). Drinking grapefruit juice with a wide variety of drugs ranging from antihistamines to blood pressure medication appears to reduce the amount of the drug your body metabolizes and eliminates. The "grapefruit effect" was first identified among people taking the antihypertensive drugs felodipine (Plendil) and nifedipine (Adalat, Procardia). It is not yet known for certain exactly what the active substance in the juice is. One possibility, however, is bergamottin, a naturally occurring chemical in grapefruit juice known to inactivate cytochrome P450 3A4, a digestive enzyme needed to convert many drugs to water-soluble substances you can flush out of your body. Without an effective supply of cytochrome P450 3A4, the amount of a drug circulating in your body may rise to dangerous levels. Reported side effects include lower blood pressure, increased heart rate, headache, flushing, and lightheadedness.

Some Drugs Known to Interact with Grapefruit Juice*

Drug Class	Generic (Brand name)
Antianxiety drug	Diazepam (Valium)
Antiarrhythmics	Amiodarone (Cordarone)
Blood-pressure drugs	Felodipine (Plendil), nicardipine (Cardene), nimodipine (Nimotop), nisoldipine (Sular), verapamil (Verelan)
Cholesterol-lowering drugs	Atorvastatin (Lipitor), lovastatin (Mevacor), simvastatin (Zocor), simvastatin/ezetimibe (Vytorin)
Immune Suppressants	Cyclosporine (Neoral), tacrolimus (Prograf)
Impotence Drug	Sildenafil (Viagra)
Pain Medication	Methadone (Dolophine, Methadose)

* This list may grow as new research appears.

Grapes

See also Raisins, Wine.

Nutritional Profile

Energy value (calories per serving): *Moderate*
Protein: *Low*
Fat: *Low*
Saturated fat: *Low*
Cholesterol: *None*
Carbohydrates: *High*
Fiber: *Low*
Sodium: *Low*
Major vitamin contribution: *Vitamin A, vitamin C*
Major mineral contribution: *Phosphorus*

About the Nutrients in This Food

Grapes are high in natural sugars, but even with the skin on they have less than one gram dietary fiber per serving. The most important nutrient in grapes is vitamin C. A serving of 10 green or red Thompson seedless grapes has 5.3 mg vitamin C (7 percent of the RDA for a woman, 6 percent of the RDA for a man).

The tart, almost sour flavor of unripened grapes comes from naturally occurring malic acid. As grapes ripen, their malic acid content declines while their sugar content rises. Ripe eating grapes are always sweet, but they have no stored starches to convert to sugars so they won't get sweeter after they are picked.

The Most Nutritious Way to Serve This Food

Fresh and ripe.

Diets That May Restrict or Exclude This Food

* * *

Buying This Food

Look for: Plump, well-colored grapes that are firmly attached to green stems that bend easily and snap back when you let them go. Green grapes should have a slightly yellow tint or a pink blush; red grapes should be deep, dark red or purple.

Avoid: Mushy grapes, grapes with wrinkled skin, and grapes that feel sticky. They are all past their prime. So are grapes whose stems are dry and brittle.

Characteristics of Different Varieties of Grapes

Red grapes

Cardinal	Large, dark red, available March–August
Emperor	Large red with seeds. September–March
Flame	Seedless, medium to large, red. June–August
Ribier	Large, blue-black, with seeds. July–February
Tokay	Large, bright red, seeds. August–November
Queen	Large, bright to dark red, seeds. June–August

White grapes

Almeria	Large, golden. August–October
Calmeria	Longish, light green. October–February
Perlette	Green, seedless, compact clusters. May–July
Thompson	Seedless, green to light gold. June–November

Source: *The Fresh Approach to Grapes* (United Fruit & Vegetable Association, n.d.).

Storing This Food

Wrap grapes in a plastic bag and store them in the refrigerator. Do not wash grapes until you are ready to use them.

Preparing This Food

To serve fresh grapes, rinse them under running water to remove debris, then drain the grapes and pick off stems and leaves.

To peel grapes (for salads), choose Catawba, Concord, Delaware, Niagara, or Scuppernong, the American varieties known as "slipskin" because the skin comes off easily. The European varieties (emperor, flame, Tokay, Muscat, Thompson) are more of a challenge. To peel them, put the grapes into a colander and submerge it in boiling water for a few seconds, then rinse or plunge them into cold water. The hot water makes cells in the grape's flesh swell, stretching the skin; the cold bath makes the cells shrink back from the skin which should now come off easily.

What Happens When You Cook This Food

See above.

How Other Kinds of Processing Affect This Food

Juice. Red grapes are colored with anthocyanin pigments that turn deeper red in acids and blue, purple, or yellowish in basic (alkaline) solutions. As a result, red grape juice will turn brighter red if you mix it with lemon or orange juice. Since metals (which are basic) would also change the color of the juice, the inside of grape juice cans is coated with plastic or enamel to keep the juice from touching the metal. Since 2000, following several deaths attributed to unpasteurized apple juice contaminated with *E. coli* O157:H7, the FDA has required that all juices sold in the United States be pasteurized to inactivate harmful organisms such as bacteria and mold.

Wine-making. Grapes are an ideal fruit for wine-making. They have enough sugar to produce a product that is 10 percent alcohol and are acidic enough to keep unwanted micro-organisms from growing during fermentation. Some wines retain some of the nutrients originally present in the grapes from which they are made. (See WINE.)

Drying. See RAISINS.

Medical Uses and/or Benefits

Lower risk of cardiovascular disease, diabetes, and some forms of cancer. Grape skin, pulp, and seed contain resveratrol, one of a group of plant chemicals credited with lowering cholesterol and thus reducing the risk of heart attack by preventing molecular fragments called free radicals from linking together to form compounds that damage body cells, leading to blocked arteries (heart disease), glucose-damaged blood vessels (diabetes), and unregulated cell growth (cancer).

The juice from purple grapes has more resveratrol than the juice from red grapes, which has more resveratrol than the juice from white grapes. More specifically, in 1998, a team of food scientists from the USDA Agricultural Research Service identified a native American grape, the muscadine, commonly used to make grape juice in the United States, as an unusually potent source of resveratrol.

Adverse Effects Associated with This Food

* * *

Food/Drug Interactions

* * *

Green Beans

(Snap beans, string beans, wax beans)

Nutritional Profile

Energy value (calories per serving): *Low*
Protein: *Moderate*
Fat: *Low*
Saturated fat: *Low*
Cholesterol: *None*
Carbohydrates: *High*
Fiber: *High*
Sodium: *Low*
Major vitamin contribution: *Vitamin A, vitamin C*
Major mineral contribution: *Iron, potassium*

About the Nutrients in This Food

Green beans and wax beans are high in dietary fiber, a moderate source of vitamin A derived from deep yellow carotenes, hidden by their green chlorophyll. Wax beans have very little vitamin A because their color comes from carotenes with little or no vitamin A activity. They have some vitamin C.

One-half cup cooked green beans has two grams dietary fiber, 437 IU vitamin A (18 percent of the RDA for a woman, 15 percent of the RDA for a man), and 6 mg vitamin C (8 percent of the RDA for a woman, 7 percent of the RDA for a man).

The Most Nutritious Way to Serve This Food

Raw, microwaved, or steamed just to the crisp-tender stage, to preserve their vitamin C.

Diets That May Restrict or Exclude This Food

* * *

Buying This Food

Look for: Firm, crisp beans with clean, well-colored green or yellow skin.

Avoid: Withered or dry beans; they have been exposed to air, heat, or sunlight and are low in vitamin A.

Storing This Food

Wrap green beans and wax beans in a plastic bag and store them in the refrigerator to protect their vitamins and keep them from drying out.

Preparing This Food

Green beans were once better known as string beans because of the "string" running down the back of the bean. Today, that string has been bred out of most green beans, but you may still find it in wax beans and in *haricots verts,* the true French green beans.

To prepare green beans and wax beans, wash them under cool running water, pick off odd leaves or stems, snip off the ends, pull the string off wax beans or *haricots verts,* and slice or sliver the beans.

What Happens When You Cook This Food

Cooking reduces the amount of vitamin C in green beans and wax beans but does not affect the vitamin A, which is insoluble in water and stable at normal cooking temperatures.

Green beans will change color when you cook them. Chlorophyll, the pigment that makes green vegetables green, is sensitive to acids. When you heat green beans, the chlorophyll in the beans will react chemically with acids in the vegetable or in the cooking water, forming pheophytin, which is brown. The pheophytin makes the beans look olive-drab.

To keep green beans green, you have to keep the chlorophyll from reacting with acids. One way to do this is to cook the beans in a large quantity of water (which will dilute the acids), but this increases the loss of vitamin C. A second alternative is to leave the lid off the pot so that the volatile acids can float off into the air. The best way may be to steam or microwave the green beans very quickly in very little water so that they hold onto their vitamin C and cook so fast that there is no time for the chlorophyll to react with the acids.

How Other Kinds of Processing Affect This Food

Canning and freezing. Commercially frozen green beans and wax beans have virtually the same nutritional value as fresh beans. Canned beans, however, usually have added salt that turns the naturally low-sodium beans into a high-sodium food. Canned green beans and wax beans have less vitamin C than fresh beans.

Medical Uses and/or Benefits

* * *

Adverse Effects Associated with This Food

* * *

Food/Drug Interactions

* * *

Greens

(Beet greens, broccoli rabe, chard [Swiss chard], collard greens, dandelion greens, kale, mustard greens, turnip greens, watercress)

See also Cabbage, Lettuce, Spinach, Turnips.

Nutritional Profile

Energy value (calories per serving): *Low*
Protein: *High*
Fat: *Low*
Saturated fat: *Low*
Cholesterol: *None*
Carbohydrates: *Moderate*
Fiber: *Moderate to high*
Sodium: *Moderate to high*
Major vitamin contribution: *Vitamin A, folate, vitamin C*
Major mineral contribution: *Calcium, iron*

About the Nutrients in This Food

Greens are the edible leafy tops of some common vegetable plants. They have moderate to high amounts of dietary fiber (one to two grams per cup of cooked greens), the insoluble cellulose and lignin in the leaf structure. Greens are also an excellent source of vitamin A, derived from deep yellow carotene pigments (including beta-carotene) hidden under their green chlorophyll, the B vitamin folate, and vitamin C.

One-half cup cooked frozen turnip greens has 2.7 g dietary fiber, 7,406 IU vitamin A (347 percent of the RDA for a woman, 250 percent of the RDA for a man), 28 mcg folate (7 percent of the RDA), 15.7 mg vitamin C (21 percent of the RDA for a woman, 17 percent of the RDA for a man), and 1.5 g iron (8 percent of the RDA for a woman, 20 percent of the RDA for a man).

The Most Nutritious Way to Serve This Food

With an iron-rich food or a food rich in vitamin C, to increase the absorption of iron.

Diets That May Restrict or Exclude This Food

Low-oxalate diet (to prevent the formation of kidney stones caused by calcium oxalate)
Low-sodium diet

Buying This Food

Look for: Fresh, crisp, clean, cold, dark green leaves. Refrigeration helps preserve vitamins A and C.

Avoid: Yellowed, blackened, wilted, or warm greens, all of which are lower in vitamins A and C.

What to Look for in Specific Greens

Broccoli rabe: Choose small, firm stalks, with very few buds and no open flowers.
Collard greens: Choose smooth, green, firm leaves.
Dandelion: Choose plants with large leaves and very thin stems but no flowers
  (flowering dandelions have tough, bitter leaves).
Kale: Choose small, deeply colored, moist leaves.
Mustard greens: Choose small, firm, tender leaves.
Swiss chard: Choose chard with crisp stalks and firm, brightly colored leaves. Chard
  is very perishable; limp stalks are past their prime.
Turnip greens: Choose small, firm, bright leaves.
Watercress: Choose crisp, bright green leaves.

Storing This Food

Refrigerate all greens, wrapped in plastic to keep them from losing moisture and vitamins. Before you store the greens, rinse them well under cool running water and discard any bruised or damaged leaves (which would continue to deteriorate even when chilled).

Preparing This Food

Rewash the greens under cool running water to flush off all sand, dirt, debris, and hidden insects.

　　If you plan to use the greens in a salad, pat them dry before you mix them with salad dressing; oil-based salad dressings will not cling to wet greens.

　　Do not tear or cut the greens until you are ready to use them; when you tear greens you damage cells, releasing ascorbic acid oxidase, an enzyme that destroys vitamin C.

What Happens When You Cook This Food

Chlorophyll, the pigment that makes green vegetables green, is sensitive to acids. When you heat greens, the chlorophyll in the leaves reacts chemically with acids in the greens or in the cooking water, forming pheophytin, which is brown. Together, the pheophytin and the yellow carotenes in dark green leaves give the cooked greens a bronze hue. Greens with few carotenes will look olive-drab.

To keep the cooked greens from turning bronze or olive, you have to prevent the chlorophyll from reacting with acids. One way to do this is to cook the greens in a large amount of water (which will dilute the acids), but this increases the loss of vitamin C. A second alternative is to leave the lid off the pot so that the volatile acids can float off into the air. The best way probably is to steam the greens in very little water, or, as researchers at Cornell University suggest, to microwave two cups of greens with about three tablespoons of water in a microwave safe plastic bag left open at the top so that steam can escape. These methods preserve vitamin C and cook the greens so fast that there is no time for the chlorophyll/acid reaction to occur.

How Other Kinds of Processing Affect This Food

Freezing. Cooked frozen greens have more fiber and vitamin A than cooked fresh greens because, ounce for ounce, they have less water and more leaf solids.

Medical Uses and/or Benefits

Lower risk of some birth defects. As many as two of every 1,000 babies born in the United States each year may have cleft palate or a neural tube (spiral cord) defect due to their mothers' not having gotten adequate amounts of folate during pregnancy. The current RDA for folate is 180 mcg for a woman and 200 mcg for a man, but the FDA now recommends 400 mcg for a woman who is or may become pregnant. Taking folate supplements before becoming pregnant and continuing through the first two months of pregnancy reduces the risk of cleft palate; taking folate through the entire pregnancy reduces the risk of neural tube defects.

Vision protection. Dark greens are a rich source of the yellow-orange carotenoid pigments lutein and zeaxanthin. Both carotenoids appear to play a role in protecting the eyes from damaging ultraviolet light, thus reducing the risk of cataracts and age-related macular degeneration, which is a leading cause of vision loss in one-third of all Americans older than 75.

Possible lower risk of heart attack. In the spring of 1998, an analysis of data from the records for more than 80,000 women enrolled in the long-running Nurses' Health Study at Harvard School of Public Health/Brigham and Women's Hospital, in Boston, demonstrated that a diet providing more than 400 mcg folate and 3 mg vitamin B$_6$ daily, either from food or supplements, might reduce a woman's risk of heart attack by almost 50 percent. Although men were not included in the study, the results were assumed to apply to them as well.

However, data from a meta-analysis published in the *Journal of the American Medical Association* in December 2006 called this theory into question. Researchers at Tulane University examined the results of 12 controlled studies in which 16,958 patients with preexisting cardiovascular disease were given either folic acid supplements or placebos ("look-alike" pills with no folic acid) for at least six months. The scientists, who found no reduction in the risk of further heart disease or overall death rates among those taking folic acid, concluded that further studies will be required to ascertain whether taking folic acid supplements reduces the risk of cardiovascular disease.

Adverse Effects Associated with This Food

Food-borne illness. According to the Centers for Disease Control and Prevention, from 1996–2005 the proportion of incidents of food-borne disease linked to leafy greens increased by 60 percent. The highest proportion of these illnesses were due to contamination by norovirus (the organism often blamed for outbreaks of gastric illness on cruise ships), followed by salmonella and *E. coli*. The illnesses were commonly associated with eating raw greens; cooking the greens to a high heat inactivates the disease-causing organisms.

Nitrates. Like beets, celery, eggplant, lettuce, radishes, and spinach, greens contain nitrates that convert naturally into nitrites in your stomach and then react with the amino acids in proteins to form nitrosamines. Although some nitrosamines are known or suspected carcinogens, this natural chemical conversion presents no known problems for a healthy adult. However, when these nitrate-rich vegetables are cooked and left to stand at room temperature, bacterial enzyme action (and perhaps some enzymes in the plants) convert the nitrates to nitrites at a much faster rate than normal. These higher-nitrite foods may be hazardous for infants; several cases of "spinach poisoning" have been reported among children who ate cooked spinach that had been left standing at room temperature.

Food/Drug Interactions

Anticoagulants Greens are rich in vitamin K, the blood-clotting vitamin produced naturally by bacteria in the intestines. Consuming large quantities of this food may reduce the effectiveness of anticoagulants (blood thinners) such as warfarin (Coumadin). One cup of drained, boiled fresh kale, for example, contains 1,062 mcg vitamin K, nearly 200 times the RDA for a healthy adult.

Guavas

Nutritional Profile

Energy value (calories per serving): *Low*
Protein: *Low*
Fat: *Low*
Saturated fat: *Low*
Cholesterol: *None*
Carbohydrates: *High*
Fiber: *Very high*
Sodium: *Low*
Major vitamin contribution: *Vitamin A, vitamin C*
Major mineral contribution: *Potassium*

About the Nutrients in This Food

The guava is very high in dietary fiber (soluble pectins), a good source of vitamin A derived from deep yellow carotenes (including beta-carotene) and, depending on the variety, an extraordinary source of vitamin C.

One fresh two-ounce (55 g) guava has three grams dietary fiber, 343 IU vitamin A (15 percent of the RDA for a woman, 12 percent of the RDA for a man), and 126 mg vitamin C (168 percent of the RDA for a woman, 140 percent of the RDA for a man), and 229 mg potassium, twice as much as two ounces of fresh orange juice.

The Most Nutritious Way to Serve This Food

Fresh. Slice off the top and eat the guava out of its skin with a spoon.

Diets That May Restrict or Exclude This Food

Low-carbohydrate, low-fiber diet

Buying This Food

Look for: Ripe guavas. Depending on the variety, the color of the skin may vary from white to yellow to dark red and the size from that of a large walnut to that of an apple. A ripe guava will yield slightly when you press it with your fingertip.

Avoid: Guavas with cracked or broken skin.

Storing This Food

Refrigerate ripe guavas.

Preparing This Food

Wash the guava under cool running water, then slice it in half and remove the seeds. Never slice or peel the fruit until you are ready to use it. When you cut into the guava and damage its cells, you activate ascorbic acid oxidase, an enzyme that oxidizes and destroys vitamin C. The longer the enzyme is working, the more vitamin the fruit will lose.

What Happens When You Cook This Food

As the guava cooks, its pectins and gums dissolve and the fruit gets softer. Cooking also destroys some water-soluble, heat-sensitive vitamin C. You can keep the loss to a minimum by cooking the guava as quickly as possible in as little water as possible. Never cook guavas (or any other vitamin C-rich foods) in a copper or iron pot; contact with metal ions hastens the loss of vitamin C.

How Other Kinds of Processing Affect This Food

Canning. Canned guavas have less vitamin A and C and more sugar (syrup) than fresh guavas do, but their flavor and texture is similar to home-cooked fruit.

Medical Uses and/or Benefits

Lowering the risk of some cancers. According to the American Cancer Society, foods rich in beta-carotene may lower the risk of cancers of the larynx, esophagus and lungs. There is no such benefit from beta-carotene supplements; indeed, one controversial study actually showed a higher rate of lung cancer among smokers taking the supplement.

Protection against heart disease. Foods high in antioxidants such as vitamin C appear to reduce the risk of heart disease. In addition, foods high in pectins appear to lower the amount of cholesterol circulating in your blood, perhaps by forming a gel in your stomach that sops up fats and keeps them from being absorbed by your body.

Potassium benefits.   Because potassium is excreted in urine, potassium-rich foods are often recommended for people taking diuretics. In addition, a diet rich in potassium (from food) is associated with a lower risk of stroke. A 1998 Harvard School of Public Health analysis of data from the long-running Health Professionals Study shows 38 percent fewer strokes among men who ate nine servings of high potassium foods a day vs. those who ate less than four servings. Among men with high blood pressure, taking a daily 1,000 mg potassium supplement—about the amount of potassium in half a guava fruit—reduced the incidence of stroke by 60 percent.

Adverse Effects Associated with This Food

* * *

Food/Drug Interactions

* * *

Honey

See also Sugar.

Nutritional Profile

Energy value (calories per serving): *High*
Protein: *Trace*
Fat: *None*
Saturated fat: *None*
Cholesterol: *None*
Carbohydrates: *High*
Fiber: *None*
Sodium: *Low*
Major vitamin contribution: *B vitamins*
Major mineral contribution: *Iron, potassium*

About the Nutrients in This Food

Honey is the sweet, thick fluid produced when bees metabolize the sucrose in plant nectar. Enzymes in the honeybee's sac split the sucrose, which is a disaccharide (double sugar), into its constituent molecules, fructose and glucose. Honey is about 80 percent fructose and glucose and 17 percent water. The rest is dextrin (formed when starch molecules are split apart), a trace of protein and small amounts of iron, potassium, and B vitamins.

Recent studies at the University of Illinois (Urbana-Champaign) and Clemson University (South Carolina) show that honey is also a source of antioxidants, substances that prevent molecule fragments from hooking up with other fragments to produce compounds that damage body cells and may cause heart disease, cancer, memory loss, and other conditions associated with aging or damaged cells. One antioxidant, pinocembrin, is found only in honey. In general, honey's antioxidant activity is linked to its color. The darker the honey, the more potent it is as an antioxidant. Two exceptions: light sweet clover honey (high in antioxidants) and dark mesquite honey (low in antioxidants).

Diets That May Restrict or Exclude This Food

Low-carbohydrate diet
Low-sugar diet

Buying This Food

Look for: Tightly sealed jars of honey. All honeys are natural products. They may be dark or light (depending on the plant from which the bees drew their nectar). Raw, unprocessed honey is thick and cloudy. Commercial honey is clear because it has been filtered. It pours more easily than raw honey because it has been heated to make it less viscous as well as to destroy potentially harmful bacteria and yeasts that might spoil the honey by turning its sugars into alcohol and other undesirable products.

The following table lists some of the plants most commonly used to make honey in the United States.

Plant	Where it grows	Color of honey	Flavor of honey
Alfalfa	Utah, Nevada, Idaho, Oregon	White or light amber	Mild
Basswood	Alabama, Texas	White	Strong, sharp
Clover	Throughout U.S.	White to amber	Mild
Orange blossom	Arizona, California, Florida, Texas	Light amber	Orangey
Sage	California	White	Mild
Tulip poplar	Southern New England, Midwest	Dark amber	Medium
Tupelo tree	Florida, Georgia	White, light amber	Mild

Source: The National Honey Board

Storing This Food

Store opened jars of honey in the refrigerator, tightly closed to keep the honey from absorbing moisture or picking up microorganisms from the air. Ordinarily, bacteria do not proliferate in honey, which is an acid solution. However, if the honey absorbs extra water or if its sugars precipitate out of solution and crystallize, the sugar/water ratio that makes honey acid will be upset and the honey will become more hospitable to microorganisms. Refrigeration offers some protection because it chills the honey and slows the growth of bacteria or mold.

Preparing This Food

To measure honey easily, coat your measuring spoon or cup with vegetable oil: the honey will slide right out of the measure. To combine honey smoothly with dry ingredients, warm it with the liquids in the recipe first. And remember to reduce the liquid in a recipe when you substitute honey for sugar. For precise amounts, check the individual recipe.

What Happens When You Cook This Food

When honey is heated, the bonds between its molecules relax and the honey becomes more liquid. If you heat it too long, however, its moisture will evaporate, the honey will become more viscous, and its sugar will burn.

In baking, honey is useful because it is more hydrophilic (water-loving) than granulated sugar. It retains moisture longer while a cake or bread is baking, and it may even extract moisture from the air into the finished product. As a result, breads and cakes made with honey stay moist longer than those made with sugar.

Honey also appears to enhance the Maillard reaction, a heat-triggered transformation of sugars that turns toast brown, caramelizes custards, and crisps the surface of meats. The Maillard reaction creates antioxidants that slow down fat's natural oxidation (rancidity). As a result, adding honey to meat dishes appears to slow the development of the characteristic warmed-over flavor associated with cooked meat that is refrigerated and then reheated. In studies at Clemson University, after two days in the refrigerator, cooked turkey roll composed of turkey pieces plus honey (15 percent by weight) showed 85 percent less fat oxidation than turkey roll made without honey.

How Other Kinds of Processing Affect This Food

* * *

Medical Uses and/or Benefits

Antioxidant activity.   Honey is rich in naturally occurring antioxidants such as the pigment beta-carotene (a precursor of vitamin A) and pinocembrin (found only in honey) that prevent molecule fragments from linking up to form compounds that damage body cells. As a rule, the darker the honey, the more potent it is as an antioxidant. Two exceptions: Light, sweet clover honey is high in antioxidants and dark mesquite honey is low.

The antibacterial activity of antioxidants may be at least partly responsible for honey's age-old reputation as a wound healer. Greek and Roman generals used it as first aid; modern medicine points to several hundred controlled studies showing that animal and human wounds heal faster, cleaner, and less painfully when dressed with sterile, medical grade honey.

Soothing dressing.   Like other sugars, honey is a demulcent, a substance that coats and soothes irritated mucous membranes. For example, warm tea with honey is often used to soothe a sore throat.

Adverse Effects Associated with This Food

Infant botulism.   *Clostridium botulinum,* the organism that produces toxins that cause *botulinum* poisoning, does not grow in the intestines of an adult or an older child. Botulism poisoning in adults and older children is caused by toxins produced when the *botulinum* spores, which are anerobic (require an airless environment), germinate in an oxygen-starved place like a sealed can of food. However, *botulinum* spores do grow in an infant's digestive tract, and infants have been poisoned by foods that have spores but no toxins. Since honey is sometimes contaminated with the *botulinum* spores, the Centers for Disease Control and the American Academy of Pediatrics recommend against feeding honey to any child younger than 12 months.

Tooth decay.   Like all sugars, honey is used by bacteria in your mouth to make tooth-eating acids.

Wild honey poisoning.   Like wild greens or wild mushrooms, wild honeys may be toxic and are best avoided in favor of the commercial product.

Food/Drug Interactions

* * *

Kiwi Fruit

(Chinese gooseberry)

Nutritional Profile

Energy value (calories per serving): *Low*
Protein: *Moderate*
Fat: *Low*
Saturated fat: *Low*
Cholesterol: *None*
Carbohydrates: *High*
Fiber: *High*
Sodium: *Low*
Major vitamin contribution: *Vitamin C*
Major mineral contribution: *Potassium*

About the Nutrients in This Food

The kiwi fruit is a high carbohydrate food, a good source of soluble dietary fiber (pectins), and an excellent source of vitamin C.

One raw, peeled three-ounce (76 g) kiwi fruit has 2.3 g dietary fiber, 71 mg vitamin C (95 percent of the RDA for a woman, 79 percent of the RDA for a man) and 237 mg potassium, 127 percent as much as three ounces of fresh orange juice.

The Most Nutritious Way to Serve This Food

Fresh sliced.

Diets That May Restrict or Exclude This Food

* * *

Buying This Food

Look for: Fruit with firm, unblemished skin. Ripe kiwi fruit is soft to the touch; those sold in American markets generally need to be ripened before eating.

Storing This Food

Set unripe kiwi fruit aside to ripen at room temperature, preferably in a brown paper bag. Do not store the fruit in a plastic bag; moisture collecting inside the plastic bag will rot the fruit before it has a chance to ripen. Refrigerate ripe kiwi fruit.

Preparing This Food

Peel and slice the fruit. Because kiwi fruits are very acidic, you can slice them in advance without fear of having the flesh turn dark.

What Happens When You Cook This Food

* * *

How Other Kinds of Processing Affect This Food

* * *

Medical Uses and/or Benefits

Antiscorbutic.   Foods high in vitamin C cure or prevent the vitamin C deficiency disease scurvy, whose symptoms include slow healing of wounds, bleeding gums, and bruising.

Protection against heart disease.   Foods high in antioxidants such as vitamin C appear to reduce the risk of heart disease. In addition, foods high in pectins appear to lower the amount of cholesterol circulating in your blood, perhaps by forming a gel in your stomach that sops up fats and keeps them from being absorbed by your body.

Enhanced absorption of iron from plant foods.   Nonheme iron, the form of iron in plant foods, is poorly absorbed because natural chemicals in the plants bind it into insoluble compounds. Vitamin C makes this iron easier to absorb, perhaps by converting it to ferrous iron.

Adverse Effects Associated with This Food

Latex-fruit syndrome.   Latex is a milky fluid obtained from the rubber tree and used to make medical and surgical products such as condoms and protective latex gloves, as well as rubber bands, balloons, and toys; elastic used in clothing; pacifiers and baby-bottle nipples; chewing gum; and various adhesives. Some of the proteins in latex are allergenic, known to cause reactions ranging from mild to potentially life-threatening. Some of the proteins found naturally in latex also occur naturally in foods from plants such as avocados, bananas, chestnuts, kiwi fruit, tomatoes, and food and diet sodas sweetened with aspartame. Persons sensitive to these foods are likely to be sensitive to latex as well. NOTE: The National Institute of Health Sciences, in Japan, also lists the following foods as suspect: Almonds, apples, apricots, bamboo shoots, bell peppers, buckwheat, cantaloupe, carrots, celery, cherries, coconut, figs, grapefruit, lettuce, loquat, mangoes, mushrooms, mustard, nectarines, oranges, passion fruit, papaya, peaches, peanuts, peppermint, pineapples, potatoes, soybeans, strawberries, walnuts, and watermelon.

Food/Drug Interactions

* * *

Kohlrabi

Nutritional Profile

Energy value (calories per serving): *Low*
Protein: *High*
Fat: *Low*
Saturated fat: *Low*
Cholesterol: *None*
Carbohydrates: *High*
Fiber: *High*
Sodium: *Low*
Major vitamin contribution: *B vitamins, vitamin C*
Major mineral contribution: *Calcium, iron, phosphorus*

About the Nutrients in This Food

Kohlrabi ("cabbage-turnip") is a cruciferous vegetable, a thick bulb-like stem belonging to the cabbage family. It is high in dietary fiber, especially the insoluble cellulose and lignin found in stems, leaves, roots, seeds and peel. Kohlrabi is an excellent source of vitamin C and potassium, with small amounts of iron.

One-half cup cooked, sliced Kohlrabi has 0.9 g dietary fiber, 45 mg vitamin C (60 percent of the RDA for a woman, 50 percent of the RDA for a man), and 0.3 mg iron (2 percent of the RDA for a woman, 4 percent of the RDA for a man).

The Most Nutritious Way to Serve This Food

Steamed just until tender, to protect the vitamin C.

Diets That May Restrict or Exclude This Food

Antiflatulence diet
Low-fiber, low-residue diet

Buying This Food

Look for: Small vegetables with fresh-looking green leaves on top.

Avoid: Very mature kohlrabi. The older the stem, the more cellulose and lignin it contains. Very old kohlrabi may have so much fiber that it is inedible.

Storing This Food

Cut off the green tops. Then, store kohlrabi in a cold, humid place (a root cellar or the refrigerator) to keep it from drying out.

Save and refrigerate the kohlrabi's green leaves. They can be cooked and eaten like spinach.

When You Are Ready to Cook This Food

Wash the kohlrabi under running water, using a vegetable brush to remove dirt and debris. Then peel the root and slice or quarter it for cooking.

What Happens When You Cook This Food

Cooking softens kohlrabi by dissolving its soluble food fibers. Like other cruciferous vegetables, kohlrabi contains natural sulfur compounds that break down into a variety of smelly chemicals (including hydrogen sulfide and ammonia) when the vegetables are heated. Kohlrabi is nowhere near as smelly as some of the other crucifers, but this production of smelly compounds is intensified by long cooking or by cooking the vegetable in an aluminum pot. Adding a slice of bread to the cooking water may lessen the odor; keeping a lid on the pot will stop the smelly molecules from floating off into the air.

How Other Kinds of Processing Affect This Food

* * *

Medical Uses and/or Benefits

Protection against certain cancers. Naturally occurring chemicals (indoles, isothiocyanates, glucosinolates, dithiolethiones, and phenols) in kohlrabi, cauliflower, Brussels sprouts, broccoli, cabbage, and other cruciferous vegetables appear to reduce the risk of some cancers, perhaps by preventing the formation of carcinogens in your body or by blocking cancer-causing substances from reaching or reacting with sensitive body tissues or by inhibiting the transformation of healthy cells to malignant ones.

All cruciferous vegetables contain sulforaphane, a member of a family of chemicals known as isothiocyanates. In experiments with laboratory rats, sulforaphane appears to increase the body's production of phase-2 enzymes, naturally occurring substances that inactivate and help eliminate carcinogens. At the Johns Hopkins University in Baltimore, Maryland, 69 percent of the rats injected with a chemical known to cause mammary cancer developed tumors vs. only 26 percent of the rats given the carcinogenic chemical plus sulforaphane.

In 1997, Johns Hopkins researchers discovered that broccoli seeds and three-day-old broccoli sprouts contain a compound converted to sulforaphane when the seed and sprout cells are crushed. Five grams of three-day-old broccoli sprouts contain as much sulforaphane as 150 grams of mature broccoli. The sulforaphane levels in other cruciferous vegetables have not yet been calculated.

Adverse Effects Associated with This Food

Enlarged thyroid gland (goiter).   Cruciferous vegetables, including kohlrabi, contain goitrin, thiocyanate, and isothiocyanate. These chemicals, known collectively as goitrogens, inhibit the formation of thyroid hormones and cause the thyroid to enlarge in an attempt to produce more. Goitrogens are not hazardous for healthy people who eat moderate amounts of cruciferous vegetables, but they may pose problems for people who have a thyroid condition or are taking thyroid medication.

Food/Drug Interactions

* * *

Lamb

(Chevon [goat meat], mutton)

Nutritional Profile*

Energy value (calories per serving): *Moderate*
Protein: *High*
Fat: *Moderate*
Saturated fat: *High*
Cholesterol: *Moderate to high*
Carbohydrates: *None*
Fiber: *None*
Sodium: *Moderate*
Major vitamin contribution: *B vitamins*
Major mineral contribution: *Iron*

About the Nutrients in This Food

Like other foods from animals, lamb is a good source of high-quality proteins with sufficient amounts of all the essential amino acids. Like other meats, it is high in fat, saturated fat, and cholesterol, an excellent source of B vitamins plus heme iron, the form of iron most easily absorbed by the body.

One three-ounce serving of roasted domestic (U.S.) lean leg of lamb has 10.6 g fat (4.3 g saturated fat, 4.65 g monounsaturated fat, 0.7 g polyunsaturated fat), 76 mg cholesterol, 1.7 mg iron (9 percent of the RDA for a woman, 21 percent of the RDA for a man), and 4 mg zinc (5 percent of the RDA for a woman, 3.6 percent of the RDA for a man).

One three-ounce serving of roasted frozen imported New Zealand leg of lamb has 11.9 g fat (5.7 g saturated fat, 4.5 g monounsaturated fat, 0.6 g polyunsaturated fat), 86 mg cholesterol, 1.8 mg iron (10 percent of the RDA for a woman, 23 percent of the RDA for a man), and 3.1 mg zinc (39 percent of the RDA for a woman, 28 percent of the RDA for a man).

The Most Nutritious Way to Serve This Food

Broiled or roasted, to allow the fat to melt and run off the meat. Soups and stews that contain lamb should be skimmed.

---

* Values are for lean roasted lamb.

With tomatoes, potatoes, and other foods rich in vitamin C to increase your body's absorption of iron from the meat.

Diets That May Restrict or Exclude This Food

Controlled fat, low-cholesterol diet
Low-protein diet (for some forms of kidney disease)

Buying This Food

Look for: Lamb that is pink to light red, with a smooth, firm texture and little fat. The color of the fat, which may vary with the breed and what the animal was fed, is not a reliable guide to quality. Meat labeled *baby lamb* or *spring lamb* comes from animals less than five months old; *lamb* comes from an animal less than a year old; *mutton* comes from an animal older than a year. The older the animal, the tougher and more sinewy the meat.

Storing This Food

Refrigerate fresh lamb immediately, carefully wrapped to prevent its drippings from contaminating other foods. Refrigeration prolongs freshness by slowing the natural multiplication of bacteria on the surface of the meat. Left on their own, these bacteria convert proteins and other substances on the surface of the meat to a slimy film and change the meat's sulfur-containing amino acids methionine and cystine into smelly chemicals called mercaptans. When the mercaptans combine with pigments in meat, they produce the greenish pigment that gives spoiled meat its characteristic unpleasant appearance.

Preparing This Food

Trim the meat carefully. By judiciously cutting away all visible fat, you can significantly reduce the amount of fat and cholesterol in each serving. Lamb and mutton are covered with a thin paperlike white membrane called a "fell." Generally, the fell is left on roasts because it acts as a natural basting envelope that makes the lamb juicier.

Do not salt lamb before you cook it; the salt will draw moisture out of the meat, making it stringy and less tender. Add salt when the meat is nearly done.

When you are done, clean all utensils thoroughly with soap and hot water. Wash your cutting board, wood or plastic, with hot water, soap, and a bleach-and-water solution. For ultimate safety in preventing the transfer of microorganisms from the meat to other foods, keep one cutting board exclusively for raw meat, fish, or poultry, and a second one for everything else. Don't forget to wash your hands.

What Happens When You Cook This Food

Cooking changes the lamb's flavor and appearance, lowers its fat and cholesterol content, and makes it safer by killing the bacteria that live naturally on the surface of raw meat.

Browning lamb before you cook it won't seal in the juices, but it will change the flavor by caramelizing proteins and sugars on the surface of the meat. Because the only sugars in lamb are the small amounts of glycogen in its muscles, we often add sugar in the form of marinades or basting liquids that may also contain acids (lemon juice, vinegar, wine, yogurt) to break down muscle fibers and tenderize the meat. (Note that browning has one minor nutritional drawback. It breaks amino acids on the surface of the meat into smaller compounds that are no longer useful proteins.)

When lamb is heated, it loses water and shrinks. Its pigments, which combine with oxygen, are denatured by the heat. They break into smaller fragments and turn brown, the natural color of well-done meat. The pigments also release iron, which accelerates the oxidation of the lamb's fat. Oxidized fat is what gives cooked meat its characteristic warmed-over flavor. Cooking and storing meat under a blanket of antioxidants—catsup or a gravy made of tomatoes, peppers, and other vitamin C-rich vegetables—reduces the oxidation of fats and the intensity of warmed-over flavor. So will reheating the meat in a microwave rather than a conventional oven.

How Other Kinds of Processing Affect This Food

Canning. Canned lamb does not develop a warmed-over flavor because the high temperatures used in canning food and alter the structure of the proteins in the meat so that the proteins act as antioxidants. Once the can is open, however, lamb fat may begin to oxidize again.

Freezing. Defrosted frozen lamb may be less tender than fresh lamb. It may also be lower in B vitamins. When you freeze lamb, the water inside its cells freezes into sharp ice crystals that can puncture cell membranes. When the lamb thaws, moisture (and some of the B vitamins) will leak out through these torn cell walls. Freezing may also cause freezer burn—dry spots left when moisture evaporates from the lamb's surface. Waxed freezer paper is designed specifically to protect the moisture in meat; plastic wrap and aluminum foil may be less effective.

Medical Uses and/or Benefits

Treating and/or preventing iron deficiency. Without meat it is virtually impossible for a woman of childbearing age to get the 18 mg iron/day she requires unless she takes an iron supplement.

Adverse Effects Associated with This Food

Increased risk of cardiovascular disease. Like other foods from animals, lamb is a significant source of cholesterol and saturated fats, which increase the amount of cholesterol circulating in your blood and raise your risk of heart disease. To reduce the risk of heart disease, the National Cholesterol Education Project recommends following the Step I and Step II diets.

The Step I diet provides no more than 30 percent of total daily calories from fat, no more than 10 percent of total daily calories from saturated fat, and no more than 300 mg of cholesterol per day. It is designed for healthy people whose cholesterol is in the range of 200–239 mg/dL.

The Step II diet provides 25–35 percent of total calories from fat, less than 7 percent of total calories from saturated fat, up to 10 percent of total calories from polyunsaturated fat, up to 20 percent of total calories from monounsaturated fat, and less than 300 mg cholesterol per day. This stricter regimen is designed for people who have one or more of the following conditions:

◆ Existing cardiovascular disease
◆ High levels of low-density lipoproteins (LDLs, or "bad" cholesterol) or low levels of high-density lipoproteins (HDLs, or "good" cholesterol)
◆ Obesity
◆ Type 1 diabetes (insulin-dependent diabetes, or diabetes mellitus)
◆ Metabolic syndrome, a.k.a. insulin resistance syndrome, a cluster of risk factors that includes type 2 diabetes (non-insulin-dependent diabetes)

Increased risk of some cancer.   According to the American Institute for Cancer Research, a diet high in red meat (beef, lamb, pork) increases the risk of developing colorectal cancer by 15 percent for every 1.5 ounces over 18 ounces consumed per week. In 2007, the National Cancer Institute released data from a survey of 500,000 people, ages 50 to 71, who participated in an eight-year AARP diet and health study identifying a higher risk of developing cancer of the esophagus, liver, lung, and pancreas among people eating large amounts of red meats and processed meats.

Decline in kidney function.   Proteins are nitrogen compounds. When metabolized, they yield ammonia that is excreted through the kidneys. In laboratory animals, a sustained high-protein diet increases the flow of blood through the kidneys, accelerating the natural age-related decline in kidney function. Some experts suggest that this may also occur in human beings.

Food/Drug Interactions

False-positive test for occult blood in the stool.   The active ingredient in the test for hidden blood in the stool is alphaguaiaconic acid, a chemical that turns blue in the presence of blood. Because the test may react to blood in meat you have eaten, producing a positive result when you do not really have any gastrointestinal bleeding, lamb and other meats are excluded from your diet for three days before this test.

Lemons

(Limes)

Nutritional Profile

Energy value (calories per serving): *Low*
Protein: *Moderate*
Fat: *Low*
Saturated fat: *Low*
Cholesterol: *None*
Carbohydrates: *High*
Fiber: *Low*
Sodium: *Low*
Major vitamin contribution: *Vitamin C*
Major mineral contribution: *Potassium*

About the Nutrients in This Food

Lemons and limes have very little sugar, no fat, and only a trace of protein, but they are high in vitamin C. One ounce fresh lemon juice has 14 mg vitamin C (19 percent of the RDA for a woman, 16 percent of the RDA for a man). One tablespoon fresh lemon juice has 7 mg vitamin C (9 percent of the RDA for a woman, 8 percent of the RDA for a man). One eight-gram lemon wedge has 2.7 mg vitamin C (4 percent of the RDA for a woman, 3 percent of the RDA for a man). One tablespoon grated lemon peel has 7.7 mg vitamin C (10 percent of the RDA for a woman, 9 percent of the RDA for a man). One ounce fresh lime juice has 9.2 mg vitamin C (12 percent of the RDA for a woman, 10 percent of the RDA for a man).

The Most Nutritious Way to Serve This Food

Fresh squeezed, in a fruit-juice drink. Fresh juice has the most vitamin C. Fruit-juice drinks (lemonade, limeade) are the only foods that use enough lemon or lime juice to give us a useful quantity of vitamin C.

Diets That May Restrict or Exclude This Food

* * *

Buying This Food

Look for: Firm lemons and limes that are heavy for their size. The heavier the fruit, the juicier it will be. The skin should be thin, smooth, and fine grained—shiny yellow for a lemon, shiny green for a lime. Deeply colored lemons and limes have a better flavor than pale ones. All lemons are egg-shaped, but the Key lime (which is the true lime) is small and round. Egg-shaped limes are hybrids.

Storing This Food

Refrigerate fresh lemons and limes. The lemons will stay fresh for a month, the limes for up to eight weeks. Sliced lemons and limes are vulnerable to oxygen, which can destroy their flavor and their vitamin C. Wrap them tightly in plastic, store them in the refrigerator, and use them as quickly as possible.

Preparing This Food

The skin of the lemon and lime are rich in essential oils that are liberated when you cut into the peel and tear open its cells. To get the flavoring oil out of the peel, grate the top, colored part of the rind (the white membrane underneath is bitter) and wrap it in cheesecloth. Then wring out the oil onto some granulated sugar, stir thoroughly, and use the flavored sugar in baking or for making drinks. You can freeze lemon and lime peel or zest (grated peel), but it will lose some flavor while frozen.

Lemons and limes are often waxed to protect them from moisture loss enroute to the store. Before you peel or grate the fruit, scrub it with a vegetable brush to remove the wax.

What Happens When You Cook This Food

Heating citrus fruits and juices reduces their supply of vitamin C, which is heat-sensitive.

How Other Kinds of Processing Affect This Food

Juice.   Since 2000, following several deaths attributed to unpasteurized apple juice contaminated with *E. coli* O157:H7, the FDA has required that all juices sold in the United States be pasteurized to inactivate harmful organisms such as bacteria and mold.

"Lemonade."   The suffix "ade" signifies that this product is not 100 percent juice and does not deliver the amounts of nutrients found in juice. NOTE: Commercial "pink lemonade" is plain lemonade colored with grape juice.

Medical Uses and/or Benefits

Antiscorbutic. Lemons and limes, which are small and travel well, were carried on board British navy ships in the 18th century to prevent scurvy, the vitamin C-deficiency disease.

Wound healing. Your body needs vitamin C in order to convert the amino acid proline into hydroxyproline, an essential ingredient in collagen—the protein needed to form skin, tendons, and bones. As a result, people with scurvy do not heal quickly, a condition that can be remedied with vitamin C, which cures the scurvy and speeds healing. Whether taking extra vitamin C speeds healing in healthy people remains to be proved.

Adverse Effects Associated with This Food

Contact dermatitis. The peel of lemon and lime contains limonene, an essential oil known to cause contact dermatitis in sensitive individuals. (Limonene is also found in dill, caraway seeds, and celery.)

Photosensitivity. Lime peel contains furocoumarins (psoralens), chemicals that are photosensitizers as well as potential mutagens and carcinogens. Contact with these chemicals can make skin very sensitive to light.

Aphthous ulcers (canker sores). Citrus fruits or juices may trigger a flare-up of canker sores in sensitive people, but eliminating these foods from the diet neither cures nor prevents canker sores.

Food/Drug Interactions

Iron supplements. Taking iron supplements with a food rich in vitamin C increases the absorption of iron from the supplement.

Lentils

See also Beans.

Nutritional Profile

Energy value (calories per serving): *Moderate*
Protein: *High*
Fat: *Low*
Saturated fat: *Low*
Cholesterol: *None*
Carbohydrates: *High*
Fiber: *Very high*
Sodium: *Moderate*
Major vitamin contribution: *Vitamin B$_6$, folate*
Major mineral contribution: *Magnesium, iron, zinc*

About the Nutrients in This Food

Lentils are seeds, a very high-fiber, low-fat, high-protein food. They are an excellent source of insoluble dietary fiber (cellulose and lignin in the seed covering) and soluble dietary fiber (pectins and gums in the bean). Their proteins are plentiful but limited in the essential amino acids methionine and cystine. Lentils are a good source of the B vitamin folate and nonheme iron, the form of iron found in plants.

One-half cup soaked lentils has 7.8 g dietary fiber, 8.9 g protein, 0.4 g fat, 179 mcg folate (45 percent of the RDA), and 3.3 mg iron (6 percent of the RDA for a woman, 41 percent of the RDA for a man).

Raw lentils contain antinutrient chemicals that inactivate enzymes you need to digest proteins and carbohydrates (starches). They also contain factors that inactivate vitamin A, and they have hemagglutinins, substances that make red blood cells clump together. Cooking lentils disarms the enzyme inhibitors and the anti-vitamin A factors, but not the hemagglutinins. However, the amount of hemagglutinins in lentils is so small that it has no measurable effect in your body.

The Most Nutritious Way to Serve This Food

Cooked, with meat, milk, cheese, or a grain (rice, pasta) to complete the proteins in the lentils.

Diets That May Restrict or Exclude This Food

Antiflatulence diet
Low-calcium diet
Low-carbohydrate diet
Low-fiber diet
Low-purine (antigout) diet

Buying This Food

Look for: Smooth-skinned, uniform, evenly colored lentils that are free of stones and debris. The good news about beans sold in plastic bags is that the transparent material gives you a chance to see the beans inside; the bad news is that pyridoxine and pyridoxal, the natural forms of vitamin B$_6$, are very sensitive to light.

Avoid: Lentils sold in bulk. The open bins expose the beans to air and light and may allow insect contamination (tiny holes in the beans indicate an insect has burrowed into or through the bean).

Storing This Food

Store lentils in air- and moistureproof containers in cool, dark cabinets where they are protected from heat, light, and insects.

Preparing This Food

Wash the lentils and pick them over carefully, discarding damaged or withered beans and any that float. The only beans light enough to float in water are those that have withered away inside. Lentils do not have to be soaked before cooking.

What Happens When You Cook This Food

When lentils are cooked in liquid, their cells absorb water, swell, and eventually rupture, so that the nutrients inside are more available to your body.

How Other Kinds of Processing Affect This Food

* * *

Medical Uses and/or Benefits

Lower risk of some birth defects. Up to two of every 1,000 babies born in the United States each year may have cleft palate or a neural tube (spinal cord) defect due to their mothers' not having gotten adequate amounts of folate during pregnancy. The current RDA for folate is 180 mcg for a woman and 200 mcg for a man, but the FDA now recommends 400 mcg for a woman who is or may become pregnant. Taking a folate supplement before becoming pregnant and continuing through the first two months of pregnancy reduces the risk of cleft palate; taking folate through the entire pregnancy reduces the risk of neural tube defects. Lentils are a significant source of folate. One-half cup cooked lentils has 178 mg folate.

Lower risk of heart attack.   In the spring of 1998, an analysis' of data from the records for more than 80,000 women enrolled in the long-running Nurses Health Study at Harvard School of Public Health/Brigham and Woman's Hospital in Boston demonstrated that a diet providing more than 400 mcg folate and 3 mg vitamin B_6 a day from either food or supplements, more than twice the current RDA for each, may reduce a woman's risk of heart attack by almost 50 percent. Although men were not included in the analysis, the results are assumed to apply to them as well. NOTE: Fruit, green leafy vegetables, beans, whole grains, meat, fish, poultry, and shellfish are good sources of vitamin B_6.

As a source of carbohydrates for people with diabetes.   Beans are digested very slowly, producing only a gradual rise in blood-sugar levels. As a result, the body needs less insulin to control blood sugar after eating beans than after eating some other high-carbohydrate foods such as bread or potato. In studies at the University of Kentucky, a bean, whole-grain, vegetable, and fruit-rich diet developed at the University of Toronto and recommended by the American Diabetic Association enabled patients with type 1 diabetes (who do not produce any insulin themselves) to cut their daily insulin intake by 38 percent. For patients with type 2 diabetes (who can produce some insulin), the bean diet reduced the need for injected insulin by 98 percent. This diet is in line with the nutritional guidelines of the American Diabetic Association, but people with diabetes should always consult their doctors and/or dietitians before altering their diet.

As a diet aid.   Although beans are very high in calories, they have so much fiber that even a small serving can make you feel full. And, since beans are insulin-sparing (because they do not cause blood-sugar levels to rise quickly), they put off the surge of insulin that makes us feel hungry again and allow us to feel full longer. In fact, research at the University of Toronto suggests the insulin-sparing effect may last for several hours after you eat the beans, perhaps until after your next meal. When subjects were given one of two breakfasts—bread and cheese or lentils—the people who ate the lentils produced 25 percent less insulin after the meal.

Adverse Effects Associated with This Food

Intestinal gas.   All dried beans, including lentils, contain raffinose and stachyose, sugars that the human body cannot digest. As a result these sugars sit in the gut, where they are fermented by the bacteria that live in our intestinal tract. The result is intestinal gas. Since the indigestible sugars are soluble in hot water, they will leach out into the water in which you cook the lentils. You can cut down on intestinal gas by draining the lentils thoroughly before you serve them.

Production of uric acid. Purines are the natural metabolic by-products of protein metabolism in the body. They eventually break down into uric acid, which can form sharp crystals that may cause gout if they collect in your joints or kidney stones if they collect in urine. Dried beans are a source of purines; eating them raises the concentration of purines in your body. Although controlling the amount of purine-producing foods in the diet may not significantly affect the course of gout, limiting these foods is still part of many gout regimens.

Food/Drug Interactions

Monoamine oxidase (MAO) inhibitors. Monoamine oxidase inhibitors are drugs used to treat depression. They inactivate naturally occurring enzymes in your body that metabolize tyramine, a substance found in many fermented or aged foods. Tyramine constricts blood vessels and increases blood pressure. If you eat a food containing tyramine while you are taking an MAO inhibitor, you cannot effectively eliminate the tyramine from your body. The result may be a hypertensive crisis. Some nutrition guides list lentils as a food to avoid while using MAO inhibitors.

Lettuce

(Arugula, butterhead [Bibb], chicory [curly endive], cos [romaine], crisphead [iceberg], endive, leaf lettuce [green, red], raddichio)

See also Greens, Spinach.

Nutritional Profile

Energy value (calories per serving): *Low*

Protein: *Low*

Fat: *Low*

Saturated fat: *Low*

Cholesterol: *None*

Carbohydrates: *High*

Fiber: *Moderate to high*

Sodium: *Low*

Major vitamin contribution: *Vitamin A, vitamin C*

Major mineral contribution: *Iron, calcium*

About the Nutrients in This Food

Lettuces are low-fiber, low-protein, virtually fat-free leafy foods whose primary nutrient contribution is vitamin A from deep yellow carotenes hidden under green chlorophyll. The darkest leaves have the most vitamin A. Lettuce also provides the B vitamin folate, vitamin C, plus small amounts of iron, calcium, and copper.

One-half cup shredded lettuce has less than one gram dietary fiber. Depending on the variety, it has 50 to 370 IU vitamin A (2 to 16 percent of the RDA for a woman, 2 to 12 percent of the RDA for a man), 14 to 39 mcg folate (4 to 10 percent of the RDA), and 2 to 3.5 mg vitamin C (3 to 5 percent of the RDA for a woman, 2 to 4 percent of the RDA for a man).

Comparing the Nutritional Value of Lettuces

◆ Looseleaf lettuce has about twice as much calcium as romaine, and nearly four times as much as iceberg.

◆ Looseleaf lettuce has about one-third more iron than romaine, nearly three times as much as iceberg, and nearly five times as much as Boston and Bibb.

Comparing the Nutritional Value of Lettuces *(Continued)*

◆ Romaine lettuce has about one-third more vitamin A than iceberg, three times as much as Boston and Bibb, and eight times as much as iceberg.

◆ Romaine lettuce has about one third more vitamin C than looseleaf, three times as much as Boston and Bibb, and six times as much as iceberg.

◆ Shredded romaine lettuce has more than twice as much folate as an equal serving of shredded iceberg, butterhead, or Boston lettuce; nearly three times as much as loose-leaf lettuce.

Source: *Composition of Foods, Vegetables and Vegetable Products,* Agriculture Handbook No. 8–11 (USDA 1984).

The Most Nutritious Way to Serve This Food

Fresh, dark leaves, torn just before serving to preserve vitamin C. Given a choice among all the varieties of lettuce, pick romaine. Overall, it has larger amounts of vitamins and minerals than any other lettuce.

Diets That May Restrict or Exclude This Food

Antiflatulence diet
Low-calcium diet
Low-carbohydrate diet
Low-fiber diet

Buying This Food

Look for: Brightly colored heads. Iceberg lettuce should be tightly closed and heavy for its size. Loose leaf lettuces should be crisp. All lettuces should be symmetrically shaped. An asymmetric shape suggests a large hidden stem that is crowding the leaves to one side or the other.

Avoid: Lettuce with faded or yellow leaves; lettuce leaves turn yellow as they age and their green chlorophyll fades, revealing the yellow carotenes underneath. Brown or wilted leaves are a sign of aging or poor storage. Either way, the lettuce is no longer at its best.

Storing This Food

Wrap lettuce in a plastic bag and store it in the refrigerator. The colder the storage, the longer the lettuce will keep. Most lettuce will stay fresh and crisp for as long at three weeks at 32°F. Raise the temperature just six degrees to 38°F (which is about the temperature inside your refrigerator), and the lettuce may wilt in a week.

Do not discard lettuce simply because the core begins to brown or small brown specks appear on the spines of the leaves. This is a natural oxidation reaction that changes the color but doesn't affect the nutritional value of the lettuce. Trim the end of the core (or remove the core from iceberg lettuce) to slow the reaction. Throw out any lettuce that feels slimy or has bright red, dark brown, or black spots. The slime is the residue of bacterial decomposition; the dark spots may be mold or rot.

Do not store unwrapped lettuce near apples, pears, melons, or bananas. These fruits release ethylene gas, a natural ripening agent that will cause the lettuce to develop brown spots.

Preparing This Food

Wash all lettuce, including lettuce sold in "pre-washed" packages of salad mix, to flush out debris.

Never slice, cut, or tear lettuce until you are ready to use it. When lettuce cells are torn, they release ascorbic acid oxidase, an enzyme that destroys vitamin C.

What Happens When You Cook This Food

Chlorophyll, the pigment that makes green vegetables green, is sensitive to acids. When you heat lettuce, the chlorophyll in its leaves will react chemically with acids in the vegetable or in the cooking water, forming pheophytin, which is brown. Together, the pheophytin and the yellow carotenes in dark green leaves will give the cooked lettuce a bronze hue. (Lighter leaves, with very little carotene, will be olive-drab.)

To keep cooked lettuce green, you have to keep the chlorophyll from reacting with acids. One way to do this is to cook the lettuce in a large quantity of water (which will dilute the acids), but this will accelerate the loss of vitamin C. A second alternative is to cook the lettuce with the lid off the pot so that the volatile acids will float off into the air. The best way may be to steam the lettuce quickly in very little water, so that it holds onto its vitamin C and cooks before the chlorophyll has time to react with the acids.

Heat also makes the water inside the lettuce cells expand. Eventually the cells rupture and the water leaks out, leaving the lettuce limp. The spines will remain stiffer because they contain more cellulose, which does not dissolve in water. Cooked lettuce has less vitamin C than fresh lettuce because heat destroys the vitamin.

How Other Kinds of Processing Affect This Food

* * *

Medical Uses and/or Benefits

Lower risk of some birth defects. Up to two of every 1,000 babies born in the United States each year may have cleft palate or a neural tube (spinal cord) defect due to their mothers' not having gotten adequate amounts of folate during pregnancy. The current RDA for folate is 180 mcg for a healthy woman and 200 mcg for a healthy man, but the FDA now recommends 400 mcg for a woman who is or may become pregnant. Taking a folate supplement before becoming pregnant and continuing through the first two months of pregnancy reduces the risk of cleft palate; taking folate through the entire pregnancy reduces the risk of neural tube defects. One cup shredded romaine lettuce has 78 mg folate.

Possible lower risk of heart attack.   In the spring of 1998, an analysis of data from the records for more than 80,000 women enrolled in the long-running Nurses' Health Study at Harvard School of Public Health/Brigham and Women's Hospital, in Boston, demonstrated that a diet providing more than 400 mcg folate and 3 mg vitamin B$_6$ daily, either from food or supplements, might reduce a woman's risk of heart attack by almost 50 percent. Although men were not included in the study, the results were assumed to apply to them as well.

However, data from a meta-analysis published in the *Journal of the American Medical Association* in December 2006 called this theory into question. Researchers at Tulane University examined the results of 12 controlled studies in which 16,958 patients with preexisting cardiovascular disease were given either folic acid supplements or placebos ("look-alike" pills with no folic acid) for at least six months. The scientists, who found no reduction in the risk of further heart disease or overall death rates among those taking folic acid, concluded that further studies will be required to ascertain whether taking folic acid supplements reduces the risk of cardiovascular disease.

Vision protection.   Dark greens are a rich source of the yellow-orange carotenoid pigments lutein and zeaxanthin. Both carotenoids appear to play a role in protecting the eyes from damaging ultraviolet light, thus reducing the risk of cataracts and age-related macular degeneration, which is a leading cause of vision loss in one-third of all Americans older than 75.

Adverse Effects Associated with This Food

Food-borne illness.   According to the Centers for Disease Control and Prevention, from 1996–2005 the proportion of incidents of food-borne disease linked to leafy greens increased by 60 percent. The highest proportion of these illnesses were due to contamination by norovirus (the organism often blamed for outbreaks of gastric illness on cruise ships), followed by salmonella and *E. coli*. The illnesses were commonly associated with eating raw greens; cooking the greens to a high heat inactivates the disease-causing organisms.

Nitrate poisoning.   Lettuce, like beets, celery, eggplant, radishes, spinach, and collard and turnip greens, contains nitrates that convert naturally into nitrites in your stomach, and then react with the amino acids in proteins to form nitrosamines. Although some nitrosamines are known or suspected carcinogens, this natural chemical conversion presents no known problems for a healthy adult. However, when these nitrate-rich vegetables are cooked and left to stand at room temperature, bacterial enzyme action (and perhaps some enzymes in the plants) convert the nitrates to nitrites at a much faster rate than normal. These higher-nitrite foods may be hazardous for infants; several cases of "spinach poisoning" have been reported among children who ate cooked spinach that had been left standing at room temperature.

Food/Drug Interactions

Anticoagulants   Some lettuces are rich in vitamin K, the blood-clotting vitamin produced naturally by bacteria in the intestines. Consuming large quantities of this food may reduce the effectiveness of anticoagulants (blood thinners) such as warfarin (Coumadin). One cup of shredded Boston or Bibb lettuce contains 56 mcg vitamin K, about 90 percent of the RDA for a healthy adult; one cup of shredded romaine lettuce contains 48 mcg vitamin K, about 80 percent of the RDA for a healthy adult.

Lima Beans

See also Beans.

Nutritional Profile

Energy value (calories per serving): *Moderate*
Protein: *High*
Fat: *Low*
Saturated fat: *Low*
Cholesterol: *None*
Carbohydrates: *High*
Fiber: *Very high*
Sodium: *Low*
Major vitamin contribution: *Vitamin B$_6$, folate*
Major mineral contribution: *Magnesium, iron, zinc*

About the Nutrients in This Food

Lima beans are seeds, a good source of starch and very high in dietary fiber, including insoluble cellulose and lignin in the seed covering and soluble pectins and gums in the bean. The lima bean's proteins are plentiful but limited in the essential amino acids methionine and cystine. Lima beans are a good source of the B vitamin folate, plus iron, and zinc.

One-half cup boiled large lima beans has 6.5 g dietary fiber, 7.4 g protein, 78 mcg folate (20 percent of the RDA), 2.2 mg iron (12 percent of the RDA for a woman, 31 percent of the RDA for a man), and 0.9 mg zinc (11 percent of the RDA for a woman, 8 percent of the RDA for a man).

Raw limas contain antinutrient chemicals that inactivate enzymes you need to digest proteins and carbohydrates (starches). They also contain factors that inactivate vitamin A, and they have hemagglutinins, substances that make red blood cells clump together. Cooking limas disarms the enzyme inhibitors and the anti-vitamin A factors, but not the hemagglutinins. However, the amount of hemagglutinins in limas is so small that it has no measurable effect in your body.

Lima beans also contain phaseolunatin, a chemical that breaks down into hydrogen cyanide when the cells of the lima bean are damaged or torn and the phaseolunatin comes into contact with an enzyme in the bean that triggers its conversion. Dark-colored lima beans and lima beans grown outside the United States may contain larger amounts of phaseolunatin than the pale American limas. Since phaseolunatin is not destroyed by cooking, there have been serious cases of poisoning among people living in the tropics, where the high-cyanide varieties of the lima beans grow. The importation of lima beans is restricted by many countries, including the United States; beans grown and sold here are considered safe.

The Most Nutritious Way to Serve This Food

Cooked, with meat, cheese, milk, or grain (pasta, rice) to complete the proteins in the beans.

The proteins in grains are deficient in the essential amino acid lysine but contain sufficient methionine and cystine; the proteins in beans are exactly the opposite. Together, these foods provide "complete" proteins with no cholesterol and very little fat.

Both iron-rich foods (meat) and foods rich in vitamin C (tomatoes, peppers, potatoes) enhance your body's ability to absorb the nonheme iron in the lima beans. The meat makes your stomach more acid, which enhances the absorption of iron, and the vitamin C may work by converting the iron in the lima beans from ferric iron (which is hard to absorb) to ferrous iron (which is absorbed more easily).

Diets That May Restrict or Exclude This Food

Antiflatulence diet
Low-calcium diet
Low-carbohydrate diet
Low-fiber diet
Low-purine (antigout) diet

Buying This Food

Look for: Well-filled, tender green pods of fresh limas. The shelled beans should be plump, with green or greenish white skin.

Avoid: Spotted or yellowing pods.

Storing This Food

Store fresh lima beans in the refrigerator.

Preparing This Food

Slice a thin strip down the side of the pod, then open the pod and remove the beans. Discard withered beans and beans with tiny holes (they show where insects have burrowed through).

What Happens When You Cook This Food

When lima beans are heated in water, their cellulose and lignin-stiffened cells absorb moisture, swell, and eventually rupture, releasing the vitamins, minerals, proteins, starch, and fiber inside. Cooking also makes lima beans safer by inactivating their antinutrients and hemagglutinins.

How Other Kinds of Processing Affect This Food

Drying. Drying reduces the moisture and concentrates the calories and nutrients in lima beans.

Canning and freezing. Frozen fresh lima beans contain about the same amounts of vitamins and minerals as fresh beans; canned lima beans are lower in vitamins but usually contain more sodium in the form of added salt.

Medical Uses and/or Benefits

Lower risk of some birth defects. Up to two of every 1,000 babies born in the United States each year may have cleft palate or a neural tube (spinal cord) defect due to their mothers' not having gotten adequate amounts of folate during pregnancy. The current RDA for folate is 180 mcg for a woman and 200 mcg for a man, but FDA now recommends 400 mcg for a woman who is or may become pregnant. Taking a folate supplement before becoming pregnant and continuing through the first two months of pregnancy reduces the risk of cleft palate; taking folate through the entire pregnancy reduces the risk of neural tube defects.

Possible lower risk of heart attack. In the spring of 1998, an analysis of data from the records for more than 80,000 women enrolled in the long-running Nurses' Health Study at Harvard School of Public Health/Brigham and Women's Hospital, in Boston, demonstrated that a diet providing more than 400 mcg folate and 3 mg vitamin B_6 daily, either from food or supplements, might reduce a woman's risk of heart attack by almost 50 percent. Although men were not included in the study, the results were assumed to apply to them as well.

However, data from a meta-analysis published in the *Journal of the American Medical Association* in December 2006 called this theory into question. Researchers at Tulane University examined the results of 12 controlled studies in which 16,958 patients with preexisting cardiovascular disease were given either folic acid supplements or placebos ("look-alike" pills with no folic acid) for at least six months. The scientists, who found no reduction in the risk of further heart disease or overall death rates among those taking folic acid, concluded that further studies will be required to ascertain whether taking folic acid supplements reduces the risk of cardiovascular disease.

To reduce the levels of serum cholesterol. The gums and pectins in dried beans appear to lower the level of cholesterol in the blood. There are currently two theories to explain how this may happen. The first theory is that the pectins in the beans form a gel in your stomach that sops up fats so that they cannot be absorbed by your body. The second is that bacteria in the gut feed on the bean fiber, producing chemicals called short-chain fatty acids that inhibit the production of cholesterol in your liver.

As a source of carbohydrates for people with diabetes.   Beans are digested very slowly, producing only a gradual rise in blood-sugar levels. As a result, the body needs less insulin to control blood sugar after eating beans than after eating some other high-carbohydrate foods (bread or potato). In studies at the University of Kentucky, researchers put diabetic patients on a bean-grains-fruit-and-vegetables diet developed at the University of Toronto and recommended by the American Diabetes Association. On the diet, patients with type 1 diabetes (whose bodies do not produce any insulin) to cut their insulin intake by 38 percent. Patients with type 2 diabetes (who can produce some insulin) were able to reduce their insulin injections by 98 percent. This diet is in line with the nutritional guidelines of the American Diabetes Association, but people with diabetes should always consult their doctors and/or dietitians before altering their diet.

As a diet aid.   Although beans are very high in calories, they have so much bulky fiber that even a small serving can make you feel full. And, since beans are insulin-sparing (because they don't cause blood-sugar levels to rise quickly), they postpone the natural surge of insulin that triggers hunger pangs. In fact, research at the University of Toronto suggests the insulin-sparing effect may last for several hours after eating beans, perhaps even until after the next meal.

Adverse Effects Associated with This Food

Intestinal gas.   All legumes (beans and peas) contain raffinose and stachyose, sugars that cannot be digested by human beings. Instead, they are fermented by bacteria living in the intestinal tract, producing the gassiness many people associate with eating beans. Since raffinose and stachyose leach out of the limas into the water when you cook lima beans, discarding the water in which you cook fresh limas beans or presoak dried ones may make them less gassy.

Allergic reaction.   According to the *Merck Manual,* legumes (including lima beans) are one of the 12 foods most likely to trigger classic food allergy symptoms: hives, swelling of the lips and eyes, and upset stomach. The others are berries (blackberries, blueberries, raspberries, strawberries), chocolate, corn, eggs, fish, milk, nuts, peaches, pork, shellfish, and wheat (see WHEAT CEREALS).

Food/Drug Interactions

Monoamine oxidase (MAO) inhibitors.   Monoamine oxidase inhibitors are drugs used to treat depression. They inactivate naturally occurring enzymes in your body that metabolize tyramine, a substance found in many fermented or aged foods. Tyramine constricts blood vessels and increases blood pressure. If you eat a food containing tyramine while you are taking an MAO inhibitor, you cannot effectively eliminate the tyramine from your body. The result may be a hypertensive crisis. Some nutrition guides list lima beans as a food to avoid while using MAO inhibitors.

Liver

Nutritional Profile*

Energy value (calories per serving): *Moderate*
Protein: *High*
Fat: *Moderate*
Saturated fat: *High*
Cholesterol: *High*
Carbohydrates: *Low*
Fiber: *None*
Sodium: *Moderate*
Major vitamin contribution: *Vitamin A, B vitamins*
Major mineral contribution: *Iron, copper*

About the Nutrients in This Food

Like meat, fish, poultry, milk, and eggs, liver is a good source of high-quality proteins with adequate amounts of all the essential amino acids. It is moderately high in fat and saturated fat and high in cholesterol.

Liver is the single best natural source of retinol ("true vitamin A").[†] It is one of the few natural sources of vitamin D, an excellent source of B vitamins, including vitamin B_{12}, which prevents or cures pernicious anemia, and an excellent source of heme iron, the form of iron most easily absorbed by your body.

One four-ounce serving of simmered beef liver has 29 g protein, 5.3 g fat (1.7 g saturated fat, 0.6 g monounsaturated fat, 0.6 g polyunsaturated fat), 396 mg cholesterol, 31,714 IU vitamin A (approximately 13 times the RDA for a woman, 11 times the RDA for a man), and 6.5 mg iron (36 percent of the RDA for a woman, 81 percent of the RDA for a man).

One four-ounce serving of simmered chicken livers has 25 g protein, 6.5 g fat (2 g saturated fat, 1.4 g monounsaturated fat, 2 g polyunsaturated fat), 563 mg cholesterol, 13,328 IU vitamin A (approximately six times the RDA for a woman, 4.5 times the RDA for a man), and 11.6 mg iron (64 percent of the RDA for a woman, 145 percent of the RDA for a man).

---

* Values are for braised beef liver.

† Carotenoids, the red and yellow pigments in some fruits and vegetables, are vitamin A precursors, chemicals that are converted to vitamin A in your body.

The Most Nutritious Way to Serve This Food

As fresh as possible. Fresh-frozen liver, if kept properly cold, may be even fresher than "fresh" liver that has never been frozen but has been sitting for a day or two in the supermarket meat case.

Diets That May Restrict or Exclude This Food

Galactose-free diet (for control of galactosemia)
Low-calcium diet
Low-cholesterol, controlled-fat diet
Low-protein, low-purine diet

Buying This Food

Look for: Liver that has a deep, rich color and smells absolutely fresh.

Storing This Food

Fresh liver is extremely perishable. It should be stored in the refrigerator for no longer than a day or two and in the freezer, at 0°F, for no longer than three to four months.

Preparing This Food

Wipe the liver with a damp cloth. If your butcher has not already done so, pull off the outer membrane, and cut out the veins. Sheep, pork, and older beef liver are strongly flavored; to make them more palatable, soak these livers for several hours in cold milk, cold water, or a marinade, then discard the soaking liquid when you are ready to cook the liver.

What Happens When You Cook This Food

When liver is heated it loses water and shrinks. Its pigments, which combine with oxygen, are denatured by the heat, breaking into smaller fragments that turn brown, the natural color of cooked meat. Since liver has virtually no collagen (the connective tissue that stays chewy unless you cook it for a long time), it should be cooked as quickly as possible to keep it from drying out.

How Other Kinds of Processing Affect This Food

* * *

Medical Uses and/or Benefits

As a source of iron. Liver is an excellent source of heme iron, the organic form of iron in meat that is absorbed approximately five times more easily than nonheme iron, the inorganic iron in plants.

Adverse Effects Associated with This Food

Increased risk of cardiovascular disease. Like other foods from animals, liver is a significant source of cholesterol and saturated fats, which increase the amount of cholesterol circulating in your blood and raise your risk of heart disease. To reduce the risk of heart disease, the National Cholesterol Education Project recommends following the Step I and Step II diets.

The Step I diet provides no more than 30 percent of total daily calories from fat, no more than 10 percent of total daily calories from saturated fat, and no more than 300 mg of cholesterol per day. It is designed for healthy people whose cholesterol is in the range of 200–239 mg/dL.

The Step II diet provides 25–35 percent of total calories from fat, less than 7 percent of total calories from saturated fat, up to 10 percent of total calories from polyunsaturated fat, up to 20 percent of total calories from monounsaturated fat, and less than 300 mg cholesterol per day. This stricter regimen is designed for people who have one or more of the following conditions:

◆ Existing cardiovascular disease
◆ High levels of low-density lipoproteins (LDLs, or "bad" cholesterol) or low levels of high-density lipoproteins (HDLs, or "good" cholesterol)
◆ Obesity
◆ Type 1 diabetes (insulin-dependent diabetes, or diabetes mellitus)
◆ Metabolic syndrome, a.k.a. insulin resistance syndrome, a cluster of risk factors that includes type 2 diabetes (non-insulin-dependent diabetes)

Vitamin A poisoning. Vitamin A is stored in the liver, so this organ is an extremely rich source of retinol, the true vitamin A. In large doses, retinol is poisonous. The RDA for a woman is 2,310 IU; for a man, 2,970. Doses of 50,000 IU a day over a period of weeks have produced symptoms of vitamin A poisoning; single doses of 2,000,000–5,000,000 IU may produce acute vitamin A poisoning (drowsiness, irritability, headache, vomiting, peeling skin). This reaction was documented in early arctic explorers who ate large amounts of polar bear liver and in people who eat the livers of large fish (shark, halibut, cod), which may contain up to 100,000 IU vitamin A per grams. In infants, as little as 7.5 to 15 mg of retinol a day for 30 days has produced vomiting and bulging fontanel. In 1980 there was a report of chronic vitamin A intoxication in infants fed 120 grams (4 ounces) of chicken liver plus vitamin supplements containing 2000 IU vitamin A, yellow vegetable and fruits, and vitamin A-enriched milk every day for four months. Liver should not be eaten every day unless specifically directed by a physician.

Production of uric acid. Purines are the natural metabolic by-products of protein metabolism in the body. They eventually break down into uric acid, which can form sharp crystals that may cause gout if they collect in your joints or kidney stones if they collect in urine. Liver is a source of purines; eating liver raises the concentration of purines in your body. Although controlling the amount of purine-producing foods in the diet may not significantly affect the course of gout, limiting foods that raise the levels of purines is still part of many gout regimens.

Food/Drug Interactions

MAO inhibitors. Monoamine oxidase (MAO) inhibitors are drugs used as antidepressants or antihypertensives. They inhibit the enzymes that break down tyramine so that it can be eliminated from your body. Tyramine, which is formed when proteins deteriorate, is a pressor amine, a chemical that constricts blood vessels and raises blood pressure. If you eat a food rich in tyramine while you are taking an MAO inhibitor, the pressor amine cannot be eliminated from your body, and the result may be a hypertensive crisis (sustained elevated blood pressure). Liver, which is extremely perishable, contains enzymes that break down its proteins quickly if the liver is not properly refrigerated or if it ages. Fresh or canned pâtés made with wine may contain more tyramine than fresh liver.

Mangoes

Nutritional Profile

Energy value (calories per serving): *Moderate*
Protein: *Low*
Fat: *Low*
Saturated fat: *Low*
Cholesterol: *None*
Carbohydrates: *High*
Fiber: *High*
Sodium: *Low*
Major vitamin contribution: *Vitamin A, vitamin C*
Major mineral contribution: *Potassium*

About the Nutrients in This Food

Mangoes are high in soluble dietary fiber (pectins in the fruit). They are an extraordinary source of vitamin A, derived from deep yellow carotenes, including beta-carotene, and an excellent source of vitamin C.

The edible part of one seven-ounce mango has 3.7 g dietary fiber (primarily the soluble fiber pectin), 1,584 IU vitamin A (69 percent of the RDA for a woman, 53 percent of the RDA for a man), 57 mg vitamin C (79 percent of the RDA for a woman, 63 percent of the RDA for a man), and 29 mg folate (7 percent of the RDA).

Unripe mangoes contain antinutrients, protein compounds that inhibit amylases (the enzymes that make it possible for us to digest starches) and catalase (the iron-containing enzyme that protects our cells by splitting potentially damaging peroxides in our body into safe water and oxygen). As the fruit ripens the enzyme inhibitors are inactivated.

The Most Nutritious Way to Serve This Food

Ripe, chilled, and freshly cut.

Diets That May Restrict or Exclude This Food

* * *

Buying This Food

Look for: Flattish, oval fruit. The skin should be yellow green or yellow green flecked with red; the riper the mango, the more yellow and red there will be. A ripe mango will give slightly when you press it with your finger.

Avoid: Mangoes with gray, pitted, or spotted skin; they may be rotten inside.

Storing This Food

Store mangoes at room temperature if they aren't fully ripe when you buy them; they will continue to ripen. When the mangoes are soft (ripe), refrigerate them and use them within two or three days. Once you have sliced a mango, wrap it in plastic and store it in the refrigerator.

Preparing This Food

Chill mangoes before you serve them. At room temperature they have a distinctly unpleasant taste and a fragrance some people compare to turpentine. The flavor of the mango doesn't develop fully until the fruit is completely ripe. If you cut into a mango and find that it's not ripe yet, poach it in sugar syrup. That way it will taste fine.

Eating a mango is an adventure. The long, oval pit clings to the flesh, and to get at the fruit you have to peel away the skin and then slice off the flesh.

What Happens When You Cook This Food

When you poach a mango, its cells absorb water and the fruit softens.

How Other Kinds of Processing Affect This Food

* * *

Medical Uses and/or Benefits

Antiscorbutics. Foods high in vitamin C cure or prevent the vitamin C deficiency disease scurvy, characterized by bleeding gums and slow healing of wounds.

Adverse Effects Associated with This Food

Contact dermatitis. The skin of the mango contains urushiol, the chemical that may cause contact dermatitis when you touch poison ivy, poison oak, and poison sumac.

Food/Drug Interactions

* * *

Melons

(Cantaloupe, casaba, honeydew, Persian, watermelon)

Nutritional Profile

Energy value (calories per serving): *Low*
Protein: *Low*
Fat: *Low*
Saturated fat: *Low*
Cholesterol: *None*
Carbohydrates: *High*
Fiber: *High*
Sodium: *Low*
Major vitamin contribution: *Vitamin A, folate, vitamin C*
Major mineral contribution: *Potassium*

About the Nutrients in This Food

All melons are rich in sugars and a good source of the soluble dietary fiber pectin. The deep-yellow melons (cantaloupe, crenshaw, Persian) are also rich in vitamin A.

One-half of a five-inch diameter cantaloupe has 2.5 g dietary fiber, 9,334 IU vitamin A (approximately four times the RDA for a woman, three times the RDA for a man), 58 mcg folate (15 percent of the RDA), and 101 mg vitamin C (approximately 1.3 times the RDA for a woman, approximately 1.1 times the RDA for a man).

One cup diced watermelon has 0.6 g dietary fiber, 865 IU vitamin A (37 percent of the RDA for a woman, 29 percent of the RDA for a man), and 12 mg vitamin C (16 percent of the RDA for a woman, 13 percent of the RDA for a man).

The Most Nutritious Way to Serve This Food

Fresh and ripe.

Diets That May Restrict or Exclude This Food

Low-carbohydrate diet
Low-fiber diet

Buying This Food

Look for: Vine-ripened melons if possible. You can identify a vine-ripened melon by check-ing the stem end. If the scar is clean and sunken, it means that the stem was pulled out of a ripe melon. Ripe melons also have a deep aroma: the more intense the fragrance, the sweeter the melon.

Cantaloupes should be round and firm, with cream-colored, coarse "netting" that stands up all over the fruit. The rind at the stem end of the melon should give slightly when you press it and there should be a rich, melony aroma. *Casabas* should have a deep-yellow rind that gives at the stem end when you press it. Ripe casabas smell pleasant and melony. *Honey-dews* should have a smooth cream-colored or a yellowish white rind. If the rind is completely white or tinged with green, the melon is not ripe. Like cantaloupes, *Persian melons* have a rind covered with "netting." As the Persian ripens, the color of its rind lightens. A ripe Persian will give when you press it. *Watermelons* should have a firm, smooth rind with a cream or yellowish undercolor. If the undercoat is white or greenish, the melon is not ripe. When you shake a ripe watermelon, the seeds inside will rattle; when you thump its rind, you should hear a slightly hollow sound.

Storing This Food

Hold whole melons at room temperature for a few days. Melons have no stored starches to convert to sugar, so they can't get sweeter once they are picked, but they will begin to soften as enzymes begin to dissolve pectin in the cell walls. As the cell walls dissolve, the melons release the aromatic molecules that make them smell sweet and ripe.

Refrigerate ripe melons to slow the natural deterioration of the fruit. Sliced melons should be wrapped in plastic to keep them from losing moisture or from absorbing odors from other foods.

Preparing This Food

In 2008, following an outbreak of food-borne illness traced to contaminated cantaloupes, the FDA released recommendations for the safe preparation of cantaloupes and other melons that minimize the chances of contaminating the fruit inside the melon with organisms on the outside of the rind. One safe method is as follows:

1. Wash the melon under running water, scrubbing the rind.
2. On a cutting board, cut the melon into large pieces with a knife and remove the central seeds, if any.
3. Wash hands with soap and water.
4. On a second cutting board, use a second knife to cut the fruit away from the rind and then into smaller pieces.
5. Refrigerate the melon pieces until ready to use.
6. Wash and dry the knives and cutting boards in hot water and soap, preferably in a dishwasher that uses hot water and dries with heat.

What Happens When You Cook This Food

* * *

How Other Kinds of Processing Affect This Food

* * *

Medical Uses and/or Benefits

Reduced risk of some cancers.   According to the American Cancer Society, foods rich in beta-carotenes may lower the risk of cancers of the larynx, esophagus and lungs. There is no similar benefit from beta-carotene supplements; indeed, one study actually showed a higher rate of lung cancer among smokers taking the supplement.

Lower risk of heart attack.   In the spring of 1998, an analysis of data from the records for more than 80,000 women enrolled in the long-running Nurses Health Study at Harvard School of Public Health/Brigham and Woman's Hospital in Boston identified the first direct link between two B vitamins and heart health. According to Eric B. Rimm, M.D., of the Harvard School of Public Health, a diet that provides more than 400 mcg folate and 3 mg vitamin B_6 a day from either food or supplements, more than twice the current RDA for each, may reduce a woman's risk of heart attack by almost 50 percent. Although men were not included in the analysis, the results are presumed to apply to them as well. Many melons are high in folate; green leafy vegetables, beans, whole grains, meat, fish, poultry, and shellfish are other good sources.

Lower risk of some birth defects.   As many as two of every 1,000 babies born in the United States each year may have cleft palate or a neural tube (spinal cord) defect due to their mothers' not having gotten adequate amounts of folate during pregnancy. The current RDA for folate is 180 mcg for a woman and 200 mcg for a man, but the FDA now recommends 400 mcg for a woman who is or may become pregnant. Taking folate supplements before becoming pregnant and continuing through the first two months of pregnancy reduces the risk of cleft palate; taking folate through the entire pregnancy reduces the risk of neural tube defects.

Adverse Effects Associated with This Food

* * *

Food/Drug Interactions

* * *

Milk, Cultured

(Acidophilus milk, buttermilk, kefir, kumiss, sour cream, yogurt)

See also Milk (fresh).

Nutritional Profile

Energy value (calories per serving): *Moderate*
Protein: *High*
Fat: *Low to high*
Saturated fat: *Low to high*
Cholesterol: *Low to high*
Carbohydrates: *Moderate*
Fiber: *None*
Sodium: *Moderate*
Major vitamin contribution: *Vitamin A, vitamin D, B vitamins*
Major mineral contribution: *Calcium*

About the Nutrients in This Food

Cultured milks are dairy products whose lactose (milk sugar) has been digested by specialized microorganisms that produce lactic acid, which thickens the milk. *Acidophilus milk* is pasteurized, whole milk cultured with *Lactobacillus acidophilus.* If you add yeast cells to acidophilus milk, the yeasts will ferment the milk, producing two low-alcohol beverages: *kefir* or *kumiss. Cultured buttermilk* is pasteurized low-fat or skim milk cultured with *Streptococcus lactis.* Sour cream is made either by culturing pasteurized sweet cream with lactic-acid bacteria or by curdling the cream with vinegar. *Yogurt* is milk cultured with *Lactobacilli bulgaricus* and *Streptococcus thermophilus.* Some yogurt also contains *Lactobacillus acidophilus.*

Like meat, fish, poultry, and eggs, cultured milks are a good source of high-quality proteins with sufficient amounts of all the essential amino acids. The primary protein in cultured milks is casein in the milk solids; the whey contains lactalbumin and lactoglobulin.

About half the calories in cultured whole milks come from milk fat, a highly saturated fat. Cultured milks made from whole fresh milk are a significant source of fat, saturated fat, and cholesterol. Cultured milks made from fresh low-fat milk or skim milk are not.

Cultured milk products made from fresh whole milk contain moderate amounts of vitamin A from carotenoids, yellow plant pigments eaten

Fat and Cholesterol Content of Cultured Milks (1 cup/8 ounces)

Milk	Total fat (g)	Saturated fat (g)	Cholesterol (mg)
Buttermilk (lowfat)	2	1.3	10
Sour cream (reduced fat / 1 tablespoon)	1.8	1.1	6
Yogurt, plain, whole milk	8	5.1	32
Yogurt, plain lowfat	3.8	2.5	15
Yogurt, plain, skim milk	0.4	0.3	5

Source: USDA Nutrient Data Laboratory. National Nutrient Database for Standard Reference. Available online. URL: www.nal.usda.gov/fnic/foodcomp/search/.

by milk cows. Because vitamin A is fat-soluble, it is removed when fat is skimmed from milk; low-fat and skim-milk products have less vitamin A than whole-milk products. For example, one cup of plain whole-milk yogurt has 243 IU vitamin A (11 percent of the RDA for a woman, 8 percent of the RDA for a man), while one cup plain lowfat yogurt has 125 IU vitamin A, and one cup plain skim-milk yogurt has only 17 IU vitamin A. Cultured milks made from vitamin D-fortified milk contain vitamin D. All milk products are good sources of B vitamins, and our best source of calcium. One cup of plain yogurt made with low-fat milk has 452 mg/calcium; one cup of non-fat buttermilk, 284 mg.

Flavored yogurt or yogurt with added fruit or preserves, is much higher in sugar and may have small amounts of fiber (from the fruit).

The Most Nutritious Way to Serve This Food

Non-fat products for adults, whole milk products for children. The American Academy of Pediatrics warns against giving children skim-milk products, which may deprive them of fatty acids essential for proper growth.

Diets That May Restrict or Exclude This Food

Controlled cholesterol, controlled saturated fat diet
Lactose intolerance diet
Sugar-free diet (flavored yogurt or yogurt made with sugared fruit)

Buying This Food

Look for: Tightly sealed, refrigerated containers that feel cold to the touch. Check the date on the container to buy the freshest product.

Storing This Food

Refrigerate all cultured milk products. At 40°F, buttermilk will stay fresh for two to three weeks, sour cream for three to four weeks, and yogurt for three to six weeks. Keep the containers tightly closed so the milks do not absorb odors from other foods.

Preparing This Food

Do not "whip" yogurt or sour cream before adding to another dish. The motion will break the curds and make the product watery.

What Happens When You Cook This Food

Cultured milk products are more unstable than plain milks; they separate quickly when heated. Stir them in gently just before serving.

How Other Kinds of Processing Affect This Food

Freezing. Ordinarily, cultured milk products separate easily when frozen. Commercially frozen yogurt contains gelatin and other emulsifiers to make the product creamy and keep it from separating. Freezing inactivates but does not destroy the bacteria in yogurt; if there were live bacteria in the yogurt when it was frozen, they will still be there when it's thawed. Nutritionally, frozen yogurt made from whole milk is similar to ice cream; frozen yogurt made from skim milk is similar to ice milk.

Medical Uses and/or Benefits

Protection against osteoporosis. The most common form of osteoporosis (literally, "bones full of holes") is an age-related loss of bone density most obvious in postmenopausal women. Starting at menopause, women may lose 1 percent a year of their bone density every year until they die. Men also lose bone, but at a slower rate. As a result, women are more likely than men to suffer bone fractures. Six of seven Americans who suffer a broken hip are women.

A life-long diet with adequate amounts of calcium can help stave off bone loss later in life. Current studies and two National Institutes of Health Conferences suggest that postmenopausal women who are not using hormone replacement therapy should get at least 1,500 mg calcium a day, the equivalent of the calcium in slightly more than three cups yogurt made with nonfat milk.

Protection against antibiotic-related illness. Gastric upset, primarily diarrhea, is a common side effect of antibiotic therapy because antibiotics eliminate beneficial bacteria in the gastrointestinal tract along with harmful microorganisms. In 2008, a report in the *British Medical Journal* confirmed earlier studies suggesting that hospitalized patients on antibiotics who were given "probiotic" cultured milks—yogurts containing beneficial microorganisms—had a significantly lower risk of developing antibiotic-related diarrhea. As an example, the following chart lists the microorganisms in the yogurts made and sold under the Dannon brand names.

Product	"Good" Microorganisms in the Yogurt
Activia	*Bifidus* Regularis, *Streptococcus thermophilus, Lactobacillus bulgaricus*
DanActive	*Lactobacillus casei* Immunitas, *Streptococcus thermophilus, Lactobacillus bulgaricus*
Light & Fit	*Lactobacillus acidophilus, Streptococcus thermophilus, Lactobacillus bulgaricus*
Danimals	*Lactobacillus* GG (LGG), *Streptococcus thermophilus, Lactobacillus bulgaricus*

Source: The Dannon Company, Inc.

Reduced risk of hypertension (high blood pressure). In 2008, a team of researchers from Brigham and Women's Hospital and the Harvard School of Public Health report in the American Heart Association journal *Hypertension* that women who consume two or more servings of fat-free milk and milk products a day reduce their risk of high blood pressure by 10 percent, compared to women who consume these products less than once a month. The finding is specific to low-fat milk products; it does not apply to milk products with higher fat content or to calcium and vitamin D supplements.

Adverse Effects Associated with This Food

Increased risk of cardiovascular disease. Like other foods from animals, whole milk is a source of cholesterol and saturated fats that increase the amount of cholesterol circulating in your blood and raise your risk of heart disease. To reduce the risk of heart disease, the National Cholesterol Education Project recommends following the Step I and Step II diets.

The Step I diet provides no more than 30 percent of total daily calories from fat, no more than 10 percent of total daily calories from saturated fat, and no more than 300 mg of cholesterol per day. It is designed for healthy people whose cholesterol is in the range of 200–239 mg/dL.

The Step II diet provides 25–35 percent of total calories from fat, less than 7 percent of total calories from saturated fat, up to 10 percent of total calories from polyunsaturated fat, up to 20 percent of total calories from monounsaturated fat, and less than 300 mg cholesterol per day. This stricter regimen is designed for people who have one or more of the following conditions:

◆ Existing cardiovascular disease
◆ High levels of low-density lipoproteins (LDLs, or "bad" cholesterol) or low levels of high-density lipoproteins (HDLs, or "good" cholesterol)
◆ Obesity
◆ Type 1 diabetes (insulin-dependent diabetes, or diabetes mellitus)
◆ Metabolic syndrome, a.k.a. insulin resistance syndrome, a cluster of risk factors that includes type 2 diabetes (non-insulin-dependent diabetes)

Allergy to milk proteins.   Milk and milk products are among the foods most often implicated as a cause of the classic symptoms of food allergy, upset stomach, hives and angioedema (swelling of the face, lips, and tongue).

Lactose intolerance.   Lactose intolerance is an inherited metabolic deficiency. People who are lactose intolerant lack sufficient amounts of lactase, the intestinal enzyme that breaks lactose into glucose and galactose, its easily digested constituents. Two-thirds of all adults, including 90 to 95 percent of all Asians, 70 to 75 percent of all African Americans, and 6 to 8 percent of northern Europeans are lactose intolerant to some extent. When they drink milk or eat milk products, the lactose remains undigested in their gut, to be fermented by bacteria that produce gas and cause bloating, diarrhea, flatulence, and intestinal discomfort.

However, the *Lactobacillus acidophilus* bacteria added to acidophilus milk and some yogurts digest lactose, converting it to ingredients lactase-deficient people may be able to consume without discomfort.

Lactose Content of Cultured Milk Products vs. Lactose in Whole Fresh Milk

Acidophilus milk	6g/cup
Buttermilk	9g/cup
Yogurt (low-fat)	12g/cup
Whole fresh milk	12g/cup

Source: Briggs, George M., and Calloway, Doris Howes, *Nutrition and Physical Fitness* (Holt, Rinehart & Winston, 1984).

Galactosemia.   Lactose, the sugar in milks, is a disaccharide ("double sugar") made of one molecule of glucose and one molecule of galactose. People with galactosemia, an inherited metabolic disorder, lack the enzymes needed to convert galactose to glucose. Babies born with galactosemia will fail to thrive and may develop brain damage or cataracts if they are given milk. To prevent this, they are kept on a milk-free diet for several years, until their bodies have developed alternative ways by which to metabolize galactose. Pregnant women who are known carriers of galactosemia may be advised to avoid milk while pregnant, lest the unmetabolized galactose in their bodies damage the fetus. Genetic counseling is available to identify galactosemia carriers.

Food/Drug Interactions

Tetracyclines (Declomycin, Minocin, Rondomycin, Terramycin, Vibramycin, et al.).   The calcium ions in milk products bind with tetracyclines to form insoluble compounds your body cannot absorb. Taking tetracyclines with acidophilus milk, buttermilk, sour cream, or yogurt makes the drugs less effective.

Milk, Fresh

(Goat's milk)

See also Milk (cultured).

Nutritional Profile*

Energy value (calories per serving): *Moderate*
Protein: *High*
Fat: *Moderate*
Saturated fat: *High*
Cholesterol: *Moderate*
Carbohydrates: *Moderate*
Fiber: *None*
Sodium: *Moderate*
Major vitamin contribution: *Vitamins A, vitamin D, B vitamins*
Major mineral contribution: *Calcium, iodine*

About the Nutrients in This Food

Like meat, fish, poultry, and eggs, milk is an excellent source of high-quality protein with sufficient amounts of all the essential amino acids. The primary protein in milk is casein in the milk solids; the whey (liquid) contains lactalbumin and lactoglobulin.

About half the calories in whole milk come from milk fat, a highly saturated fat that is lighter than water, rises to the top, and can be skimmed off as cream. Homogenized milk is whole milk that has been processed through machinery that breaks its fat globules into fragments small enough to remain suspended in the liquid rather than floating to the top. Whole milk is high in cholesterol.

Whole milk, which get its creamy color comes from beta-carotene and other yellow pigments in foods eaten by milk cows and goats, is a naturally excellent source of vitamin A. Because vitamin A is fat-soluble, it is lost when milk is skimmed. Low-fat and nonfat milks are fortified with added vitamin A; all fresh cow's milk sold in the United States is fortified with vitamin D. Milk is a good source of B vitamins, including vitamin B_6, a "visible vitamin" whose green pigment is masked by the carotenes in whole milk. When the fat is removed, B_6 gives skimmed milk its greenish blue cast.

---

* Values are for whole milk

Milk is our best source of calcium. Even though some plant foods such as beans have more calcium per ounce, the calcium in plants is bound into insoluble compounds by phytic acids while the calcium in milk is completely available to our bodies. No calcium is lost when milk is skimmed.

Iodine and copper are unexpected bonuses in milk. The iodine comes from supplements given the milk cows and perhaps, from iodates and iodophors used to clean the machinery in milk-processing plants; milk picks up copper from the utensils in which it is pasteurized.

One cup whole milk has eight grams protein, eights gram total fat (4.5 g saturated fat), 24 mg cholesterol, 249 IU vitamin A, and 276 mg calcium.

One cup 1-percent (lowfat) milk with added vitamin A has eight grams protein, 476 IU vitamin A, and 290 mg calcium.

One cup nonfat milk with added vitamin A has eight grams protein, 0.2 g total fat (0.1 g saturated fat), 5 mg cholesterol, 500 IU vitamin A, and 306 mg calcium.

The Most Nutritious Way to Serve This Food

In general, nutrition experts recommend low- or non-fat milk for adults, but whole milk for very young children. In fact, the American Academy of Pediatrics warns specifically that giving infants or very young children low- or non-fat milks deprives them of fatty acids essential for proper growth and development.

Diets That May Restrict or Exclude This Food

Lactose- and galactose-free diet
Low-calcium diet
Low-cholesterol, controlled-fat diet

Buying This Food

Look for: Tightly sealed, dry, refrigerated cartons that feel cold to the touch. Check the date on the carton and pick the latest one you can find.

Storing This Food

Refrigerate fresh milk and cream in tightly closed containers to keep the milk from picking up odors from other foods in the refrigerator. Never leave milk cartons standing at room temperature.

Protect milk from bright light, including direct sunlight, daylight, and fluorescent light, whose energy can "cook" the milk and change its taste by altering the structure of its protein molecules. Light may also destroy riboflavin (vitamin B$_2$) and vitamin B$_6$. Milk stored in glass bottles exposed to direct sunlight may lose as much as 70 percent of its riboflavin in just two hours. Opaque plastic cartons reduce the flow of light into the milk but do not block it completely.

Preparing This Food

Chill, pour, and serve. *Never* pour unused milk or cream back into the original container. Doing that might introduce bacteria that can contaminate all the other milk in the bottle or carton.

What Happens When You Cook This Food

When milk is warmed, its tightly-curled protein molecules relax and unfold, breaking internal bonds (bonds between atoms on the same molecule) and forming new, intermolecular bonds between atoms on neighboring molecules. The newly linked protein molecules create a network with water molecules caught in the net. As the milk cooks, the network tightens, squeezing out the water molecules and forming the lumps we call curds.

Casein, the proteins that combine with calcium to form the "skin" on top of hot milk, will also form curds if you make the milk more acid by adding lemon juice, fruit, vegetables, vinegar, or wine. Whey proteins do not coagulate when you make the milk more acid, but they precipitate (fall to the bottom of the pot) when the milk is heated to a temperature above 170°F. If the bottom of the pot gets hotter, the whey proteins will scorch and the milk will smell burnt.

How Other Kinds of Processing Affect This Food

Freezing. Milk that has been frozen and defrosted has less vitamin C and B vitamins than fresh milk. Freezing also changes the taste and texture of milk. First, it breaks up milk's protein molecules. When the milk is defrosted, they clump together so that the milk no longer tastes perfectly smooth. Second, freezing slows but does not stop the natural oxidation of milk's fat molecules. The longer milk is frozen, the more fat molecules will oxidize and the stronger the milk will taste.

Drying. Dried milk tastes cooked because it has been heated to evaporate its moisture. Unopened packages of dried milk should be stored in a cool, dry cabinet where they may hold their flavor and nutrients for several months. Once dried milk is opened, it should be stored in a tightly closed container to keep out the moisture that will encourage bacterial growth and change the flavor of the milk. Once the dried milk is reconstituted, it should be refrigerated.

Condensed and evaporated milk. Evaporated and condensed milks have been cooked to evaporate moisture; condensed milk has added sugar. Both evaporated and condensed milk have a cooked flavor. They also have less vitamin C and vitamin B_6 than fresh milk.

Unopened cans of condensed or evaporated milk should be stored in a cool, dark cabinet. Unopened cans of evaporated milk will keep for one month at 90°F, one to two years at 70°F, and two years or more at 39°F. At the same temperatures, unopened cans of condensed milk will keep for three months, four to nine months, and two years. Once a can of milk is opened, the milk should be poured into a clean container and refrigerated.

Heat treatments that make milk safer.   Raw (unpasteurized) milk may contain a variety of microorganisms, including pathogenic and harmless bacteria, plus yeasts and molds that are destroyed when the milk is pasteurized (heated to 145°F for 30 minutes or 160°F for 15 seconds). Ultrapasteurized milk has been heated to 280°F for two seconds or more. The higher temperature destroys more microorganisms than pasteurization and prolongs the shelf life of the milk and cream (which must be refrigerated). Ultra-high-temperature sterilization heats the milk to 280°–302°F for two to six seconds. The milk or cream is then packed into presterilized containers and aseptically sealed so that bacteria that might spoil the milk cannot enter. Aseptically packaged milk, which is widely available in Europe, can be stored on an unrefrigerated grocery or kitchen shelf for as long as three months without spoiling or losing any of its vitamins. None of these treatments will protect milk indefinitely, of course. They simply put off the milk's inevitable deterioration by reducing the initial microbial population.

Medical Uses and/or Benefits

Protection against osteoporosis.   The most common form of osteoporosis (literally, "bones full of holes") is an age-related loss of bone density most obvious in postmenopausal women. Starting at menopause, women may lose 1 percent of bone density every year for the rest of their lives. Men also lose bone, but at a slower rate. As a result, women are more likely to suffer bone fractures; six of seven Americans who suffer a broken hip are women.

A lifelong diet with adequate amounts of calcium can help stave off bone loss later in life. Current studies and two National Institutes of Health Conferences suggest that postmenopausal women who are not using hormone replacement therapy should get at least 1,500 mg calcium a day, the amount of calcium in five glasses of nonfat milk.

Reduced risk of hypertension (high blood pressure).   In 2008, a team of researchers from Brigham and Women's Hospital and the Harvard School of Public Health report in the American Heart Association journal *Hypertension* that women who consume two or more servings of fat-free milk and milk products a day reduce their risk of high blood pressure by 10 percent, compared to women who consume these products less than once a month. The finding is specific to low-fat milk products; it does not apply to milk products with higher fat content or to calcium and vitamin D supplements.

Use as contrast medium.   Patients undergoing a CT scan or X-ray of the gastrointestinal tract to diagnose disorders such as Crohn's disease, diverticulitis, or tumors are often given an oral "contrast agent," a barium suspension (barium particles in liquid) that pools in the intestines to outline any abnormalities on the resulting image. A report from researchers at St. Luke's–Roosevelt Hospital Center in New York, published in the May 2008 issue of the *American Journal of Roentgenology* (the journal of the American Roentgen Ray Society), says that giving patients whole milk instead of barium is as effective in showing abnormalities, is less expensive, and leads to fewer adverse effects.

Protection against rickets. Virtually all fresh sweet milk in this country is fortified with vitamin D to prevent the vitamin D–deficiency disease rickets.

Reduce symptoms of PMS. A 1998 study at St. Luke's–Roosevelt Hospital Center in New York City suggests that 1,200 mg calcium supplements a day can alleviate the symptoms of premenstrual syndrome. The study did not measure the effect of calcium from foods.

Adverse Effects Associated with This Food

Increased risk of cardiovascular disease. Like other foods from animals, whole milk is a source of cholesterol and saturated fats that raise your risk of heart disease. To reduce the risk of heart disease, the National Cholesterol Education Project recommends following the Step I and Step II diets.

The Step I diet provides no more than 30 percent of total daily calories from fat, no more than 10 percent of total daily calories from saturated fat, and no more than 300 mg of cholesterol per day. It is designed for healthy people whose cholesterol is in the range of 200–239 mg/dL.

The Step II diet provides 25–35 percent of total calories from fat, less than 7 percent of total calories from saturated fat, up to 10 percent of total calories from polyunsaturated fat, up to 20 percent of total calories from monounsaturated fat, and less than 300 mg cholesterol per day. This stricter regimen is designed for people who have one or more of the following conditions:

- Existing cardiovascular disease
- High levels of low-density lipoproteins (LDLs, or "bad" cholesterol) or low levels of high-density lipoproteins (HDLs, or "good" cholesterol)
- Obesity
- Type 1 diabetes (insulin-dependent diabetes, or diabetes mellitus)
- Metabolic syndrome, a.k.a. insulin resistance syndrome, a cluster of risk factors that includes type 2 diabetes (non-insulin-dependent diabetes)

Lactose intolerance. Lactose intolerance—the inability to digest the sugar in milk—is not an allergy. It is an inherited metabolic deficiency that affects two-thirds of all adults, including 90 to 95 percent of all Asians, 70 to 75 percent of all blacks, and 6 to 8 percent of Caucasians. These people do not have sufficient amounts of lactase, the enzyme that breaks lactose (a disaccharide) into its easily digested components, galactose and glucose. When they drink milk, the undigested sugar is fermented by bacteria in the gut, causing bloating, diarrhea, flatulence, and intestinal discomfort. Some milk is now sold with added lactase to digest the lactose and make the milk usable for lactase-deficient people.

Galactosemia. Lactose, the sugar in milks, is a disaccharide ("double sugar") made of one molecule of glucose and one molecule of galactose. People with galactosemia, an inherited metabolic disorder, lack the enzymes needed to convert galactose to glucose. Babies born with galactosemia will fail to thrive and may develop brain damage or cataracts if they are given milk. To prevent this, they are kept on a milk-free diet for several years, until their bodies have developed alternative ways by which to metabolize galactose. Pregnant women who are known carriers of galactosemia may be advised to avoid milk while pregnant, lest the unmetabolized galactose in their bodies damage the fetus. Genetic counseling is available to identify galactosemia carriers.

Allergic reaction. According to the *Merck Manual,* milk is one of the 12 foods most likely to trigger classic food allergy symptoms: hives, swelling of the lips and eyes, and upset stomach. The others are berries (blackberries, blueberries, raspberries, strawberries), chocolate, corn, eggs, fish, legumes (green peas, lima beans, peanuts, soybeans), nuts, peaches, pork, shellfish, and wheat (see WHEAT CEREALS).

Food poisoning. Raw (unpasteurized) milk may be contaminated with *Salmonella* and/or *Listeria* organisms. Poisoning with *Salmonella* organisms may cause nausea, vomiting, and diarrhea—which can be debilitating and potentially serious in infants, the elderly, and people who are ill. *Listeria* poisoning is a flulike illness that may be particularly hazardous for pregnant women or invalids who are at risk of encephalitis, meningitis, or infections of the bloodstream. *Listeria* may also be found in milk foods made from infected raw milk. *Salmonella* will also grow in pasteurized milk if the milk is not refrigerated.

Food/Drug Interactions

Tetracyclines. The calcium ions in milk bind to tetracyclines, such as Declomycin, Minocin, Rondomycin, Terramycin, and Vibramycin, forming insoluble compounds your body cannot absorb. Taking tetracyclines with milk makes them less effective.

Antacids containing calcium carbonate. People who take calcium carbonate antacids with homogenized milk fortified with vitamin D (which facilitates the absorption of calcium) may end up with milk-alkali syndrome, a potentially serious kidney disorder caused by the accumulation of excessive amounts of calcium in the blood. Milk-alkali syndrome, which is rare, subsides gradually when the patient stops taking either the antacid or the milk.

Mushrooms

Nutritional Profile

Energy value (calories per serving): *Low*
Protein: *High*
Fat: *Low*
Saturated fat: *Low*
Cholesterol: *None*
Carbohydrates: *High*
Fiber: *High*
Sodium: *Low*
Major vitamin contribution: *B vitamins, folate*
Major mineral contribution: *Potassium*

About the Nutrients in This Food

Mushrooms are high in dietary fiber, both insoluble cellulose in the outer skin and pectins in the flesh. They have traces of protein and small amounts of the B vitamin folate.

One-half cup cooked fresh mushrooms has 2 g dietary fiber, 2 g protein, and 14 mcg folate (4 percent of the RDA).

The Most Nutritious Way to Serve This Food

Fresh, in salads.

Diets That May Restrict or Exclude This Food

* * *

Buying This Food

Look for: Smooth, plump, uniformly cream-colored button mushrooms. The cap should be closed tightly, hiding the gills. As mushrooms age, they turn darker; they also lose moisture and shrink, which is why the caps spring open, revealing the pink or tan gills. (Black gills are also an indication of age.) Older mushrooms are more intensely flavored than young ones, but they also have a shorter shelf life. And they also have less sugar than truly fresh mushrooms. By the fourth day after mushrooms are picked, about half their sugar and starch will have turned to chitin, a polymer (a compound with many molecules) similar to cellulose. That is why older mushrooms are "crisper" than fresh ones.

Look for dried mushrooms in tightly sealed packages.

Avoid: Any wild mushrooms. Stick to commercially grown mushrooms from reputable growers.

Storing This Food

Refrigerate fresh mushrooms in containers that allow air to circulate among the mushrooms. The aim is to prevent moisture from collecting on the mushrooms; damp mushrooms deteriorate quickly. Mushrooms should never be stored in plastic bags.

Preparing This Food

Rinse the mushrooms under cold running water and rub them dry with a soft paper towel or scrub them with a soft mushroom brush to remove dirt on the cap.

You can clean mushrooms quickly simply by peeling the cap, but that will make them less tasty. The mushroom's flavor comes from an unusually large amount of glutamic acid in the skin. Glutamic acid is the natural version of the flavor enhancer we know as MSG (monosodium glutamate).

Slicing mushrooms hastens the loss of riboflavin. According to the United Fresh Fruit and Vegetable Association, boiled whole mushrooms may retain as much as 82 percent of their riboflavin, sliced mushrooms only 66 percent. Slicing also changes the color of mushrooms. When you cut the mushroom, you tear its cells, releasing polyphenoloxidase, an enzyme that hastens the oxidation of phenols in the mushroom, producing brownish particles that make the white mushroom dark. You can slow this natural reaction (but not stop it entirely) by coating the mushrooms with an acid—lemon juice, vinegar, or a salad dressing that contains one or the other.

Button mushrooms lose moisture and shrink when you cook them. If you choose to cut off their stems before you cook them, leave a small stub to help the mushroom hold its shape.

Dried mushrooms must be soaked and rinsed as directed on the package.

What Happens When You Cook This Food

The B vitamins in mushrooms are all water-soluble. They will leach out into the cooking water, which should be added to your recipe along with the mushrooms.

Cooking toughens the stem of button mushrooms but does not affect their nutritional value since riboflavin is not destroyed by heat and remains stable in a neutral solution or an acid one such as a tomato sauce or a stew with tomatoes and bell peppers.

How Other Kinds of Processing Affect This Food

Canning. Canned mushrooms with their liquid may contain up to 100 times as much sodium as fresh mushrooms. Riboflavin, the most important nutrient in mushrooms, is not destroyed by heat, but it will leach out into the salty liquid. Riboflavin is sensitive to light; mushrooms in glass jars should be stored in a cool, dark cabinet.

Drying. Dried mushrooms should be sold and stored in a tightly closed package that protects the mushrooms from moisture, and they should be kept in a cool, dark place out of direct sunlight. They should be stored in the refrigerator only if the refrigerator is less humid than the kitchen cabinet. Properly stored dried mushrooms may remain usable for as long as six months. To use dried mushrooms, cover them with boiling water and let them stand for about 15 minutes. Then rinse them thoroughly to get rid of sand and debris in the folds of the mushroom.

Medical Uses and/or Benefits

* * *

Adverse Effects Associated with This Food

Mushroom poisoning. About 100 of the more than 1,000 varieties of mushrooms are poisonous. In the United States, nearly 90 percent of all mushroom poisoning is due to two species of *Amanita* mushrooms, *Amanita muscaria* and *Amanita phalloides*. *Amanita muscaria* contains muscarine, a parasympathetic-nervous-system poison that can cause tearing, salivation, sweating, vomiting, cramps and diarrhea, dizziness, confusion, coma, and convulsions. These symptoms may show up anywhere from a few minutes to two hours after you eat the mushrooms. Muscarine poisoning is potentially fatal. Phalloidin, the toxin in *Amanita phalloide* mushrooms, is a liver poison whose symptoms include all those attributed to muscarine poisoning, plus jaundice from liver damage. These symptoms may not show up until two to three days after you eat the mushrooms. Phalloidin is a potentially lethal poison; the death rate for phalloidin poisoning is 50 percent.

Food/Drug Interactions

False-positive test for occult blood in the stool. The active ingredient in the guaiac slide test for hidden blood in feces is alphaguaiaconic acid, a chemical that turns blue in the presence of blood. Alphaguaiaconic acid also turns blue in the presence of peroxidase, a chemical that occurs naturally in mushrooms. Eating mushrooms in the 72 hours before taking the guaiac test may produce a false-positive result in people who not actually have any blood in their stool.

Alcohol/disulfiram interaction. Disulfiram (Antabuse) is a drug used to treat alcoholism. It causes flushing, difficulty in breathing, nausea, chest pain, vomiting and rapid heart beat if taken with alcohol. Some mushrooms, including the cultivated edible varieties, may contain naturally-occurring disulfiram. If taken with alcohol, these mushrooms may cause symptoms of a disulfiram-alcohol reaction in sensitive individuals. Since disulfiram lingers in your system, the symptoms may appear half an hour after you drink alcohol, even if you ate the mushrooms as much as four or five days ago.

Nuts

(Almonds, Brazil nuts, cashews, chestnuts, macadamias, pecans, pistachios, walnuts)

See also Coconuts, Peanuts, Vegetable oils.

Nutritional Profile

Energy value (calories per serving): *High*
Protein: *Moderate*
Fat: *High*
Saturated fat: *High*
Cholesterol: *None*
Carbohydrates: *Low*
Fiber: *Very high*
Sodium: *Low**
Major vitamin contribution: *Vitamin E, folate*
Major mineral contribution: *Iron, phosphorus*

About the Nutrients in This Food

Nuts are a very high-fiber, high-fat, high-protein food. They have insoluble dietary fiber (cellulose and lignin in the papery "skin") and soluble gums and pectins in the nut. Their oils are composed primarily of unsaturated fatty acids, a good source of vitamin E, but nuts have so much fat that even a small serving is high in saturated fat. Nut's proteins are plentiful but limited in the essential amino acid lysine.

Nuts are an excellent source of B vitamins, particularly folate. Plain raw or roasted nuts are low in sodium; salted nuts are a high-sodium food.

For example, one-half cup dry-roasted unsalted almonds has eight grams dietary fiber, 36 g total fat (2.7 g saturated fat, 23.2 g monounsaturated fat, 8.7 g polyunsaturated fat), 15 g protein, and 23 mcg folate (6 percent of the RDA).

---

* Unsalted nuts. Salted nuts are high in sodium.

Folate Content of ½ Cup Nuts

Nut*	Folate (mcg)	%RDA†
Almonds	44	22–24
Cashew	47.9	24–27
Filberts/hazelnuts	10.6	5–6
Macadamia oil-roasted	10.6	5–6
Pistachios	37.8	19–21
Walnuts black, dried	40.9	20–23

* Dry-roast, unless otherwise noted
† The lower number is for men; the higher, for women

Source: USDA Nutrient Database: www.nal.usda.gov/fnic/cgi-bin/nut_search.pl, *Nutritive Value of Foods,* Home and Garden Bulletin No. 72 (USDA, 1989).

The Most Nutritious Way to Serve This Food

With peanuts or with beans. Both are legumes, which provide the essential amino acid lysine needed to "complete" the proteins in nuts. Adding raisins adds iron.

Diets That May Restrict or Exclude This Food

Antiflatulence diet
Low-calcium diet
Low-fat diet
Low-fiber, low-residue diet
Low-oxalate diet (for people who form calcium oxalate kidney stones; almonds and cashews)
Low-protein diet
Low-sodium diet (salted nuts)

Buying This Food

Look for: Fresh nuts with clean, undamaged shells. The nuts should feel heavy for their size; nuts that feel light may be withered inside.

Choose crisp, fresh shelled nuts. They should taste fresh and snap when you bite into them. As nuts age, their oils oxidize and become rancid; old nuts will have an "off" flavor. If nuts sold in bulk are exposed to air, heat, and light, their fats will oxidize more quickly than the fats in packaged nuts. Check the date on the bottom of the can or jar to be sure packaged nuts are fresh.

Avoid: Moldy, shriveled, or discolored nuts. The molds that grow on nuts may produce potentially carcinogenic aflatoxins that have been linked to liver cancer.

Storing This Food

Store nuts in a cool, dry, dark place in a container that protects them from the air, heat, light, and moisture. The unsaturated fats in nuts are very sensitive to oxygen. When nuts are exposed to air, the fat molecules link up with oxygen atoms, and the nuts "spoil"—turn rancid. Protecting nuts from air, heat, and light slows the rancidity reaction.

Pack nuts in a moistureproof container and store them in the freezer if you don't plan to use them right away. The cold will slow down the oxidation of fats and the nuts will stay fresh longer. For example, shelled pecans stay fresh up to one year in the freezer against about two months on a cool, dark kitchen shelf.

Check the nuts occasionally; throw out any moldy nuts or any that have shriveled.

Do not shell nuts until you are ready to use them. The shell is a natural protective shield.

Preparing This Food

Almonds.   To peel shelled almonds, boil the nuts, drain them, and plunge them into cold water. The skin should slip off easily.

Brazil nuts.   Brazil nuts are easy to open if you chill them first. To slice shelled Brazil nuts, boil the nuts in water for five minutes, then cool and slice. Or you can shave them into slivers with a potato peeler.

Cashews.   Always cook raw cashews before you shell them. Between the shell and the raw nut is a thin layer of urushiol, the irritating oil also found in poison oak and poison ivy. The oil is inactivated by heat.

Chestnuts.   Slice an X in the flat end of the chestnut and peel off the heavy outer skin. To remove the thin inner skin, bake the chestnuts on a cookie sheet in a 400°F oven for about twenty minutes or cover them with boiling water and simmer them for fifteen minutes. Then drain the nuts and slip off the skins.

Macadamia nuts.   To open macadamia nuts, wrap them, one at a time, in a heavy cloth napkin or towel, put the package on a wooden breadboard, and hit the nut with a hammer.

Pecans and walnuts.   Crack the nut with a nutcracker.

Pistachios.   Open the nuts with your fingers, not your teeth.

What Happens When You Cook This Food

* * *

How Other Kinds of Processing Affect This Food

Vacuum packaging.   Canned nuts and nuts in glass jars stay fresh longer than nuts sold in bulk because they are protected from the oxygen that combines with oils and turns them rancid. Nuts in sealed cans and jars may stay fresh for as long as a year if stored in a cool, dark place. Once the can or jar is opened, the oils will begin to oxidize and eventually become rancid.

Medical Uses and/or Benefits

Lower risk of some birth defects. As many as two of every 1,000 babies born in the United States each year may have cleft palate or a neural tube (spinal cord) defect due to their mothers' not having gotten adequate amounts of folate during pregnancy. The current RDA for folate is 180 mcg for a woman and 200 mcg for a man, but the FDA now recommends 400 mcg for a woman who is or may become pregnant. Taking folate supplements before becoming pregnant and continuing through the first two months of pregnancy reduces the risk of cleft palate; taking folate through the entire pregnancy reduces the risk of neural tube defects.

Lower levels of cholesterol. Although nuts are high in fat, they are low in saturated fat and, as plant foods, have no cholesterol at all. Several recent studies have shown that eating nuts lowers blood levels of cholesterol and low-density lipoproteins (LDLs, or "bad" cholesterol) while raising blood levels of high-density lipoproteins (HDLs, or "good" cholesterol).

At Loma Linda University (California), volunteers with mildly elevated cholesterol levels were given two diets. First they tried the American Heart Association (AHA) Step I diet, the low-fat, controlled-cholesterol regimen generally used as a first step in reducing cholesterol levels. Then, they got the same diet with one small adjustment: 20 percent of its daily calories came from a handful of nuts (almonds, pecans, or walnuts) mixed into cereals, salads, and entries such as pasta. The result: While the AHA Step I diet lowered total cholesterol 5.2 percent, when volunteers added nuts their cholesterol levels fell as much as 11.3 percent. Even better, while LDLs dropped 6.1 percent on the AHA diet, they fell a whopping 16.5 percent with pecans. This is significant because the National Cholesterol Education Program estimates that your risk of heart attack declines 1.5 percent for every 1 percent drop in LDLs. Loma Linda researchers had similar results with the diets that included almonds or walnuts.

Adverse Effects Associated with This Food

Allergic reaction. According to the *Merck Manual,* nuts are one of the 12 foods most likely to trigger classic food allergy symptoms: hives, swelling of the lips and eyes, and upset stomach. The others are berries (blackberries, blueberries, raspberries, strawberries), chocolate, corn, eggs, fish, legumes (green peas, lima beans, peanuts, soybeans), milk, peaches, pork, shellfish, and wheat (see WHEAT CEREALS).

Flare-up of aphthous ulcers (canker sores). Eating nuts may trigger an episode of canker sores in susceptible people, but avoiding nuts will not prevent or cure an attack.

Food/Drug Interactions

False-positive urine test for carcinoid syndrome. Carcinoid tumors, which may arise from the tissues of the endocrine or gastrointestinal systems, secrete serotonin, a nitrogen compound that makes blood vessels expand or contract. The test for these tumors measures the amount of serotonin in the blood. Eating walnuts, which are high in serotonin, in the 72 hours before taking the test for a carcinoid tumor may cause a false-positive result, suggesting that you have the tumor when in fact you do not. (Other foods high in serotonin are avocados, bananas, eggplant, plums, pineapple, and tomatoes.)

Oats (Oatmeal)

See also Wheat cereals.

Nutritional Profile

Energy value (calories per serving): *Moderate*
Protein: *Moderate*
Fat: *Low*
Saturated fat: *Low*
Cholesterol: *None*
Carbohydrates: *High*
Fiber: *High*
Sodium: *Low*
Major vitamin contribution: *B vitamins*
Major mineral contribution: *Iron, potassium*

About the Nutrients in This Food

What we call *oats* is actually oatmeal, oats that have been rolled (ground) into a meal, then steamed to break down some of their starches, formed into flakes, and dried. Steel-cut oats have been ground in a special steel machine; oat flour is finely ground oatmeal.

Unlike cows and other ruminants, human beings cannot break through the cellulose and lignin covering on raw grain to reach the nutrients inside. Cooking unprocessed oats to the point where they are useful to human beings can take as long as 24 hours. The virtue of rolled oats is that they have been precooked and can be prepared in five minutes or less. Instant oatmeals, like other "instant" cereals, are treated with phosphates to allow them to absorb water more quickly.

Oatmeal is a high-carbohydrate food, rich in starch and high in dietary fiber, with insoluble cellulose and lignin in the bran and soluble gums (such as the beta-glucans that gives cooked oatmeal its characteristic sticky texture) in the grain.

The proteins in oats are limited in the essential amino acid lysine. Oats have up to five times as much fat as rye and wheat plus an enzyme that speeds the oxidation of fats. Rolling and steaming oats to make oatmeal inactivates the enzyme and retards rancidity.

Oatmeal is a good source of nonheme iron, the form of iron found in plants. Plain uncooked oatmeal has no sodium, but water in which it is cooked may make the finished cereal a high-sodium food.

One-half cup plain oatmeal has two grams dietary fiber, one gram fat (0.2 g saturated fat), and 0.79 mg iron (5.3 percent of the RDA for a woman of childbearing age).

The Most Nutritious Way to Serve This Food

With a low-fat source of high-quality protein, such as low-fat milk, low- or nonfat cheese.

Diets That May Restrict or Exclude This Food

Gluten-restricted, gliadin-free diet
Low-carbohydrate diet
Low-fiber, low-residue diet
Low-sodium diet

Buying This Food

Look for: Tightly sealed boxes or canisters.

Avoid: Bulk cereals; grains in open bins may be exposed to moisture, mold, and insect contamination.

Storing This Food

Keep oats in air- and moistureproof containers to protect them from potentially toxic fungi that grow on damp grains. Properly stored and dry, rolled oats may keep for as long as a year. Whole-grain oats (oats with the outer fatty covering) may oxidize and become rancid more quickly.

Preparing This Food

* * *

What Happens When You Cook This Food

Starch consists of molecules of the complex carbohydrates amylose and amylopectin packed into a starch granule. As you heat oatmeal in liquid, its starch granules absorb water molecules, swell, and soften. When the temperature of the liquid reaches approximately 140°F, the amylose and amylopectin molecules inside the granules relax and unfold, breaking some of their internal bonds (bonds between atoms on the same molecule) and forming new bonds between atoms on different molecules. The result is a network that traps and holds water molecules, making the starch granules even more bulky and thickening the liquid. Eventually the starch granules rupture, releasing the nutrients inside so that they can be absorbed more easily by the body. Oatmeal also contains hydrophilic (water-loving) gums and pectins, including beta-glucans, that attract and hold water molecules, immobilizing them so that the liquid thickens. The beta-glucans give oatmeal its characteristic sticky texture.

Ounce for ounce, cooked oatmeal has smaller amounts of vitamins and minerals than dry oatmeal simply because so much of its weight is now water. The single exception is sodium. Plain, uncooked oatmeal, with no additives, has no sodium; cooked oatmeal, made with water or milk, does.

How Other Kinds of Processing Affect This Food

* * *

Medical Uses and/or Benefits

A lower risk of some kinds of cancer. In 1998, scientists at Wayne State University in Detroit conducted a meta-analysis of data from more than 30 well-designed animal studies measuring the anti-cancer effects of wheat bran, the part of grain with highest amount of the insoluble dietary fibers cellulose and lignin. They found a 32 percent reduction in the risk of colon cancer among animals fed wheat bran; now they plan to conduct a similar meta-analysis of human studies. Like wheat bran, whole oats are a good source of insoluble dietary fiber. NOTE: The amount of fiber per serving listed on a food package label shows the total amount of fiber (insoluble and soluble).

Early in 1999, however, new data from the long-running Nurses Health Study at Brigham Women's Hospital/Harvard University School of Public Health showed that women who ate a high-fiber diet had a risk of colon cancer similar to that of women who ate a low fiber diet. Because this study contradicts literally hundreds of others conducted over the past thirty years, researchers are awaiting confirming evidence before changing dietary recommendations.

However, early the following year, new data from the long-running Nurses' Health Study at Harvard School of Public Health and Brigham and Women's Hospital, in Boston, showed no difference in the risk of colon cancer between women who ate a high-fiber diet and those who did not. Nonetheless, many nutrition researchers remain wary of ruling out a protective effect for dietary fiber. They note that there are different kinds of dietary fiber that may have different effects, that most Americans do not consume a diet with the recommended amount of dietary fiber, and that gender, genetics, and various personal health issues may also affect the link between dietary fiber and the risk of colon cancer.

NOTE: The current recommendations for dietary fiber consumption are 25 grams per day for women younger than 50, and 21 grams per day for women older than 50; 38 grams per day for men younger than 50, and 30 grams per day for men older than 50.

To reduce cholesterol levels in the blood. Foods high in soluble gums and pectins appear to lower the amount of cholesterol and low-density lipoproteins (LDLs), the particles that carry cholesterol into your arteries, in your blood, a task beta-glucans performs more effectively than any other soluble fiber. There are currently two theories to explain how soluble fibers work. The first is that the pectins in the oats may form a gel in your stomach that sops up fats keep them from being absorbed by your body. The second is that bacteria in the gut may feed on the fiber in the oats and produce short chain fatty acids that inhibit the production of cholesterol in your liver.

A 1990 study at the University of Kentucky showed that adding $1/2$ cup oat bran (measured when dry) to you daily diet can reduce levels of LDLs by as much as 25 percent. A second study, with 220 healthy people, at the Medical School of Northwestern University, showed that people with cholesterol levels of 200 mg/dL could reduce total cholesterol an average 9.3 percent by following a low-fat, low-cholesterol diet supplemented by two ounces of oats or oat bran. The oats were given credit for about one-third of the drop in cholesterol levels; the rest went to the low-fat, low-cholesterol diet.

In 1997, the Food and Drug Administration approved the use on labels of health claims for oats such as: "Soluble fiber from foods such as oat bran, as part of a diet low in saturated fat and cholesterol, may reduce the risk of heart disease."

Calming effect. Your mood is affected by naturally occurring chemicals called neurotransmitters that allow cells in your brain to transmit impulses from one to the other. Tryptophan, an amino acid, is the most important constituent of serotonin, a "calming" neurotransmitter. Foods such as oatmeal, which are high in complex carbohydrates, may help move tryptophan into your brain, increasing your ability to use serotonin.

As a source of carbohydrates for people with diabetes. Cereal grains are digested very slowly, producing only a gradual rise in the level of sugar in the blood. As a result, the body needs less insulin to control blood sugar after eating plain, unadorned cereal grains than after eating some other high-carbohydrate foods (bread or potato). In studies at the University of Kentucky, a whole-grain, bean, vegetable, and fruit-rich diet developed at the University of Toronto and recommended by the American Diabetes Association enabled patients with type 1 diabetes (who do not produce any insulin themselves), to cut their daily insulin intake by 38 percent. For patients with type 2 diabetes (who can produce some insulin), the bean diet reduced the need for injected insulin by 98 percent. This diet is in line with the nutritional guidelines of the American Diabetes Association, but people with diabetes should always check with their doctor and/or dietitian before altering their diet.

Adverse Effects Associated with This Food

Gliadin intolerance. Celiac disease is an intestinal allergic disorder whose victims are sensitive to gluten and gliadin, proteins in wheat and rye. People with celiac disease cannot digest the nutrients in these grains; if they eat foods containing gluten, they may suffer anemia, weight loss, bone pain, swelling, and skin disorders. Oats contain small amounts of gliadin. Corn flour, potato flour, rice flour, and soy flour are all gluten- and gliadin-free.

Food/Drug Interactions

* * *

Okra

Nutritional Profile

Energy value (calories per serving): *Low*
Protein: *High*
Fat: *Low*
Saturated fat: *Low*
Cholesterol: *None*
Carbohydrates: *High*
Fiber: *High*
Sodium: *Low*
Major vitamin contribution: *Vitamin A, folate, vitamin C*
Major mineral contribution: *Potassium*

About the Nutrients in This Food

Okra, the vegetable, is the unripe seed capsule of the okra plant, a starchy food high in soluble dietary fiber. It is a good source of vitamin A from deep yellow carotenes (plant pigments) hidden under its green chlorophyll, the B vitamin folate and vitamin C.

A serving of eight cooked okra pods has two grams dietary fiber, 241 IU vitamin A (10 percent of the RDA for a woman, 8 percent of the RDA for a man), 39 mcg folate (10 percent of the RDA), and 13.9 mg vitamin C (19 percent of the RDA for a woman, 15 percent of the RDA for a man).

The Most Nutritious Way to Serve This Food

In a soup or stew.

Diets That May Restrict or Exclude This Food

* * *

Buying This Food

Look for: Young, green tender pods of okra no more than 4 inches long.

Storing This Food

Keep okra in the refrigerator.

Preparing This Food

Wash the okra under cold running water, then use it whole or sliced thickly.

What Happens When You Cook This Food

When okra is heated in water, its starch granules absorb water molecules and swell. Eventually, they rupture, releasing amylose and amylopectin molecules as well as gums and pectic substances, all of which attract and immobilize water molecules, thickening the soup or stew.

How Other Kinds of Processing Affect This Food

Canning and freezing. Canned and frozen okra have less vitamin C per serving than fresh okra.

Medical Uses and/or Benefits

Lower risk of some birth defects. As many as two of every 1,000 babies born in the United States each year may have cleft palate or a neural tube (spinal cord) defect due to their mothers' not having gotten adequate amounts of folate during pregnancy. The current RDA for folate is 180 mcg for a woman and 200 mcg for a man, but the FDA now recommends 400 mcg for a woman who is or may become pregnant. Taking folate supplements before becoming pregnant and continuing through the first two months of pregnancy reduces the risk of cleft palate; taking folate through the entire pregnancy reduces the risk of neural tube defects.

Possible lower risk of heart attack. In the spring of 1998, an analysis of data from the records for more than 80,000 women enrolled in the long-running Nurses' Health Study at Harvard School of Public Health/Brigham and Women's Hospital, in Boston, demonstrated that a diet providing more than 400 mcg folate and 3 mg vitamin B_6 daily, either from food or supplements, might reduce a woman's risk of heart attack by almost 50 percent. Although men were not included in the study, the results were assumed to apply to them as well.

However, data from a meta-analysis published in the *Journal of the American Medical Association* in December 2006 called this theory into question. Researchers at Tulane University examined the results of 12 controlled studies in which 16,958 patients with preexisting cardiovascular disease were given either folic acid supplements or placebos ("look-alike" pills with no folic acid) for at least six months. The scientists, who found no reduction in the risk of further heart disease or overall death rates among those taking folic acid, concluded that further studies will be required to prove that taking folic acid supplements reduces the risk of cardiovascular disease.

To reduce the levels of serum cholesterol.   Eating foods rich in gums and pectins appears to lower the levels of serum cholesterol. There are currently two theories to explain how this may happen. The first theory is that the pectins form a gel in your stomach that sops up fats and keeps them from being absorbed by your body. The second is that bacteria in the gut feed on the gums and pectins, producing short-chain fatty acids that inhibit the production of cholesterol in your liver.

Adverse Effects Associated with This Food

* * *

Food/Drug Interactions

* * *

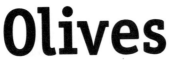

Olives

See also Vegetable oils.

Nutritional Profile

Energy value (calories per serving): *Moderate*
Protein: *Low*
Fat: *High*
Saturated fat: *Low*
Cholesterol: *None*
Carbohydrates: *Low*
Fiber: *High*
Sodium: *High*
Major vitamin contribution: *Vitamin E*
Major mineral contribution: *Iron*

About the Nutrients in This Food

Olives come in two basic colors, green and black. The green are picked before they ripen; the black are picked ripe and dipped in an iron solution to stabilize their color. After harvesting, all green olives and most black olives are soaked in a mild solution of sodium hydroxide, then washed thoroughly in water to rid them of oleuropein, a naturally bitter carbohydrate. (The exceptions are salt-cured black Greek and Italian olives, which retain their oleuropein.) Green olives are sometimes fermented before being packed in brine; black olives aren't, which is why they taste milder.

Greek and Italian olives are black olives that taste sharp because they have not been soaked to remove their oleuropein. They are salt-cured and sold in bulk, covered with olive oil that protects them from oxygen and helps preserve them.

Olives are a high-fiber, high-fat food that derive 69 to 78 percent of their calories from olive oil, a predominantly unsaturated fat.

A serving of five olives, green or black, weighing 19 to 22 g, has 2 g fat (0.3 g saturated fat). A serving of ripe olives has one gram dietary fiber; green olives, less than one gram.

The Most Nutritious Way to Serve This Food

Plain olives have less sodium than salt-cured olives.

Diets That May Restrict or Exclude This Food

Low-fat diet
Low-sodium diet

Buying This Food

Look for: Tightly sealed bottles or cans. Small olives are less woody than large ones. Green olives have a more astringent taste than black olives. Greek olives, available only in bulk, have a sharp, spicy taste. Pitted olives are the best buy if you want to slice the olives into a salad, otherwise olives with pits are less-expensive and a better buy.

Storing This Food

Store unopened cans or jars of olives on a cool, dry shelf. Once you open a can of olives, take the olives out of the can and refrigerate them in a clean glass container.

Preparing This Food

Olives will taste less salty if you bathe them in olive oil before you use them.

What Happens When You Cook This Food

* * *

How Other Kinds of Processing Affect This Food

Pressing. Olives are pressed to produce olive oil, one of the few vegetable oils with a distinctive flavor and aroma. Olive oils are graded according to the pressing from which they come and the amount of free oleic acid they contain. (The presence of free oleic acid means that the oil's molecules have begun to break down.) Virgin olive oil is oil from the first pressing of the olives. Pure olive oil is a mixture of oils from the first and second pressings. Virgin olive oil may contain as much as 4 percent free oleic acid. Fine virgin olive oil may contain 3 percent free oleic acid, superfine virgin olive oil 1.5 percent, and extra virgin olive oil 1 percent.

Olive oil is a more concentrated source of alpha-tocopherol (vitamin E) than olives. Because it is high in unsaturated fatty acids, whose carbon atoms have double bonds that can make room for more oxygen atoms, olive oil oxidizes and turns rancid fairly quickly if exposed to heat or light. To protect the oil, store it in a cool, dark cabinet.

Medical Uses and/or Benefits

Lower levels of low-density lipoproteins (LDLs). Olive oil is 95 percent monounsaturated fatty acids, fats that reduce blood levels of LDLs that carry cholesterol into your arteries.

Adverse Effects Associated with This Food

* * *

Food/Drug Interactions

* * *

Onions

(Chives, leeks, scallions [green onions], shallots)

See also Garlic.

Nutritional Profile

Energy value (calories per serving): *Low*
Protein: *Moderate*
Fat: *Low*
Saturated fat: *Low*
Cholesterol: *None*
Carbohydrates: *High*
Fiber: *Moderate*
Sodium: *Low*
Major vitamin contribution: *Folate, vitamin C*
Major mineral contribution: *Calcium, iron*

About the Nutrients in This Food

All onions are high in dietary fiber and a good source of the B vitamin folate and vitamin C. Immature onions—known as *scallions,* if they are picked before the bulbs have fully developed, or *green onions* or *spring onions,* if they are picked with large bulbs—have moderate amounts of vitamin A derived from deep yellow carotenes masked by green chlorophyll pigments in the green tops. Red onions are colored with red anthocyanins; shallots, yellow onions, white onions, and the white bulbs of the leeks, green onions, ramps [wild leeks], and scallions are colored with creamy pale yellow anthoxan-thins. Neither anthocyanin nor anthoaxanthins provide vitamin A.

One-half cup chopped white or yellow onion has 1.4 g dietary fiber and 5.9 mg vitamin C (13 percent of the RDA for a woman, 14 percent of the RDA for a man).

One-half cup chopped green onions, a.k.a. scallions (bulb and leaves), has 1.3 g dietary fiber, 498 IU vitamin A (22 percent of the RDA for a woman, 17 percent of the RDA for a man), and 9.4 mg vitamin C (13 percent of the RDA for a woman, 10 percent of the RDA for a man).

The Most Nutritious Way to Serve This Food

Whole fresh green onions or green onions chopped (green portions and all) and added to a salad or other dish.

Diets That May Restrict or Exclude This Food

Antiflatulence diet
Low-fiber diet

Buying This Food

Look for: Firm, clean shallots; yellow, white, or red onions with smooth, dry, crisp skin free of any black mold spots. Leeks and green onions should have crisp green tops and clean white bulbs.

Avoid: Onions that are sprouting or soft or whose skin is wet—all signs of internal decay.

Storing This Food

Store shallots and red, yellow, and white onions in a cool cabinet room or root cellar where the temperature is 60°F or lower and there is plenty of circulating air to keep the onions dry and prevent them from sprouting. Properly stored, onions should stay fresh for three to four weeks; at 55°F they may retain all their vitamin C for as long as six months.

Cut the roots from green onions, scallions, and leeks; trim off any damaged tops; and refrigerate the vegetables in a tightly closed plastic bag. Check daily and remove tops that have wilted.

Preparing This Food

When you cut into an onion, you tear its cell walls and release a sulfur compound called pro-panethial-S-oxide that floats up into the air. The chemical, identified in 1985 by researchers at the University of St. Louis (Missouri), turns into sulfuric acid when it comes into contact with water, which is why it stings if it gets into your eyes. You can prevent this by slicing fresh onions under running water, diluting the propanethial-S-oxide before it can float up into the air.

Another way to inactivate propanethial-S-oxide is to chill the onion in the refrigerator for an hour or so before you slice it. The cold temperature slows the movement of the atoms in the sulfur compound so that they do not float up into the air around your eyes.

To peel the brown papery outer skin from an onion or a shallot, heat the vegetable in boiling water, then lift it out with a slotted spoon and put it in cold water. The skin should come off easily.

What Happens When You Cook This Food

Heat converts an onion's sulfurous flavor and aroma compounds into sugars, which is why cooked onions taste sweet. When you "brown" onions, the sugars and amino acids on their surface caramelize to a deep rich brown and the flavor intensifies. This browning of sugars and amino acids is called the Maillard reaction, after the French chemist who first identified it.

Onions may also change color when cooked. Onions get their creamy color from anthoxanthins, pale-yellow pigments that turn brown if they combine with metal ions. (That's why onions discolor if you cook them in an aluminum or iron pot or slice them with a carbon-steel knife.) Red onions contain anthocyanin pigments that turn redder in acid (lemon juice, vinegar) and bluish in a basic (alkaline) solution. And the chlorophyll molecules that make the tops of green onions green are sensitive to acids. When heated, chlorophyll reacts with acids in the vegetable or in the cooking water to produce pheophytin, which is brown. The pheophytin makes green onion tops olive-drab. To keep green onions green, you have to reduce the interaction between the chlorophyll and the acids. You can do this by leaving the top off the pot so that the acids float off into the air or by steaming the onions in little or no water or by cooking them so quickly that there is no time for the reaction to occur.

How Other Kinds of Processing Affect This Food

Drying. Drying onions into flakes removes the moisture and concentrate the nutrients. Ounce for ounce, dried onions have approximately nine times the vitamin C, eight times the thiamin, ten times the riboflavin, nine times the niacin, five times the iron, and eleven times as much potassium as fresh onions.

Medical Uses and/or Benefits

* * *

Adverse Effects Associated with This Food

Halitosis.   The onion's sulfur compounds can leave a penetrating odor on your breath unless you brush after eating. Fresh onions are smellier than cooked ones, since cooking breaks down the sulfur compounds.

Food/Drug Interactions

Anticoagulants Green Onions are rich in vitamin K, the blood-clotting vitamin produced naturally by bacteria in the intestines. Consuming large quantities of this food may reduce the effectiveness of anticoagulants (blood thinners) such as warfarin (Coumadin). One chopped, raw green onion (top and bulbs) contains 207 mcg vitamin K, more than three times the RDA for a healthy adult.

Oranges

Nutritional Profile

Energy value (calories per serving): *Low*
Protein: *Low*
Fat: *Low*
Saturated fat: *Low*
Cholesterol: *None*
Carbohydrates: *High*
Fiber: *High*
Sodium: *Low*
Major vitamin contribution: *Folate, vitamin C*
Major mineral contribution: *Potassium*

About the Nutrients in This Food

Oranges are high in sugars and soluble dietary fiber (pectins), one of the best sources of vitamin C, which is concentrated in the white tissue just under the skin, and an excellent source of the B vitamin folate.

One cup fresh orange juice (with pulp) has 0.5 g dietary fiber, 74 mcg folate (19 percent of the RDA), 124 mg vitamin C (1.5 times the RDA for a woman, 1.4 times the RDA for a man), and 496 mg potassium.

One small orange, 2.4-inch diameter, has 2.3 g dietary fiber, 29 mcg folate (7 percent of the RDA), 51 mg vitamin C (68 percent of the RDA for a woman, 57 percent of the RDA for a man), and 178 mg potassium.

The Most Nutritious Way to Serve This Food

Freshly sliced, quartered, or squeezed.

Diets That May Restrict or Exclude This Food

* * *

Buying This Food

Look for: Firm fruit that is heavy for its size; the heavier the orange, the juicier it is likely to be. The skin on juice oranges (Valencias from Florida) should be thin, smooth, and fine-grained. The skin on navel oranges, the large seedless "eating orange," is thicker; it comes off easily when you peel the orange.*

Storing This Food

Refrigerate oranges if you plan to keep them for longer than a week or two.

Refrigerate fresh orange juice in a tightly closed glass bottle. The key to preserving vitamin C is to protect the juice from heat and air (which might seep in through plastic bottles). The juice should fill the bottle as high as possible, so that there is very little space at the top for oxygen to gather. Stored this way, the juice may hold its vitamin C for two weeks. Frozen juice should be kept frozen until you are ready to use it; once reconstituted, it should be handled like fresh juice.

Preparing This Food

Oranges may be waxed to prevent moisture loss and protect them in shipping. If you plan to grate orange rind and use it for flavoring, scrub the orange first to remove the wax. Do not grate deeper than the colored part of the skin; if you hit the white underneath, you will be getting bitter-tasting components in with the rind.

Orange peel contains volatile fragrant oils whose molecules are liberated when the skin is torn and its cell walls ruptured. These molecules are also more fragrant at room temperature than when cold. "Eating oranges" have a much truer aroma and flavor if you let them come to room temperature before peeling and serving.

What Happens When You Cook This Food

Heat destroys the vitamin C but not the flavoring oils in an orange. When oranges or orange peel are cooked, they add flavor but no noticeable amounts of vitamin C.

How Other Kinds of Processing Affect This Food

Commercially prepared juices. How well a commercial orange juice holds its vitamin C depends on how it is prepared, stored, and packaged. Sealed cans of orange juice stored in

---

* Oranges look most appetizing when they are a deep, vibrant orange, but on the tree a mature orange is usually green-skinned. It will turn orange only if it is chilled and the cold temperature destroys green chlorophyll pigments, allowing the yellow carotenoids underneath to show through. In a warm climate, like the Mideast, oranges are always green, but in the United States oranges are green only if they are picked in the fall before the first cold snap or if they are picked early in the spring when the tree is flooded with chlorophyll to nourish the coming new growth. Green oranges will also change color if they are exposed to ethylene gas which, like cold, breaks down the chlorophyll in the orange's skin. (Ethylene is a natural chemical found in all fruits that encourages them to ripen.) Oranges may also be dyed with food coloring.

the refrigerator may lose only 2 percent of their vitamin C in three months. Prepared, pasteurized "fresh" juices in glass bottles hold their vitamin C better than the same juice sold in plastic bottles or waxed paper cartons that let oxygen pass through. Oranges are not a natural source of calcium, but some orange juices are calcium-fortified.

Canned oranges and orange juice retain most of their vitamin C. As soon as the can is opened, the oranges or juice should be removed and transferred to a glass containers to prevent the fruit or juice from absorbing lead used to seal the can. The absorption of lead is triggered by oxygen, which enters the can when the seal is broken. No lead is absorbed while the can is intact.

Since 2000, following several deaths attributed to unpasteurized apple juice contaminated with *E. coli* O157:H7, the FDA has required that all juices sold in the United States be pasteurized to inactivate harmful organisms such as bacteria and mold.

Drying. Orange peel may be dried for use as a candy or flavoring. Dried orange peel may be treated with sulfites (sodium sulfite, sodium bisulfite, and the like) to keep it from darkening. In sensitive people, sulfites can trigger serious allergic reactions, including potentially fatal anaphylactic shock.

Medical Uses and/or Benefits

Lower cholesterol levels. Oranges are high in pectin, which appears to slow the body's absorption of fats and lower cholesterol levels. There are currently two theories about how this happens. The first is that the pectins dissolve into a gel that sops up fats in your stomach so that your body cannot absorb them. The second is that bacteria in the gut digest the fiber and then produce short chain fatty acids that slow down the liver's natural production of cholesterol.

Possible lower risk of heart attack. In the spring of 1998, an analysis of data from the records for more than 80,000 women enrolled in the long-running Nurses' Health Study at Harvard School of Public Health/Brigham and Women's Hospital, in Boston, demonstrated that a diet providing more than 400 mcg folate and 3 mg vitamin B6 daily, either from food or supplements, might reduce a woman's risk of heart attack by almost 50 percent. Although men were not included in the study, the results were assumed to apply to them as well.

However, data from a meta-analysis published in the *Journal of the American Medical Association* in December 2006 called this theory into question. Researchers at Tulane University examined the results of 12 controlled studies in which 16,958 patients with preexisting cardiovascular disease were given either folic acid supplements or placebos ("look-alike" pills with no folic acid) for at least six months. The scientists, who found no reduction in the risk of further heart disease or overall death rates among those taking folic acid, concluded that further studies will be required to determine whether taking folic acid supplements reduces the risk of cardiovascular disease.

Lower risk of stroke. Various nutrition studies have attested to the power of adequate potassium to keep blood pressure within safe levels. For example, in the 1990s, data from the long-running Harvard School of Public Health/Health Professionals Follow-Up Study of male doctors showed that a diet rich in high-potassium foods such as bananas, oranges, and plantain may reduce the risk of stroke. In the study, the men who ate the higher number of potassium-rich foods (an average of nine servings a day) had a risk of stroke 38 percent lower than that of men who consumed fewer than four servings a day. In 2008, a similar survey at the Queen's Medical Center (Honolulu) showed a similar protective effect among men and women using diuretic drugs (medicines that increase urination and thus the loss of potassium).

Protection against some cancers.   According to the American Cancer Society, a diet high in foods rich in antioxidant vitamin C may reduce your risk of some cancers, such as cancer of the respiratory tract. In addition, oranges contain D-limonene, an aromatic compound found in citrus oils. D-limonene is a monoterpene, a member of a family of chemicals that appears to reduce the risk of some cancers, perhaps by preventing the formation of carcinogens in your body or by blocking carcinogens from reaching or reacting with sensitive body tissues or by inhibiting the transformation of healthy cells to malignant ones.

Lower risk of some birth defects.   Up to two of every 1,000 babies born in the United States each year may have cleft palate or a neural tube (spinal cord) defect due to their mothers' not having gotten adequate amounts of folate during pregnancy. The current RDA for folate is 180 mcg for a woman and 200 mcg for a man, but the FDA now recommends 400 mcg for a woman who is or may become pregnant. Taking a folate supplement before becoming pregnant and through the first two months of pregnancy reduces the risk of cleft palate; taking folate through the entire pregnancy reduces the risk of neural tube defects.

Potassium benefits.   Because potassium is excreted in urine, potassium-rich foods are often recommended for people taking diuretics. In addition, a diet rich in potassium (from food) is associated with a lower risk of stroke. A 1998 Harvard School of Public Health analysis of data from the long-running Health Professionals Study shows 38 percent fewer strokes among men who ate nine servings of high potassium foods a day vs. those who ate fewer than four servings. Among men with high blood pressure, taking a daily 1,000 mg potassium supplement—about the amount of potassium in two cups orange juice—reduced the incidence of stroke by 60 percent.

Antiscorbutics.   All citrus fruits are excellent sources of vitamin C, used to cure or prevent the vitamin C–deficiency disease scurvy. Your body also needs vitamin C in order to convert the amino acid proline into hydroxyproline, an essential ingredient in collagen, the protein needed to form skin, tendons, and bones. People with scurvy do not heal quickly, a condition that can be cured by feeding them foods rich in vitamin C. Whether taking extra vitamin C speeds healing in healthy people remains to be proved. Oranges and other citrus fruits also contain rutin, hesperidin, and other natural chemicals known collectively as flavonoids ("bioflavonoids"). In experiments with laboratory animals, flavonoids appear to strengthen capillaries, the tiny blood vessels just under the skin. To date this effect has not been demonstrated in human beings.

Enhanced absorption of iron from plant foods.   Nonheme iron, the inorganic form of iron found in plant foods, is poorly absorbed by the body because it is bound into insoluble compounds by natural chemicals in the plants. Vitamin C appears to make nonheme iron more available to your body, perhaps by converting it from ferric iron to ferrous iron, which is more easily absorbed. Eating vitamin C–rich foods along with plant foods rich in iron can increase the amount of iron you get from the plant—the nutritional justification for a breakfast of orange juice and cereal or bread. (See also BEANS, BREAD, FLOUR, OATS, WHEAT CEREAL.)

Adverse Effects Associated with This Food

Flare-up of aphthous ulcers.   In sensitive people, eating citrus fruits may trigger an attack of aphthous ulcers (canker sores), but eliminating citrus fruit from the diet neither cures nor prevents canker sores.

Contact dermatitis.   Although there is ample anecdotal evidence to suggest that many people are sensitive to natural chemicals in an orange's flesh or peel, the offending substances have never been conclusively identified.

Food/Drug Interactions

Aspirin and other nonsteroidal anti-inflammatory drugs (ibuprofen, naproxen, and others).   Taking aspirin with acidic foods and drinks such as oranges or orange juice may make the drugs more irritating to the stomach.

False-negative test for hidden blood in the stool.   The active ingredient in the guaiac slide test for hidden blood in feces is alphaguaiaconic acid, a chemical that turns blue in the presence of blood. Citrus fruits or vitamin supplements containing more than 250 mg ascorbic acid may produce excess ascorbic acid in the feces, which inhibits the ability of alphaguaiaconic acid to react with blood may produce a false-negative test result that fails to disclose the presence of a tumor in the colon.

Papaya

Nutritional Profile

Energy value (calories per serving): *Low*
Protein: *Low*
Fat: *Low*
Saturated fat: *Low*
Cholesterol: *None*
Carbohydrates: *High*
Fiber: *Very high*
Sodium: *Low*
Major vitamin contribution: *Vitamins A, folate, vitamin C*
Major mineral contribution: *Potassium*

About the Nutrients in This Food

Papayas (a.k.a. paw-paws) are high in soluble dietary fiber (gums and pectins) with moderate amounts of vitamin A, as well as an excellent source of the B vitamin folate and vitamin C.

Half of one five-inch long papaya has 2.8 g dietary fiber, 1,663 IU vitamin A (22 percent of the RDA for a woman, 56 percent of the RDA for a man), 58 mcg folate (15 percent of the RDA), and 94 mg vitamin C (1.3 times the RDA for a woman, 100 percent of the RDA for man).

Unripe papayas and the leaves of the papaya plant contain a papain, a proteolytic (protein-dissolving) enzyme that breaks long protein molecules into smaller fragments. You can tenderize meat by cooking it wrapped in papaya leaves or by dusting it with a meat tenderizer of commercially extracted papain dried to a powder. (Soybeans, *haricots verts,* garden peas, broad beans, wheat flours, and egg white all contain proteins that inactivate papain.)

The Most Nutritious Way to Serve This Food

Fresh, sliced.

Diets That May Restrict or Exclude This Food

* * *

Buying This Food

Look for: Medium-size, pear-shaped fruit whose skin is turning yellow. The yellower the skin, the riper the fruit. Papayas ripen from the bottom up, toward the stem. Always look for fruit that is yellow at least halfway up.

Storing This Food

Store papayas at room temperature until they are fully ripe, which means that they have turned golden all over and are soft enough to give when you press the stem end.

Store ripe papayas in the refrigerator.

Preparing This Food

Wash the papaya under cool running water, then cut it in half, spoon out the seeds, and sprinkle it with lemon or lime juice.

The seeds of the papaya taste like peppercorns. They can be dried and ground as a seasoning or simply sprinkled, whole, on a salad.

What Happens When You Cook This Food

* * *

How Other Kinds of Processing Affect This Food

Extraction of papain.   Commercial meat tenderizers contain papain extracted from fresh papaya and dried to a powder. The powder is a much more efficient tenderizer than either fresh papaya or papaya leaves. At the strength usually found in these powders, papain can "digest" (tenderize) up to 35 times its weight in meat. Like bromelain (the proteolytic enzyme in fresh pineapple) and ficin (the proteolytic enzyme in fresh figs), papain breaks down proteins only at a temperature between 140°F and 170°F. It won't work when the temperature is higher or lower.

Medical Uses and/or Benefits

Lower risk of some birth defects.   Up to two or every 1,000 babies born in the United States each year may have cleft palate or a neural tube (spinal cord) defect due to their mothers' not having gotten adequate amounts of folate during pregnancy. The current RDA for folate is 180 mcg for a woman and 200 mcg for a man, but the FDA now recommends 400 mcg for a woman who is or may become pregnant. Taking a folate supplement before becoming pregnant and through the first two months of pregnancy reduces the risk of cleft palate; taking folate through the entire pregnancy reduces the risk of neural tube defects.

Possible lower risk of heart attack.   In the spring of 1998, an analysis of data from the records for more than 80,000 women enrolled in the long-running Nurses' Health Study at Harvard School of Public Health/Brigham and Women's Hospital, in Boston, demonstrated that a diet providing more than 400 mcg folate and 3 mg vitamin B_6 daily, either from food or supplements, might reduce a woman's risk of heart attack by almost 50 percent. Although men were not included in the study, the results were assumed to apply to them as well.

However, data from a meta-analysis published in the *Journal of the American Medical Association* in December 2006 called this theory into question. Researchers at Tulane University examined the results of 12 controlled studies in which 16,958 patients with preexisting cardiovascular disease were given either folic acid supplements or placebos ("look-alike" pills with no folic acid) for at least six months. The scientists, who found no reduction in the risk of further heart disease or overall death rates among those taking folic acid, concluded that further studies will be required to determine whether taking folic acid supplements reduces the risk of cardiovascular disease.

Adverse Effects Associated with This Food

Irritated skin.   Because it can break down proteins, papain (and/or fresh papayas) may cause dermatitis, including a hivelike reaction. This is not an allergic response: it can happen to anyone.

Food/Drug Interactions

Monoamine oxidase (MAO) inhibitors.   Monoamine oxidase inhibitors are drugs used to treat depression. They inactivate naturally occurring enzymes in your body that metabolize tyramine, a substance found in many fermented or aged foods. Tyramine constricts blood vessels and increases blood pressure. One by-product of papain's breaking up long-chain protein molecules to tenderize meat is the production of tyramine. If you eat a food such as papain-tenderized meat while you are taking an MAO inhibitor, you cannot effectively eliminate the tyramine from your body. The result may be a hypertensive crisis.

Parsnips

Nutritional Profile

Energy value (calories per serving): *Moderate*
Protein: *Moderate*
Fat: *Low*
Saturated fat: *Low*
Cholesterol: *None*
Carbohydrates: *High*
Fiber: *High*
Sodium: *Low*
Major vitamin contribution: *Folate, vitamin C*
Major mineral contribution: *Potassium, calcium*

About the Nutrients in This Food

Parsnips are roots high in starch and dietary fiber, including insoluble cellulose and soluble gums and pectins. They are an excellent source of the B vitamin folate and a good source of vitamin C.

One-half cup cooked, sliced parsnips has 3 g dietary fiber, 25 mcg folate (11 percent of the RDA), and 10 mg vitamin C (13 percent of the RDA for a woman, 11 percent of the RDA for a man).

The Most Nutritious Way to Serve This Food

Boiled and drained.

Diets That May Restrict or Exclude This Food

Low-fiber diet

Buying This Food

Look for: Smooth, well-shaped, cream or tan small-to-medium roots. The larger the root, the woodier and coarser it will be.

Avoid: Discolored parsnips. Parsnips that are darker in spots may have been frozen on the way to market. Gray spots or soft spots warn of rot inside the root.

Storing This Food

Keep parsnips cold and humid so they won't dry out. Store them in a root cellar or in the refrigerator. In storage, parsnips will convert some of their starch to sugar. As a rule of thumb, the sweeter the parsnip, the longer it has been stored.

Preparing This Food

Scrub the parsnips with a vegetable brush under cool running water or simply peel them—but not until you are ready to use them. When you peel or slice a parsnip, you tear its cell walls, releasing polyphenoloxidase, an enzyme that hastens the combination of oxygen with phenols in the parsnips, turning the vegetable brown. You can slow this reaction (but not stop it completely) by dipping raw peeled or sliced parsnips into an acid solution (lemon juice and water, vinegar and water). Polyphenoloxidase also works more slowly in the cold, but storing peeled parsnips in the refrigerator is much less effective than an acid bath.

You can keep parsnips from darkening in a stew by blanching them before you add them to the dish. Boil the unpeeled parsnips for about 15 minutes to inactivate the polyphenoloxidase, then add them to the stew. If you prefer, you can freeze blanched parsnips for future use.

What Happens When You Cook This Food

Heat dissolves the pectic substances in the parsnip's cell walls, making the vegetable softer. At the same time, the parsnip's starch granules absorb water, swell, and eventually rupture, releasing nutrients inside and making the vegetables easier to digest.

How Other Kinds of Processing Affect This Food

Freezing. When parsnips are frozen, liquids inside the vegetable's cell form ice crystals that may tear the cells, allowing moisture to escape when you thaw the parsnips. As a result, when roots like carrots, potatoes, and parsnips are frozen and thawed, their texture is mushy rather than crisp.

Medical Uses and/or Benefits

Lower risk of some birth defects. As many as two of every 1,000 babies born in the United States each year may have cleft palate or a neural tube (spinal cord) defect due to their mothers' not having gotten adequate amounts of folate during pregnancy. The current RDA for folate is 180 mcg for a woman and 200 mcg for a man, but the FDA now recommends 400 mcg for a woman who is or may become pregnant. Taking folate supplements before becoming pregnant and continuing through the first two months of pregnancy reduces the risk of cleft palate; taking folate through the entire pregnancy reduces the risk of neural tube defects.

Possible lower risk of heart attack. In the spring of 1998, an analysis of data from the records for more than 80,000 women enrolled in the long-running Nurses' Health Study at Harvard School of Public Health/Brigham and Women's Hospital, in Boston, demonstrated that a diet providing more than 400 mcg folate and 3 mg vitamin B_6 daily, either from food or supplements, might reduce a woman's risk of heart attack by almost 50 percent. Although men were not included in the study, the results were assumed to apply to them as well.

However, data from a meta-analysis published in the *Journal of the American Medical Association* in December 2006 called this theory into question. Researchers at Tulane University examined the results of 12 controlled studies in which 16,958 patients with preexisting cardiovascular disease were given either folic acid supplements or placebos ("look-alike" pills with no folic acid) for at least six months. The scientists, who found no reduction in the risk of further heart disease or overall death rates among those taking folic acid, concluded that further studies will be required to determine whether taking folic acid supplements reduces the risk of cardiovascular disease.

Adverse Effects Associated with This Food

Photosensitivity. Like celery and parsley, parsnips contain psoralens, natural chemicals that make the skin sensitive to light. Psoralens are not inactivated by cooking; they are present in both raw and cooked parsnips.

In laboratory animals, psoralens applied to the skin are known to trigger cancers when the animals are exposed to light. Among human beings, their only documented side effect is the skin inflammation common among food workers who handle and process vegetables without wearing protective gloves. In 1981, however, scientists at the U.S. Department of Agriculture's Veterinary Toxicology and Entomology Research Laboratory in College Station, Texas, suggested that detailed epidemiological studies might link physiological effects to eating parsnips as well as handling them. The connection remains to be proved.

Food/Drug Interactions

* * *

Pasta

See also Flour.

Nutritional Profile

Energy value (calories per serving): *Moderate*
Protein: *Moderate*
Fat: *Low*
Saturated fat: *Low*
Cholesterol: *None*
Carbohydrates: *High*
Fiber: *Low to High*
Sodium: *Low*[*]
Major vitamin contribution: *B vitamins*
Major mineral contribution: *Iron*

About the Nutrients in This Food

The basic ingredients in pasta are water plus flour or semolina (the coarsely milled inner part of the wheat kernel called the endosperm). *Whole wheat pasta,* which is darker than ordinary pasta, is made with whole wheat flour. *Egg noodles* are made with flour and water plus eggs. *Spinach pasta* adds dried spinach for taste and color. *High-protein pasta* is fortified with soy flour. *Light pasta* is treated to absorb more water than regular pasta. *Imitation pasta* is made with flour ground from Jerusalem artichokes rather than wheat. *Rice noodles* are made with rice flour, *cellophane noodles* with flour ground from sprouted mung beans.

All pasta is high-carbohydrate (starch) food. Since semolina is virtually all protein, the more semolina the pasta contains, the more protein it provides. The proteins in pasta are considered "incomplete" because they are deficient in the essential amino acids in lysine and isoleucine. Pasta made without eggs has no fat and no cholesterol.

All pasta is a good source of the B vitamins thiamin (vitamin B_1) and riboflavin (vitamin B_2). Pasta made with flour also contains nonheme iron, the inorganic form of iron found in plants, which is harder for your body to absorb than the iron in foods of animal origin.

---

[*] Dry pasta.

One serving (two ounces, dry) enriched spaghetti has 1.8 g dietary fiber, 7.9 g protein, 0.9 g total fat, no cholesterol, and 1.9 mg iron (11 percent of the RDA for a woman, 23 percent of the RDA for a man).

One serving (two ounces, dry) enriched egg noodles has two grams dietary fiber, eight grams protein, 2.5 g total fat, 48 mg cholesterol, and 2.3 mg iron (13 percent of the RDA for a woman, 29 percent of the RDA for a man).

The Most Nutritious Way to Serve This Food

With meat, eggs, or milk products (cheese), which supply lysine and isoleucine to "complement" the proteins in the pasta.

With beans or peas. Grains are deficient in the essential amino acids lysine and isoleucine but contain sufficient amounts of tryptophan, methionine, and cystine. Beans and peas are just the opposite. Together, their proteins are complementary.

With a food rich in iron (meat) or a food rich in vitamin C (tomatoes). Both enhance your body's ability to absorb the iron in pasta. The meat makes your stomach produce more acid (which favors the absorption of iron); the vitamin C converts the iron from ferric iron (which is hard to absorb) to ferrous iron (which is more available to your body).

Diets That May Restrict or Exclude This Food

Gluten-restricted, gliadin-free diet (all pastas made with wheat flour)

Buying This Food

Look for: Tightly sealed packages. If you can see into the box, pick the pasta that looks smooth and shiny. Dry or dusty pasta is stale; so is pasta that is crumbling. The yellower the pasta, the more durum wheat it contains. (Egg noodles get their yellow from eggs.) Whole wheat pasta is brown.

Storing This Food

Store pasta in air- and moistureproof glass or plastic containers. Pasta will stay fresh for about a year, egg noodles for six months.

Preparing This Food

To cook pasta most efficiently, start with salted water. At sea level, water boils at 212°F (100°C), the temperature at which its molecules have enough energy to escape from the surface as steam. If you add salt, the water molecules will need to pick up more energy to push the salt molecules aside and escape from the surface. In effect, adding salt forces the water to boil at a higher temperature, which means the pasta will cook more quickly.

The water should be boiling furiously before you add the pasta so that it can penetrate the pasta's starch granules as fast as possible. Add the pasta slowly so that the water continues to boil and the pasta cooks evenly.

What Happens When You Cook This Food

Starch consists of molecules of the complex carbohydrates amylose and amylopectin packed into a starch granule. When you boil pasta, water molecules force their way into the starch granules. When the water reaches a temperature of approximately 140°F, the amylose and amylopectin molecules inside the starch granules relax and unfold, forming new bonds between atoms on different molecules and creating a network inside the starch granule that traps water molecules. The granules bulk up and the pasta gets thicker. In fact, the starch granules can hold so much water that plain flour-and-water pastas like spaghetti, macaroni, and lasagna will actually double in size.

The longer you cook the pasta, the more likely it is that the starch granules will absorb too much water and rupture, releasing some of their starch and making the pasta sticky. One way to keep the pieces of pasta from sticking together is to cook them in a large pot, which gives them room to boil without hitting their neighbors. Or you might add a tablespoon of olive oil to make the pasta slick enough to slide apart. If you plan to refrigerate the cooked pasta, drain it, rinse it in warm water (to wash off the starch on the outside), and toss it with olive oil.

How Other Kinds of Processing Affect This Food

Canning and freezing. When pasta is canned or frozen in sauce, its starch granules continue to absorb the liquid and the pasta becomes progressively more limp.

Medical Uses and/or Benefits

A lower risk of some kinds of cancer. In 1998, scientists at Wayne State University in Detroit conducted a meta-analysis of data from more than 30 well-designed animal studies measuring the anti-cancer effects of wheat bran, the part of grain with highest amount of the insoluble dietary fibers cellulose and lignin. They found a 32 percent reduction in the risk of colon cancer among animals fed wheat bran; now they plan to conduct a similar meta-analysis of human studies. Pasta made with whole grain wheat is a good source of wheat bran. NOTE: The amount of fiber per serving listed on a food package label shows the total amount of fiber (insoluble and soluble).

Early in 1999, however, new data from the long-running Nurses Health Study at Brigham Women's Hospital/Harvard University School of Public Health showed that women who ate a high-fiber diet had a risk of colon cancer similar to that of women who ate a low-fiber diet. Because this study contradicts literally hundreds of others conducted over the past thirty years, researchers are awaiting confirming evidence before changing dietary recommendations.

However, early the following year, new data from the long-running Nurses' Health Study at Harvard School of Public Health and Brigham and Women's Hospital, in Boston, showed no difference in the risk of colon cancer between women who ate a high-fiber diet and those who did not. Nonetheless, many nutrition researchers remain wary of ruling out a protective effect for dietary fiber. They note that there are different kinds of dietary fiber that may have different effects, that most Americans do not consume a diet with the recommended amount of dietary fiber, and that gender, genetics, and various personal health issues may also affect the link between dietary fiber and the risk of colon cancer. NOTE: The current recommendations for dietary fiber consumption are 25 grams per day for women younger than 50, and 21 grams per day for women older than 50; 38 grams per day for men younger than 50, and 30 grams per day for men older than 50.

As a source of increased energy for athletes. When we eat carbohydrates, our bodies break them down into glycogen, which is stored in our muscles. When we need energy we convert the stored glycogen to glucose, the fuel on which our bodies run. Athletes who engage in the kind of strenuous exercise that can lead to exhaustion in 45 minutes need more glycogen than people who lead sedentary lives. Without the extra glycogen, they will run out of energy in midgame or midmarathon. One way to increase the amount of glycogen in the muscles is to increase the amount of high-carbohydrate foods, such as pasta, in the diet, a regimen known as carbohydrate loading. The classic carbohydrate-loading diet developed in Scandinavia in the 1960s calls for two days on a very low-carbohydrate diet plus very heavy exercise to deplete the muscles' normal store of glycogen, followed by three days of very little exercise and a diet which is 70 to 90 percent carbohydrates. Because so many athletes are reluctant to stop exercising for three days before an event, a modified version of this regime, developed at Ball State University in Indiana, suggests two days on a normal diet with normal to heavy exercise, then three days on a diet very high in carbohydrates while exercise tapers down to nothing on the day before the event. According to a number of studies by sports-medicine researchers, both versions of the carbohydrate-loading diet appear to increase the amount of glycogen in the athlete's muscles and thus to increase long-term stamina.

As a source of carbohydrates for people with diabetes. Pasta is digested very slowly, producing only a gradual rise in blood-sugar levels. As a result, the body needs less insulin to control blood sugar after eating pasta than after eating some other high-carbohydrate foods (rice, bread, or corn). In studies at the University of Kentucky, a bean, whole-grain, vegetable, and fruit-rich diet developed at the University of Toronto and recommended by the American Diabetes Association enabled patients with type 1 diabetes (who do not produce any insulin themselves) to cut their daily insulin intake by 38 percent. For patients with type 2 diabetes (who can produce some insulin), the bean diet reduced the need for injected insulin by 98 percent. This diet is in line with the nutritional guidelines of the American Diabetes Association, but people with diabetes should always consult their doctor and/or dietitian before altering their diet.

Calming effect. Your mood is affected by naturally occurring chemicals called neurotransmitters that allow cells in your brain to transmit impulses from one to the other. Tryptophan, an amino acid, is the most important constituent of serotonin, a "calming" neurotransmitter. High-carbohydrate foods like pasta help move tryptophan into your brain, increasing your ability to use serotonin. Eating pasta can be a soothing, calming act.

Adverse Effects Associated with This Food

Food allergy. According to the *Merck Manual,* wheat is among the foods most often implicated as a cause of the classic food allergy symptoms—upset stomach, hives, skin rashes, angioedema (swelling of the face, eyes, and lips). For more information, see under WHEAT CEREALS.

Gluten intolerance (celiac disease). Celiac disease is an intestinal allergic disorder that results in an inability to absorb the nutrients in gluten and gliadin. People with celiac disease cannot absorb the nutrients in wheat or wheat products, such as pasta. Corn flour, potato flour, rice flour, and soy flour are gluten- and gliadin-free. So are pasta products made of flour ground from Jerusalem artichokes.

Food/Drug Interactions

* * *

Peaches

(Nectarines)

Nutritional Profile

Energy value (calories per serving): *Low*
Protein: *Moderate*
Saturated fat: *Low*
Fat: *Low*
Cholesterol: *None*
Carbohydrates: *High*
Fiber: *Moderate*
Sodium: *Low (fresh or dried fruit)*
      High (dried fruit treated with sodium sulfur compounds)
Major vitamin contribution: *Vitamin A*
Major mineral contribution: *Potassium*

About the Nutrients in This Food

Peaches and nectarines (a.k.a. "peaches without fuzz") have moderate amounts of dietary fiber, insoluble cellulose in the skin and soluble pectins in the fruit. They have moderate to high amounts of vitamin A derived from deep yellow carotenes, including beta-carotene in the flesh, and are a good source of vitamin C.

One fresh peach (2.75-inch diameter) has 2.2 g dietary fiber, 489 IU vitamin A (21 percent of the RDA for a woman, 16 percent of the RDA for a man), and 9.9 mg vitamin C (13 percent of the RDA for a woman, 11 percent of the RDA for a man).

One fresh nectarine (2.5-inch diameter) has 2.4 g dietary fiber, 471 IU vitamin A (20 percent of the RDA for a woman, 16 percent of the RDA for a man), and 7.7 mg vitamin C (10 percent of the RDA for a woman, 9 percent of the RDA for a man).

Like apple seeds and apricot pits, the leaves and bark of the peach tree as well as the "nut" inside the peach pit contain amygdalin, a naturally occurring cyanide/sugar compound that breaks down into hydrogen cyanide in your stomach. Accidentally swallowing one peach pit is not a serious hazard for an adult, but cases of human poisoning after eating peach pits have been reported (see APPLES).

The Most Nutritious Way to Serve This Food

Fresh and ripe.

Diets That May Restrict or Exclude This Food

* * *

Buying This Food

Look for: Peaches and nectarines with rich cream or yellow skin. The red "blush" characteristic of some varieties of peaches is not a reliable guide to ripeness. A better guide is the way the fruit feels and smells. Ripe peaches and nectarines have a warm, intense aroma and feel firm, with a slight softness along the line running up the length of the fruit.

Avoid: Green or hard unripe peaches and nectarines. As peaches and nectarines ripen enzymes convert their insoluble pectic substances to soluble pectins and decrease their concentration of bitter phenols. The longer the peach is left on the tree, the lower the concentration of phenols will be, which is why late-season peaches and nectarines are the sweetest. Once you pick the peach or nectarine, the enzyme action stops completely. The fruit may shrivel, but it cannot continue to ripen.

Storing This Food

Store firm ripe peaches and nectarines at room temperature until they soften. Once they have softened, put them in the refrigerator. The cold will stop the enzymatic action that dissolves pectins in the fruit and softens it.

　　The pectin in freestone peaches is more soluble than the pectin in cling peaches, so ripe freestones are softer than ripe cling peaches (which stay firm even when cooked). NOTE: The names "freestone" and "cling" indicate the ease with which the fruit separates from the pit.

Preparing This Food

To peel peaches, immerse them in hot water for a few seconds, then lift them out and plunge them into cold water. The hot water destroys a layer of cells under the skin, allowing the skin to slip off easily.

　　Don't peel or slice peaches and nectarines until you are ready to use them. When you cut into them, you tear their cell walls, releasing polyphenoloxidase, an enzyme that promotes the oxidation of phenols, forming brownish compounds that darken the fruit. You can slow the reaction (but not stop it completely) by chilling the fruit or by dipping it in an acid solution (lemon juice and water or vinegar and water) or by mixing the sliced peaches and nectarines into a fruit salad with citrus fruits.

What Happens When You Cook This Food

When you cook peaches, pectins in the cell walls dissolve and the fruit softens. As noted above, cling peaches will stay firmer than freestones. Cooking peaches and nectarines also destroys polyphenoloxidase and keeps the fruit from darkening.

How Other Kinds of Processing Affect This Food

Drying. Drying removes water and concentrates the peach flesh. Ounce for ounce, dried peaches have up to three times as much vitamin A as fresh peaches. One fresh peach weighing 87 g (about three ounces) has 470 IU vitamin A. A similar serving of uncooked dried peaches has approximately 1,880 IU. Like other dried fruits, dried peaches may be treated with sulfites (sodium sulfite) that inhibit polyphenoloxidase and keep the peaches from darkening. People who are sensitive to sulfites may suffer serious allergic reactions, including potentially lethal anaphylactic shock, if they eat dried peaches treated with these compounds.

Medical Uses and/or Benefits

* * *

Adverse Effects Associated with This Food

Allergic reaction. According to the *Merck Manual,* peaches are one of the 12 foods most likely to trigger classic food allergy symptoms: hives, swelling of the lips and eyes, and upset stomach. The others are berries (blackberries, blueberries, raspberries, strawberries), chocolate, corn, eggs, fish, legumes (green peas, lima beans, peanuts, soybeans), milk, nuts, pork, shellfish, and wheat (see WHEAT CEREALS).

Sulfite allergies. See *How other kinds of processing affect this food,* above.

Food/Drug Interactions

* * *

Peanuts

Nutritional Profile*

Energy value (calories per serving): *Moderate to high*
Protein: *High*
Fat: *High*
Saturated fat: *High*
Cholesterol: *None*
Carbohydrates: *Low*
Fiber: *High*
Sodium: *Low*
Major vitamin contribution: *Vitamin E, folate*
Major mineral contribution: *Iron, potassium*

About the Nutrients in This Food

Peanuts are not nuts. They are legumes (beans and peas), unusual in that they store their energy as fat rather than starch.

Peanuts are high in dietary fiber, including insoluble cellulose and lignin in their papery "skin" and soluble gums and pectins in the nuts. They are high in fat, primarily (86 percent) unsaturated fatty acids. Their proteins are plentiful but limited in the essential amino acids tryptophan, methionine, and cystine. Peanuts are an excellent source of vitamin E (from polyunsaturated fatty acids).

Peanuts are an excellent source of vitamin E. Raw peanuts, with the skin on, are a good source of thiamin (vitamin B_1), but much of the thiamin, as well as vitamin B_6, is lost when peanuts are roasted. All peanuts are a good source of riboflavin (vitamin B_2) and folate. They are high in potassium. Ounce for ounce, they have nearly three times as much potassium as fresh oranges. They are also a good source of nonheme iron, the iron in plant foods, and zinc.

One ounce dry-roasted unsalted peanuts has 2.3 g dietary fiber, 14.1 g total fat (2g saturated fat, 7 g monounsaturated fat, 4.4 polyunsaturated fat), 6.7 g protein, 41 mcg folate (10 percent of the RDA), 0.6 mg iron (3 percent of the RDA for a woman, 8 percent of the RDA for a man), and 0.9 mg zinc (11 percent of the RDA for a woman, 8 percent of the RDA for a man).

---

* Values are for dry-roasted, unsalted peanuts.

The Most Nutritious Way to Use This Food

With grains. The proteins in peanuts and other legumes are deficient in the essential amino acids tryptophan, methionine, and cystine but contain sufficient amounts of the essential amino acids lysine and isoleucine. The proteins in grains are exactly the opposite. Together they complement each other and produce "complete" proteins, which is the reason a peanut-butter sandwich is nutritionally sound.

With meat or a food rich in vitamin C. Both will increase the absorption of iron from the peanuts. Meat increases the acidity of the stomach (iron is absorbed better in an acid environment); vitamin C may change the iron in the peanuts from ferrous iron (which is hard to absorb) to ferric iron (which is easier to absorb).

Diets That May Restrict or Exclude This Food

Low residue diet
Low-purine (antigout diet)
Low-sodium diet (salted peanuts, peanut butters)

How to Buy This Food

Look for: Tightly sealed jars or cans of processed peanuts. Peanuts are rich in polyunsaturated fatty acids that combine easily with oxygen and turn rancid if the peanuts are not protected from air and heat.

Choose unshelled loose peanuts rather than shelled ones. The shell is a natural shield against light and air.

Storing This Food

Store shelled or unshelled peanuts in a cool, dark cabinet. Keep them dry to protect them against mold. If you plan to hold them for longer than a month, refrigerate them in a tightly closed container.

Preparing This Food

Pick over the peanuts and discard any that are moldy and may be contaminated with carcinogenic toxins called aflatoxins.

What Happens When You Cook This Food

Heat destroys the thiamin (vitamin B_1) in peanuts. Roasted peanuts are much lower in thiamin than fresh peanuts.

How Other Kinds of Processing Affect This Food

Peanut butter.   Peanut butters generally have more fat, saturated fat, salt (sodium), and sugar than plain peanuts, with as much fiber and potassium per serving as plain peanuts, but less folate. Two tablespoons (one ounce) chunky-style peanut butter has an average 2.11 g fiber, 239 mg potassium, and 29.44 mcg folate.

Medical Uses and/or Benefits

Lower risk of cardiovascular disease, diabetes, and some forms of cancer.   Grape skin, pulp, and seed, and wines made from grapes, contain resveratrol, one of a group of plant chemicals credited with lowering cholesterol and thus reducing the risk of heart attack by preventing molecular fragments called free radicals from linking together to form compounds that damage body cells leading to blocked arteries, glucose-damaged blood vessels (diabetes), and unregulated cell growth (cancer). Peanuts also contain resveratrol. In fact, a 1998 analysis from the USDA Agricultural Research Service in Raleigh, North Carolina, shows that peanuts have 1.7 to 3.7 mcg resveratrol per gram of peanuts vs. 0.6 to 8.0 mcg resveratrol per gram of red wine.

Possible lower risk of heart attack.   In the spring of 1998, an analysis of data from the records for more than 80,000 women enrolled in the long-running Nurses' Health Study at Harvard School of Public Health/Brigham and Women's Hospital, in Boston, demonstrated that a diet providing more than 400 mcg folate and 3 mg vitamin B_6 daily, either from food or supplements, might reduce a woman's risk of heart attack by almost 50 percent. Although men were not included in the study, the results were assumed to apply to them as well.

However, data from a meta-analysis published in the *Journal of the American Medical Association* in December 2006 called this theory into question. Researchers at Tulane University examined the results of 12 controlled studies in which 16,958 patients with preexisting cardiovascular disease were given either folic acid supplements or placebos ("look-alike" pills with no folic acid) for at least six months. The scientists, who found no reduction in the risk of further heart disease or overall death rates among those taking folic acid, concluded that further studies will be required to ascertain whether taking folic acid supplements reduces the risk of cardiovascular disease.

Lower cholesterol levels.   A 1998 study at the University of Rochester, Pennsylvania State University, and the Bassett Research Institute suggests that a diet high in monounsaturated fatty acids from peanut oil and peanut butter reduces levels of cholesterol and low density lipoproteins (LDLs) without increasing levels of triglycerides (another form of fat considered an independent risk factor for heart disease).

Lower risk of some birth defects.   As many as two of every 1,000 babies born in the United States each year may have cleft palate or a neural tube (spinal cord) defect due to their mothers' not having gotten adequate amounts of folate during pregnancy. The current RDA for folate is 180 mcg for a woman and 200 mcg for a man, but the FDA now recommends 400 mcg for a woman who is or may become pregnant. Taking folate supplements before becoming pregnant and continuing through the first two months of pregnancy reduces the risk of cleft palate; taking folate through the entire pregnancy reduces the risk of neural tube defects.

Adverse Effects Associated with This Food

Allergic reaction. According to the *Merck Manual,* peanuts are one of the 12 foods most likely to trigger classic food allergy symptoms: hives, swelling of the lips and eyes, and upset stomach. The others are berries (blackberries, blueberries, raspberries, strawberries), chocolate, corn, eggs, fish, milk, nuts, peaches, pork, shellfish, and wheat (see WHEAT CEREALS). NOTE: In 1998, USDA advised pregnant or breast-feeding women who suffer from eczema, hay fever, asthma, or other allergies or whose partner or children have allergies not to eat peanuts because children exposed to peanuts while in the womb or nursing are at higher risk of developing serious allergies to peanuts.

Production of uric acid. Purines are the natural metabolic by-products of protein metabolism in the body. They eventually break down into uric acid, which may form sharp crystals that may cause gout if they collect in your joints or kidney stones if they collect in urine. Fresh and roasted peanuts are a source of purines; eating them raises the concentration of purines in your body. Although controlling the amount of purine-producing foods in the diet may not significantly affect the course of gout (which is treated with medication such as allopurinol, which inhibits the formation of uric acid), limiting these foods is still part of many gout regimens.

Food/Drug Interactions

* * *

Pears

Nutritional Profile

Energy value (calories per serving): *Moderate*
Protein: *Low*
Fat: *Low*
Saturated fat: *Low*
Cholesterol: *None*
Carbohydrates: *High*
Fiber: *High*
Sodium: *Low (fresh or dried fruit)*
       High (dried fruit treated with sodium sulfur compounds)
Major vitamin contribution: *Vitamin C*
Major mineral contribution: *Potassium*

About the Nutrients in This Food

Pears are high in dietary fiber, with insoluble cellulose in the skin, lignin in the tiny gritty particles in the fruit flesh, plus soluble pectins. They are high in sugars and have moderate amounts of vitamin C, concentrated in the skin. Their most important mineral is potassium.

One six-ounce fresh pear, with skin, has 5.5 g dietary fiber and 7.5 mg vitamin C (10 percent of the RDA for a woman, 8 percent of the RDA for a man).

Like apple seeds and peach pits, the seeds of pears contain amygdalin, a cyanide/sugar compound that breaks down into hydrogen cyanide in your stomach. Accidentally swallowing a pear seed is not necessarily hazardous for an adult, but there have been reports of serious poisoning among people who have eaten several apple seeds (see APPLES).

The Most Nutritious Way to Use This Food

Fresh and ripe, with the skin (for the extra fiber and vitamin C).

Diets That May Restrict or Exclude This Food

* * *

Buying This Food

Look for: Large, firm, ripe pears. Most fruit and vegetables get softer after they are picked because their pectic enzymes begin to dissolve the pectin in their cell walls. With pears, this reaction occurs if the pear is left on the tree to ripen, which is why tree-ripened pears sometimes taste mushy. The best-tasting pears are ones that are picked immature and allowed to ripen in storage or on your grocer's shelf.

Look for bright, clear-colored pears. Anjou pears are yellow to green (with some russet shades) and have a bland, buttery flesh. Bartletts are clear golden or yellow with a reddish blush and sweet, juicy flesh. Boscs are russet, sweet and juicy. Round Comice pears have a yellow green skin and fine, juicy flesh. Red Seckel pears are firm and aromatic. Anjou, Bartlett, and Bosc are good eating and cooking pears; Comice and Seckel pears are for eating.

Avoid: Cut, shriveled, or bruised pears. They are probably discolored inside.

Storing This Food

Store pears at room temperature for a few days if they are not fully ripe when you buy them. Pears ripen from inside out, so you should never let a pear ripen until it is really soft on the surface. A ripe pear will yield when you press it lightly with your palm.

Do not store pears in sealed plastic bags either in or out of the refrigerator. Without oxygen circulating freely around the pear, the fruit will begin to "breathe" internally, creating compounds that turn the core brown and make brownish spots under the skin.

Preparing This Food

Handle pears with care; never peel or slice them until you are ready to use them. When you bruise a pear or slice into it, you tear its cells, releasing polyphenoloxidase, an enzyme that hastens the oxidation of phenols in the fruit, producing clumps of brownish compounds that darken the pear's flesh. You can slow this natural reaction (but not stop it completely) by chilling the pears, brushing the cut surface with an acid solution (lemon juice and water, vinegar and water), or mixing the peeled, sliced fruit into a fresh fruit salad with citrus fruits full of vitamin C, a natural antioxidant.

What Happens When You Cook This Food

Like other fruits and vegetables, pears have cell walls made of cellulose, hemicellulose, and pectic substances. As the fruit cooks and its pectins dissolve, it gets softer. But no amount of cooking will dissolve the lignin particles in the pear flesh. In fact, the softer the pear, the easier it is to taste the lignin particles.

How Other Kinds of Processing Affect This Food

Drying. Dried pears have more fiber and potassium but less vitamin C than fresh pears. One-half of a dried pear (2 ounces) has 5.7 g fiber, 405 mg potassium, and 5.32 mg vitamin C. Fresh pears are sometimes treated with sulfur compounds such as sulfur dioxide to inactivate polyphenoloxidase and keep the pears from darkening when they are exposed to air while drying. People who are sensitive to sulfites may suffer serious allergic reactions, including anaphylactic shock, if they eat these treated dried pears.

Sealed packages of dried pears may be stored at room temperature for up to six months. Once the package is opened, the pears should be refrigerated in a tightly closed container that will protect them from air and moisture.

Medical Uses and/or Benefits

Potassium replacement. Pears are a moderately good source of potassium. One 3.5-ounce Bartlett has about as much the potassium as three ounces of fresh orange juice. Foods rich in potassium are sometimes prescribed for people taking diuretics that lower the body's level of potassium, which is excreted in urine. However, there is some question as to whether potassium gluconate, the form of potassium found in pears and other fresh fruit, is as useful to the body as potassium citrate and potassium chloride, the forms of potassium given to laboratory animals in the experiments which showed that people taking diuretic drugs would benefit from potassium supplements.

Adverse Effects Associated with This Food

Sulfite allergies. See *How other kinds of processing affect this food.*

Food/Drug Interactions

* * *

Peas

(Snow pea pods [sugar peas], split peas)

See also Beans.

Nutritional Profile

Energy value (calories per serving): *Moderate*
Protein: *High*
Fat: *Low*
Saturated fat: *Low*
Cholesterol: *None*
Carbohydrates: *High*
Fiber: *High*
Sodium: *Low*
Major vitamin contribution: *Vitamin A, folate, vitamin C*
Major mineral contribution: *Iron*

About the Nutrients in This Food

Like most legumes (beans and peas), fresh green peas are a high-fiber, high-carbohydrate, low-fat, high-protein food.

Peas are a good source of dietary fiber, both insoluble cellulose in the skin and soluble gums and pectins in the pea. They start out high in sugar but convert their sugars to starch as they age. A few hours after picking, as much as 40 percent of the sugar in peas may have turned to starch. The proteins in peas are plentiful but limited in the essential amino acids tryptophan, methionine, and cystine.

Peas have moderate amounts of vitamin A derived from deep yellow carotenes, including beta-carotene, masked by their green chlorophyll. They are also a good source of the B vitamin folate, vitamin C, and non-heme iron, the form of iron found in plants.

Fresh peas, sometimes known as garden peas, are peas straight from the pod. *Petits pois* is a French term for "small peas," peas that are mature but not yet full size. Dried peas are whole peas minus the natural moisture, with more nutrients per gram than fresh peas; they must be soaked before cooking. Split peas are dried peas that have been boiled, skinned, and split in half so they can be cooked without soaking. Pea pods are very young pods with only a hint of peas inside.

One-half cup of cooked fresh peas has 3.7 g dietary fiber, 0.3 g total fat, 4 g protein, 554 IU vitamin A (24 percent of the RDA for a woman, 19 percent of the RDA for a man), and 63 mcg folate (16 percent of the RDA).

One-half cup of boiled split peas has eight grams dietary fiber, 0.4 g total fat, eight grams protein, seven IU vitamin A (negligible amount), and 63 mcg folate (16 percent of the RDA).

The Most Nutritious Way to Use This Food

With grains. The proteins in peas and other legumes are deficient in the essential amino acids tryptophan, methionine, and cystine but contain sufficient amounts of the essential amino acids lysine and isoleucine. The proteins in grains are exactly the opposite. Together, they complement each other and produce "complete" proteins.

Diets That May Restrict or Exclude This Food

Low-residue diet
Low-purine (antigout) diet

How to Buy This Food

Look for: Fresh, firm bright green pods, loose fresh peas, or snow pea pods. The pods should feel velvety; fresh pea pods should look full, with round fat peas inside.

Avoid: Flat or wilted fresh pea pods (the peas inside are usually immature), fresh pea pods with gray flecks (the peas inside are usually overly mature and starchy), or yellowed fresh or snow pea pods.

Storing This Food

Refrigerate fresh peas in the pod and use them quickly. As peas age their sugars turn to starch; the older the peas, the less sweet. Snow pea pods should also be stored in the refrigerator.

Do not wash pea pods before you store them. Damp pods are likely to mold.

Preparing This Food

To prepare fresh peas, wash the pods, cut off the end, pull away the string running down the side, and shell the peas. To prepare snow pea pods, wash them under cold running water, pull away the string, snip off the ends, then stir-fry or boil quickly to keep them crisp.

What Happens When You Cook This Food

Chlorophyll, the pigment that makes green vegetables green, is sensitive to acids. When you heat green peas, the chlorophyll in the peas reacts chemically with the acids in the vegetable or in the cooking water, forming pheophytin, which is brown. The pheophytin turns the cooked peas olive-drab.

To keep cooked peas green, you have to keep the chlorophyll from reacting with acids. One way to do this is to cook the peas in lots of water, which will dilute the acids. A second alternative is to leave the lid off the pot when you cook the peas so that the volatile acids can float off into the air. Or you can steam the peas in very little water or stir-fry them so fast that they cook before the chlorophyll has time to react with the acids. No matter how you cook the peas, save the cooking liquid. It contains the peas' water-soluble B vitamins.

How Other Kinds of Processing Affect This Food

Drying. Fresh green garden peas are immature seeds. The peas used to make dried split peas are mature seeds, may have twice as much starch as fresh peas, and are an extremely good source of protein. A cup and a half of dried split peas, which will weigh about 14 ounces (400 grams) when cooked, has 20 to 25 grams protein, half the RDA for a healthy adult. Split peas don't have to be soaked before cooking; in fact, soaking drains the B vitamins. When buying split peas, look for well-colored peas in a tightly sealed box or bag. Store the peas in an air- and moistureproof container in a cool, dry cupboard. When you are ready to use them, pick the peas over, discarding any damaged, broken, or withered ones along with any pebbles or other foreign matter.

Dried split peas contain hemagglutinens, naturally occurring chemicals that cause red blood cells to clump together. Although the hemagglutinens in peas are not inactivated by cooking, they are not known to cause any ill effects in the amounts we usually eat.

Medical Uses and/or Benefits

Lower levels of cholesterol. Foods high in soluble gums and pectins appear to lower the amount of cholesterol in the blood and offer some protection against heart disease. There are currently two theories to explain how this may happen. The first theory is that the pectins may form a gel in your stomach that sops up fats and keeps them from being absorbed by your body. The second is that bacteria in the gut may feed on fiber in the peas, producing short chain fatty acids that inhibit the production of cholesterol in your liver.

As a source of carbohydrates for people with diabetes. Legumes are digested very slowly, producing only a gradual rise on blood-sugar levels. As a result, the body needs less insulin to control blood sugar after eating beans than after eating some other high-carbohydrate foods (bread or potato). In studies at the University of Kentucky, a diet rich in beans, whole-grains, vegetables, and fruit developed at the University of Toronto enabled patients with type 1 diabetes (who do not produce any insulin themselves) to cut their daily insulin intake by 38 percent. For patients with type 2 diabetes (who can produce some insulin) the diet reduced the need for injected insulin by 98 percent. This diet is in line with the nutritional guidelines of the American Diabetes Association, but people with diabetes should always consult with their doctors and/or dietitians before altering their diet.

Adverse Effects Associated with This Food

Allergic reaction. According to the *Merck Manual,* legumes (peas, beans, peanuts) are one of the 12 foods most likely to trigger classic food allergy symptoms: hives, swelling of the lips and eyes, and upset stomach. The others are berries (blackberries, blueberries, raspberries, strawberries), chocolate, corn, eggs, fish, milk, nuts, peaches, pork, shellfish, and wheat (see WHEAT CEREALS).

Production of uric acid. Purines are the natural metabolic by-products of protein metabolism in the body. They eventually break down into uric acid, forming sharp crystals that may cause gout if they collect in your joints or kidney stones if they collect in urine. Fresh and dried peas are a source of purines; eating them raises the concentration of purines in your body. Although controlling the amount of purine-producing foods in the diet may not significantly affect the course of gout (which is treated with medication such as allopurinol, which inhibits the formation of uric acid), limiting these foods is still part of many gout regimens.

Food/Drug Interactions

Monoamine oxidase (MAO) inhibitors. Monoamine oxidase inhibitors are drugs used to treat depression. They inactivate naturally occurring enzymes in your body that metabolize tyramine, a substance found in many fermented or aged foods. Tyramine constricts blood vessels and increases blood pressure. If you eat a food containing tyramine while you are taking an MAO inhibitor, you cannot effectively eliminate the tyramine from your body. The result may be a hypertensive crisis. Some nutrition guides advise avoiding dried split peas while using MAO inhibitors.

Peppers

(Bell peppers, chili peppers, jalapeño peppers, pimentos)

Nutritional Profile

Energy value (calories per serving): *Low*

Protein: *Moderate*

Fat: *Low*

Saturated fat: *Low*

Cholesterol: *None*

Carbohydrates: *High*

Fiber: *Moderate*

Sodium: *Low*

Major vitamin contribution: *Vitamin A, folate (sweet peppers), vitamin C*

Major mineral contribution: *Iron, potassium*

About the Nutrients in This Food

Sweet peppers, also known as bell peppers, are green when immature and red, yellow, or purple when ripe. *Hot peppers* are distinguished from sweet peppers by their shape (they are longer and skinnier) and by their burning taste. Like bell peppers, jalapeños, chili peppers, and cayennes will turn red as they ripen.

Sweet peppers with the skin on have about one gram dietary fiber per pepper (insoluble cellulose and lignin in the peel, soluble pectins in the flesh). Peppers have moderate to high amounts of vitamin A derived from yellow carotenes (including beta-carotene). The amount of vitamin A increases as the pepper ripens; sweet red bell peppers have nearly 10 times as much vitamin A as green ones. Peppers are also a good source of vitamin C.

Fresh peppers hold their nutrients well, even at room temperature. For example, green peppers stored at room temperature retained 85 percent of their vitamin C after 48 hours.

Peppers are members of the nightshade family, Solanacea. Other members of this family are eggplant, potatoes, tomatoes, and some mushrooms. Nightshade plants produce natural toxins called glycoalkaloids. The toxin in pepper is solanine. It is estimated that an adult would have to eat 4.5 pounds of peppers at one sitting to get a toxic amount of this glycoalkaloid.

Vitamin A and Vitamin C Content of Peppers

Pepper	Serving	Vitamin A (IU)	Vitamin C (mg)
Bell pepper (green, raw)	1 medium	440	95
Bell pepper (red, raw)	1 medium	3,726	152
Hot green chili (canned)	½ cup	88	23.8
Hot red chili (canned)	½ cup	8.87	46.2
Jalapeño (canned)	½ cup	1,156	6.8
Chili powder	1 teaspoon	771	2

Source: USDA Nutrient Data Laboratory. National Nutrient Database for Standard Reference. Available online. URL: http://www.nal.usda.gov/fnic/foodcomp/search/.

The Most Nutritious Way to Serve This Food

Bell peppers: Fresh sliced or chopped on a salad.

Hot peppers: Seeded, in a soup or stew.

Diets That May Restrict or Exclude This Food

Antiflatulence diet
Bland diet

Buying This Food

Look for: Firm peppers that feel thick and fleshy. Their skin should be brightly colored green, red, yellow, or purple.

Avoid: Dull-colored peppers; they may be immature. If the skin is wrinkled, the peppers have lost moisture; soft spots suggest decay inside.

Storing This Food

Refrigerate fresh peppers in the vegetable crisper to preserve their moisture and vitamin C.

Preparing This Food

Sweet bell peppers.   Wash the peppers under cold running water, slice, and remove the seeds and membranes (which are irritating). If you plan to cook the peppers, peel them; the skin will otherwise curl up into a hard, unpalatable strip. Immerse the pepper in hot water, then lift it out and plunge it into cold water. The hot water bath damages a layer of cells under the skin so that the skin is very easy to peel off. Roasting the peppers produces the same result.

Hot peppers. NEVER HANDLE ANY VARIETY OF HOT PEPPERS WITH YOUR BARE HANDS. Hot peppers contain large amounts of the naturally occurring irritants capsaicin (pronounced cap-say-i-sun), nordyhydrocapsaicin, and dihydrocapsaicin. These chemicals cause pain by latching on to special sites called receptors on the surface of nerve cells, opening small channels in the cells that permit calcium particles to flood in. The calcium particles trigger the pain reaction. Exposure to high temperatures, like a burn, produces the same effect.

Capsaicins irritate the lining of your mouth and esophagus (which is why they cause heartburn). They can burn unprotected skin and mucous membranes. Capsaicins dissolve in milk fat and alcohol, but not water. They cannot simply be washed off your hands.

NOTE: Capsaicin extracted from hot peppers and applied to the skin as the active ingredient in a cream or ointment is an effective over-the-counter pain remedy. In addition, in a 1991 study at the University of Florence (Italy), 39 men and women suffering from cluster headaches (a form of migraine) obtained relief by squirting a capsaicin-containing solution into the nostril on the headache side of the face. WARNING: *THE CAPSAICIN USED TO RELIEVE PAIN IS A PURIFIED, MEDICAL-GRADE PRODUCT EXTRACTED FROM PEPPERS. HOT PEPPERS THEM-SELVES DO NOT RELIEVE PAIN AND SHOULD NEVER BE APPLIED TO SKIN OR MUCOUS MEMBRANES.*

What Happens When You Cook This Food

Chlorophyll, the pigment that makes green vegetables green, is sensitive to acids. When you heat green peppers, the chlorophyll in the flesh will react chemically with acids in the pepper or in the cooking water, forming pheophytin, which is brown. The pheophytin makes a cooked pepper olive-drab or (if the pepper has a lot of yellow carotenes) bronze.

To keep cooked green peppers green, you have to keep the chlorophyll from reacting with acids. One way to do this is to cook peppers in a large quantity of water (which dilutes the acids), but this increases the loss of vitamin C. A second alternative is to cook them in a pot with the lid off so that the volatile acids float off into the air. Or you can stir-fry the peppers, cooking them so fast that there is almost no time for the chlorophyll/acid reaction to occur.

When long cooking is inevitable, as with stuffed sweet green peppers, the only remedy is to smother the peppers in sauce so that it doesn't matter what color the peppers are. (Red and yellow peppers won't fade; their carotenoid pigments are impervious to heat.)

Because vitamin C is sensitive to heat, cooked peppers have less than fresh peppers. But peppers have so much vitamin C to begin with that even cooked peppers are a good source of this nutrient.

How Other Kinds of Processing Affect This Food

* * *

Medical Uses and/or Benefits

Relieving the congestion of a cold. Hot spices, including hot pepper, irritate the mucous membranes lining your nose and throat and the bronchi in your lungs, making the tissues "weep." The water secretions may make it easier for you to cough up mucus or blow your nose, thus helping to relieve your congestion for a while.

Adverse Effects Associated with This Food

Irritant dermatitis. See *Preparing this food (Hot peppers),* above.

Painful urination. The irritating oils in peppers are eliminated through urination. They may cause temporary irritation of the urinary tract.

Food/Drug Interactions

* * *

Persimmons

Nutritional Profile

Energy value (calories): *Moderate*
Protein: *Low*
Fat: *Low*
Saturated fat: *Low*
Cholesterol: *None*
Carbohydrates: *High*
Fiber: *High*
Sodium: *Low*
Major vitamin contribution: *Vitamin A, vitamin C*
Major mineral contribution: *Potassium*

About the Nutrients in This Food

The Japanese persimmon (also known as *kaki*) is high in dietary fiber (soluble pectins in the flesh). It is an excellent source of vitamin A from yellow carotenes (including beta-carotene), with small amounts of the B vitamin folate, plus vitamin C.

One Japanese persimmon (2.5-inch diameter) has six grams dietary fiber, 2,733 IU vitamin A (1.2 times the RDA for a woman, 92 percent of the RDA for a man), and 12.6 mg vitamin C (17 percent of the RDA for a woman, 14 percent of the RDA for a man).

The smaller, more seedy American persimmon has about nine times as much vitamin C, but similar amounts of other nutrients.

The Most Nutritious Way to Serve This Food

Fresh and ripe.

Diets That May Restrict or Exclude This Food

* * *

Buying This Food

Look for: Firm, plump fruit with brightly colored, smooth unbroken skin. The bright green stem cap should be firmly anchored to the fruit.

Storing This Food

Let persimmons ripen at room temperature until they are soft, then store them in the refrigerator. Oriental persimmons, which are more astringent than the American varieties, will lose some of their sharpness if you store them in a plastic bag with an apple. The apple releases ethylene gas, which ripens and mellows the persimmon.

Preparing This Food

Wash the persimmon and pull off its stem cap. Then peel and slice the persimmon or put it through a food mill to mash the flesh and remove the seeds.

What Happens When You Cook This Food

* * *

How Other Kinds of Processing Affect This Food

* * *

Medical Uses and/or Benefits

* * *

Adverse Effects Associated with This Food

* * *

Food/Drug Interactions

* * *

Pineapple

Nutritional Profile

Energy value (calories per serving): *Low*

Protein: *Low*

Fat: *Low*

Saturated fat: *Low*

Cholesterol: *None*

Carbohydrates: *High*

Fiber: *High*

Sodium: *Low (fresh or dried fruit)*
      High (dried fruit treated with sodium sulfur compounds)

Major vitamin contribution: *Vitamin C*

Major mineral contribution: *Potassium*

About the Nutrients in This Food

Pineapples are high in dietary fiber, primarily soluble pectins and gums. Their most important nutrient is vitamin C.

One cup fresh pineapple chunks has 2.3 g dietary fiber and 79 mg vitamin C (slightly more than the RDA for a woman, 88 percent of the RDA for a man).

One-half cup canned unsweetened pineapple juice with added vitamin C has 54.8 mg vitamin C (72 percent of the RDA for a woman, 60 percent of the RDA for a man).

The pineapple fruit and the stem of the pineapple plant contain bromelain, a proteolytic ("protein-dissolving") enzyme, similar to papain (in unripe papayas) and ficin (in fresh figs). Bromelain is a natural meat tenderizer that breaks down the protein molecules in meat when you add the fruit to a stew or baste a roast with the juice.

Diets That May Restrict or Exclude This Food

* * *

Buying This Food

Look for: Large pineapples. The leaves in the crown on top should be fresh and green, the pineapple should feel heavy for its size (which means it's

298

juicy), it should have a rich pineapple aroma, and you should hear a solid "thunk" when you tap a finger against the side. While the pineapple's shell generally loses chlorophyll and turns more golden as the fruit ripens, some varieties of pineapple have more chlorophyll and stay green longer than others, so the color of the shell is not a reliable guide to ripeness.

Storing This Food

Store pineapples either at room temperature or in the refrigerator. Neither will have any effect on the sweetness of the fruit. Fruits and vegetables get sweeter after they are picked by converting stored starches to sugars. Since the pineapple has no stored starch and gets its sugar from its leaves, it is as sweet as it ever will be on the day it is picked. It will get softer while stored, though, as its pectic enzymes break down pectins in its cell walls.

Preparing This Food

To sweeten and soften fresh pineapple, peel and slice the fruit (or cut it into chunks), sprinkle it with sugar, and chill it in the refrigerator. The sugar and water on the pineapple's surface is a denser solution than the liquid inside the pineapple's cells. As a result liquid flows out of the cells. Without liquid to hold them rigid, the cell walls will collapse inward and the pineapple will be softer. This physical phenomenon—the flow of liquids across a membrane from a less dense to a more dense environment—is called osmosis.

What Happens When You Cook This Food

As you cook pineapple, the pectic substances in its cell walls dissolve and the pineapple softens.

If you add fresh pineapple to gelatin, the bromelain will digest the proteins in the gelatin and the dish won't "set." However, bromelain only works at a temperature between 140°F and 170°F; it is destroyed by boiling. For the maximum effect in stewing, set the heat at simmer. To add fresh pineapple to a gelatin mold, boil the fruit first.

How Other Kinds of Processing Affect This Food

Drying.   Drying concentrates the calories and nutrients in pineapple. Fresh pineapple may be treated with a sulfur compound such as sulfur dioxide to protect its vitamin C and keep it from darkening as it dries. In people sensitive to sulfites, these compounds may provoke serious allergic reactions, including potentially fatal anaphylactic shock.

Juice.   Since 2000, following several deaths attributed to unpasteurized apple juice contaminated with *E. coli* O157:H7, the FDA has required that all juices sold in the United States be pasteurized to inactivate harmful organisms such as bacteria and mold.

Medical Uses and/or Benefits

* * *

Adverse Effects Associated with This Food

Dermatitis. Bromelain, which breaks down proteins, may cause irritant dermatitis. Pineapples may also cause allergic dermatitis. (Irritant dermatitis may occur in anyone who touches a pineapple; allergic dermatitis occurs only in an individual who is sensitive to a particular substance.)

Sulfur allergies. See *How other kinds of processing affect this food,* above.

Food/Drug Interactions

False-positive test for carcinoid tumors. Carcinoid tumors, which may arise from tissues in the endocrine or gastrointestinal system, secrete serotonin, a natural chemical that makes blood vessels expand or contract. Because serotonin is excreted in urine, these tumors are diagnosed by measuring serotonin levels by products in the urine. Pineapples contain large amounts of serotonin; eating them in the three days before a test for an endocrine tumor might produce a false-positive result, suggesting that you have the tumor when in fact you don't. (Other foods high in serotonin are avocados, bananas, eggplant, plums, tomatoes, and walnuts.)

Plantain

Nutritional Profile

Energy value (calories per serving): *Low*
Protein: *Low*
Fat: *Low*
Saturated fat: *Low*
Cholesterol: *None*
Carbohydrates: *High*
Fiber: *High*
Sodium: *Low*
Major vitamin contribution: *B vitamins, vitamin C*
Major mineral contribution: *Potassium, magnesium*

About the Nutrients in This Food

Plantains are a variety of banana, but unlike "eating bananas," they do not convert their starches to sugar as they mature. Even ripe plantains must be cooked before serving.

The plantain is classified botanically as a vegetable; the banana is classified as a fruit. Nutritionally, the plantain has up to 14 times as much vitamin A, two times as much vitamin C, and one-third more potassium than the banana.

One-half cup boiled plantain slices has 2 g dietary fiber, 700 IU vitamin A (30 percent of the RDA for a woman, 24 percent of the RDA for a man), 8.4 mg vitamin C (11 percent of the RDA for a woman, 9 percent of the RDA for a man), and 358 mg potassium (72 percent as much potassium as eight ounces fresh orange juice).

NOTE: Unripe plantains, like unripe bananas, contain proteins that inhibit the actions of amylase, an enzyme required to digest starch and other complex carbohydrates.

The Most Nutritious Way to Serve This Food

Cooked.

Diets That May Restrict or Exclude This Food

Controlled potassium diet

Buying This Food

Look for: Large, firm plantains with green peel flecked with some brown spots. The riper the plantain, the blacker its skin.

Avoid: Plantains with soft spots under the skin.

Storing This Food

Store plantains at room temperature or refrigerate.

Preparing This Food

Cut off the ends of the plantain, slice down through the peel and remove it in strips, under running water to prevent the plantain from staining your hands.

What Happens When You Cook This Food

When you cook a plantain the starch granules in its flesh will swell and rupture. The fruit softens and its nutrients become easier to absorb.

How Other Kinds of Processing Affect This Food

* * *

Medical Uses and/or Benefits

Potassium benefits.   Because potassium is excreted in urine, potassium-rich foods are often recommended for people taking diuretics. In addition, a diet rich in potassium (from food) is associated with a lower risk of stroke. A 1998 Harvard School of Public Health analysis of data from the long-running Health Professionals Study shows 38 percent fewer strokes among men who ate nine servings of high-potassium foods a day vs. those who ate less than four servings. Among men with high blood pressure, taking a daily 1,000 mg potassium supplement—about the amount of potassium in $1^1/_2$ cups sliced plantain—reduced the incidence of stroke by 60 percent.

Lower risk of stroke.   Various nutrition studies have attested to the power of adequate potassium to keep blood pressure within safe levels. For example, in the 1990s, data from the long-running Harvard School of Public Health/Health Professionals Follow-Up Study of male doctors showed that a diet rich in high-potassium foods such as bananas, oranges, and plantain may reduce the risk of stroke. In the study, the men who ate the higher number of potassium-rich foods (an average of nine servings a day) had a risk of stroke 38 percent lower than that of men who consumed fewer than four servings a day. In 2008, a similar survey at the Queen's Medical Center (Honolulu) showed a similar protective effect among men and women using diuretic drugs (medicines that increase urination and thus the loss of potassium).

Improved mood. Bananas and plantains are both rich in serotonin, dopamine, and other natural mood-elevating neurotransmitters—natural chemicals that facilitate the transmission of impulses among nerve cells.

Adverse Effects Associated with This Food

Digestive problems. Unripe plantains, like unripe bananas, contain proteins that inhibit the actions of amylase, an enzyme required to digest starch and other complex carbohydrates.

Food/Drug Interactions

False-positive test for carcinoid tumors. Carcinoid tumors, which may arise from tissues of the endocrine system, the intestines, or the lungs, secrete serotonin, a natural chemical that makes blood vessels expand or contract. Because serotonin is excreted in urine, these tumors are diagnosed by measuring the levels of serotonin by-products in the urine. Plantains contain large amounts of serotonin; eating them in the three days before a test for an endocrine tumor might produce a false positive result, suggesting that you have the tumor when in fact you don't. Other foods high in serotonin are avocados, bananas, eggplant, pineapple, plums, tomatoes, and walnuts.

Plums

See also Prunes.

Nutritional Profile

Energy value (calories per serving): *Moderate*
Protein: *Low*
Fat: *Low*
Saturated fat: *Low*
Cholesterol: *None*
Carbohydrates: *High*
Fiber: *Moderate*
Sodium: *Low*
Major vitamin contribution: *Vitamin A, vitamin C*
Major mineral contribution: *Potassium*

About the Nutrients in This Food

Plums have moderate amounts of dietary fiber and a little vitamin A. They are a good source of vitamin C.

One fresh plum ($2^1/_8$-inch diameter) has one gram dietary fiber, 228 IU vitamin A (10 percent of the RDA for a woman, 8 percent of the RDA for a man), and 6 mg vitamin C (8 percent of the RDA for a woman, 7 percent of the RDA for a man).

Like apple seeds, apricot pits, and peach pits, the seed inside a plum pit contains amygdalin, a naturally occurring cyanide compound (see APPLES).

The Most Nutritious Way to Serve This Food

Fresh and ripe, with the peel.

Diets That May Restrict or Exclude This Food

* * *

Buying This Food

Look for: Firm, brightly colored fruit that are slightly soft to the touch, yielding a bit when you press them with your finger.

Comparing Varieties of Plums

Damson	Dark skin and flesh (for preserves only)
Friar	Dark red skin, deep yellow flesh
Greengage	Green yellow skin and yellow flesh
Italian ("prune" plums)	Small, oval, with blue purple skin and firm golden flesh
Laroda	Large; yellow skin with a red blush and yellow flesh
Red beauty	Bright red skin, firm yellow flesh
Santa Rosa	Red purple skin, yellow flesh (very tart)

Sources: "Guide to Selection and Care of Fresh Fruit" and "The fresh approach to plums," United Fresh Fruit and Vegetable Association (n.d.); Rombauer, Irma S. and Becker, Marion Rombauer, *The Joy of Cooking* (Indianapolis: Bobbs-Merrill, 1984).

Storing This Food

Store firm plums at room temperature. Plums have no stored starch to convert to sugars, so they won't get sweeter after they are picked, but they will soften as their pectic enzymes dissolve some of the pectin stiffening their cell walls. When the plums are soft enough, refrigerate them to stop the enzyme action.

Preparing This Food

Wash and serve fresh plums or split them, remove the pit, and slice the plums for fruit salad. Plums can be stewed in the skin; if you prefer them skinless, put them in boiling water for a few minutes, then lift them out with a slotted spoon and plunge them into cold water. The hot water will damage a layer of cells under the skin, the plum will swell, and its skin will split and peel off easily.

What Happens When You Cook This Food

When you cook a plum, its water-soluble pectins and hemicellulose will dissolve and the flesh will soften.

Cooking may also change the color of red, purple, or blue red plums containing anthocyanin pigments that are sensitive to acids or bases (alkalis). The colors get more intensely red or purple in acids (lemon juice) and less so in bases (baking soda). Cooking plums (which are acid) in an aluminum pot can create acid/metal compounds that discolor either the pot or the plum.

How Other Kinds of Processing Affect This Food

Drying. See PRUNES.

Medical Uses and/or Benefits

* * *

Adverse Effects Associated with This Food

* * *

Food/Drug Interactions

False-positive test for carcinoid tumors. Carcinoid tumors, tumors that may arise from tissues of the endocrine or gastrointestinal systems, secrete serotonin, a chemical that makes blood vessels expand or contract. Because serotonin is excreted in urine, these tumors are diagnosed by measuring the serotonin levels in the patient's urine. Plums contain large amounts of serotonin. Eating plums in the 72 hours before the test might give a false-positive result, suggesting that you have an endocrine tumor when in fact you do not. (Other foods rich in serotonin include avocados, bananas, eggplant, pineapple, tomatoes, and walnuts.)

Pomegranates

Nutritional Profile

Energy value (calories per serving): *Moderate*
Protein: *Low*
Fat: *Low*
Saturated fat: *Low*
Cholesterol: *None*
Carbohydrates: *High*
Fiber: *Low*
Sodium: *Low*
Major vitamin contribution: *Vitamin C*
Major mineral contribution: *Potassium*

About the Nutrients in This Food

The juice of the pomegranate, obtained by crushing the jelly clinging to the pomegranate seeds, has moderate amounts of vitamin C and is high in potassium.

One fresh pomegranate has one gram dietary fiber, 9.4 mg vitamin C (13 percent of the RDA for a woman, 10 percent of the RDA for a man), and 399 mg potassium, 80 percent of the potassium in an eight-ounce cup of fresh orange juice.

The Most Nutritious Way to Serve This Food

Fresh cut or juiced.

Diets That May Restrict or Exclude This Food

* * *

Buying This Food

Look for: A pomegranate that feels heavy for its size (which means it's juicy). The rind should be bright red.

Avoid: Pale pomegranates or pomegranates that look dry or wrinkled.

Storing This Food

Store pomegranates in the refrigerator and use within a week.

Preparing This Food

Slice through the stem end of the pomegranate and pull off the top—carefully, to avoid splashing red pomegranate juice all over yourself. Then slice the pomegranate into wedges and pull the wedges apart. Once you cut the pomegranate apart you can handle it in one of two ways, the messy way and the neat way. The messy way is to pull the seeds out of the pomegranate, crush them in your teeth to get the juice, and then spit out the crushed seeds. The neat way is to put the seeds through a strainer, collect the juice, and discard the seeds.

What Happens When You Cook This Food

* * *

How Other Kinds of Processing Affect This Food

Freezing. You can freeze a whole pomegranate or just its seeds. To eat, just thaw.

Medical Uses and/or Benefits

Lower risk of stroke. Various nutrition studies have attested to the power of adequate potassium to keep blood pressure within safe levels. For example, in the 1990s, data from the long-running Harvard School of Public Health/Health Professionals Follow-Up Study of male doctors showed that a diet rich in high-potassium foods such as bananas, oranges, and plantain may reduce the risk of stroke. In the study, the men who ate the higher number of potassium-rich foods (an average of nine servings a day) had a risk of stroke 38 percent lower than that of men who consumed fewer than four servings a day. In 2008, a similar survey at the Queen's Medical Center (Honolulu) showed a similar protective effect among men and women using diuretic drugs (medicines that increase urination and thus the loss of potassium).

Lower levels of cholesterol. Pomegranate liquid is rich in polyphenols, antioxidant compounds that help lower "bad" cholesterol. Nutrition researchers at the Technion Faculty of Medicine and Rambam Medical Center in Haifa (Israel) rate pomegranate juice higher in polyphenols than red wine, blueberry juice, cranberry juice, green tea, black tea, and orange juice.

Potassium replacement. Because potassium is excreted in urine, potassium-rich foods are often recommended for people who are taking diuretic drugs.

Adverse Effects Associated with This Food

* * *

Food/Drug Interactions

* * *

Pork

Nutritional Profile[*]

Energy value (calories per serving): *Moderate*
Protein: *High*
Fat: *Moderate*
Saturated fat: *High*
Cholesterol: *Moderate*
Carbohydrates: *None*
Fiber: *None*
Sodium: *Moderate*
Major vitamin contribution: *B vitamins*
Major mineral contribution: *Iron*

About the Nutrients in This Food

Like beef, fish, poultry, eggs, and milk products, pork provides high-quality proteins with sufficient amounts of all the essential amino acids. Pork fat is slightly less saturated than beef fat, but it has about the same amount of cholesterol per serving. Pork is a good source of B vitamins and heme iron, the form of iron most easily absorbed by your body.

One broiled boneless five-ounce top loin pork chop has 4.7 g total fat (1.6 g saturated fat), 70 mg cholesterol, and 0.7 mg iron (4 percent of the RDA for a woman, 9 percent of the RDA for a man).

The Most Nutritious Way to Serve This Food

Lean pork, thoroughly cooked.

Diets That May Restrict or Exclude This Food

Controlled-fat, low-cholesterol diet
Low-protein diet

---

* Values are for lean broiled meat.

Buying This Food

Look for: Firm, fresh pork that is light pink or reddish and has very little visible fat. If there are any bone ends showing, they should be red, not white; the whiter the bone ends, the older the animal from which the meat was taken.

Avoid: Packages with a lot of liquid. Meat that has lost moisture is likely to be dry and tough.

Storing This Food

Refrigerate fresh pork immediately. Refrigeration prolongs the freshness of pork by slowing the natural multiplication of bacteria on the surface of meat. Left to their own devices, these bacteria convert proteins and other substances on the surface of the meat to a slimy film and, eventually, they will convert the meat's sulfur-containing amino acids methionine and cystine into smelly chemicals called mercaptans. When the mercaptans combine with myoglobin, they produce the greenish pigment that gives spoiled meat its characteristic unpleasant appearance.

Refrigeration slows this whole chain of events so that fresh roasts and chops usually stay fresh for three to five days. For longer storage, store the pork in the freezer where the very low temperatures will slow the bacteria even more.

Store unopened smoked or cured pork products in the refrigerator in the original wrapper and use according to the date and directions on the package.

Preparing This Food

Trim the pork carefully. You can significantly reduce the amount of fat and cholesterol in each serving by judiciously cutting away all visible fat.

Do not add salt to the pork before you cook it; the salt will draw moisture out of the meat, making it stringy and tough. Add salt near the end of the cooking process.

When you are done, clean all utensils thoroughly with soap and hot water. Wash your cutting board, wood or plastic, with hot water, soap, and a bleach-and-water solution. For ultimate safety in preventing the transfer of microorganisms from meat to other foods, keep one cutting board exclusively for raw meat, fish, or poultry, and a second one for everything else.

What Happens When You Cook This Food

Cooking changes the way pork looks and tastes, alters its nutritional value, makes it safer, and extends its shelf life.

Browning meat before you cook it does not seal in the juices, but it does change the flavor by caramelizing proteins and sugars on the surface. Because the only sugars that occur naturally in pork are the small amounts of glycogen in its muscles, we add sugars in the form of marinades or basting liquids that may also contain acids (vinegar, lemon juice, wine) to break down muscle fibers and tenderize the meat. Browning has one minor nutritional drawback. It breaks amino acids on the surface of the meat into smaller compounds that are no longer useful proteins.

When pork is heated, it loses water and shrinks. Its pigments, which combine with oxygen, are denatured (broken into smaller fragments) by the heat and turn brown, the natural color of cooked meat. This color change is more dramatic in beef (which starts out red) than in pork (which starts out gray pink). In fact, you can pretty much judge beef's doneness from its color, but you must use a meat thermometer to measure the internal temperature of the meat before you can say it is thoroughly cooked.

Pork is considered done (and safe to eat) when it reaches an average uniform internal temperature of 170°F, hot enough to kill *Trichinella spiralis,* the organism that causes trichinosis.[*]

Killing these organisms is one obvious benefit of heating pork thoroughly. Another is that heat liquifies the fat on the meat so that it simply runs off the meat. The unsaturated fatty acids that remain in the meat, continue to oxidize as the meat cooks. Oxidized fats give cooked meat a characteristic warmed-over flavor. You can reduce the warmed-over flavor by cooking and storing the meat under a blanket of catsup or a gravy made from tomatoes, peppers, and other vitamin C–rich vegetables, all natural antioxidants that slow the oxidation of the fats.

How Other Kinds of Processing Affect This Food

Freezing. Freezing changes the flavor and texture of fresh pork. When fresh pork is frozen, the water in its cells turn into ice crystals that can tear the cell walls so that liquids leak out when the pork is thawed. That's why defrosted pork, like defrosted beef, veal, or lamb, may be drier and less tender than fresh meat.

Curing, smoking, and aging. Curing preserves meat by osmotic action. The dry salt or a salt solution draws liquid out the cells of the meat and the cells of any microorganisms living on the meat.[†] *Smoking*—hanging meat over an open fire—gives meat a rich, "smoky" flavor

---

[*] Cooking pork in a microwave oven requires careful attention to the temperature. In 1982, researchers at Iowa State University found live trichinae in nine of 51 experimentally infected samples of pork that had been cooked in different brands and models of microwave ovens according to directions from the manufacturers and from the Pork Producers Council. In each case, while the internal temperature of the meat rose to 170°F, moisture evaporating on the surface of the meat kept the temperature there too low to kill the trichinae. In a second study, in 1983, the researchers recommended that pork cooked in a microwave oven be cooked in a special transparent plastic cooking bag to prevent the evaporation of moisture on the surface of the meat. Subsequent laboratory tests at Iowa showed that pork roasts microwaved in these bags reached temperatures high enough to kill trichinae on all surfaces of the meat.

[†] Osmosis is the physical phenomenon by which liquids flow across a membrane, like a cell wall, from a less dense to a more dense environment. Since salt or salty liquid is denser than the liquid inside cells, it pulls out moisture. Pork becomes dryer, and the microorganisms, which cannot live without water, died after preparing the meat. Irradiation destroys the thiamin (vitamin B_1) in fresh pork.

that varies with the wood used in the fire. Meats smoked over an open fire are exposed to carcinogenic chemicals in the smoke, including a-benzopyrene. Meats treated with artificial smoke flavoring are not, since the flavoring is commercially treated to remove tar and a-benzopyrene. Cured and smoked meats sometimes have less moisture and proportionally more fat than fresh meat. They are also saltier. *Aging*—letting the meat hang exposed to air—further reduces the moisture content and shrinks the meat.

Irradiation.   Irradiation makes meat safer by exposing it to gamma rays, high-energy ionizing radiation, the kind of radiation that kills living cells including potentially hazardous microorganisms. The process does not change the way meat looks, feels, or tastes, nor does it make the food radioactive. But it does change the structure of some naturally occurring chemicals in meat, breaking molecules apart to form new compounds called "radiolytic products" (abbreviated as RP). About 90 percent of these compounds are also found in non-irradiated foods. The rest, called "unique radiolytic products" (URP), are found only in irradiated foods (including meat). In 1985, the Food and Drug Administration approved the use of low doses of radiation to kill *Trichinella spiralis,* the organism in pork that causes trichinosis. Today, irradiation is an approved technique in more than 37 countries around the world, including the United States. NOTE: Irradiation reduces the amount of thiamin (vitamin B_1) in pork. (See above, *Preparing this food.*)

Medical Uses and/or Benefits

* * *

Adverse Effects Associated with This Food

Trichinosis.   Trichinosis comes from eating improperly cooked meat contaminated with cysts of *Trichinella spiralis,* a parasitic roundworm found in meat-eating animals. Meat-fed hogs are not the only source of trichinosis; Arctic explorers have gotten trichinosis from polar bear meat. About 10 to 100 cases of trichinosis from pork are reported each year in the United States; many mild cases, with symptoms similar to those of a mild flu, undoubtedly remain undiagnosed. See *What happens when you cook this food,* above.

Increased risk of cardiovascular disease.   Like other foods from animals, pork is a source of cholesterol and saturated fats, which increase the amount of cholesterol circulating in your blood and raise your risk of heart disease. To reduce the risk of heart disease, the National Cholesterol Education Project recommends following the Step I and Step II diets.

The Step I diet provides no more than 30 percent of total daily calories from fat, no more than 10 percent of total daily calories from saturated fat, and no more than 300 mg of cholesterol per day. It is designed for healthy people whose cholesterol is in the range of 200–239 mg/dL.

The Step II diet provides 25–35 percent of total calories from fat, less than 7 percent of total calories from saturated fat, up to 10 percent of total calories from polyunsaturated fat, up to 20 percent of total calories from monounsaturated fat, and less than 300 mg cholesterol per day. This stricter regimen is designed for people who have one or more of the following conditions:

- Existing cardiovascular disease
- High levels of low-density lipoproteins (LDLs, or "bad" cholesterol) or low levels of high-density lipoproteins (HDLs, or "good" cholesterol)
- Obesity
- Type 1 diabetes (insulin-dependent diabetes, diabetes mellitus)
- Metabolic syndrome, a.k.a. insulin resistance syndrome, a cluster of risk factors that includes type 2 diabetes (non-insulin-dependent diabetes)

Decline in kidney function. Proteins are nitrogen compounds. When metabolized, they yield ammonia that is excreted through the kidneys. In laboratory animals, a sustained high-protein diet increases the flow of blood through the kidneys, accelerating the natural age-related decline in kidney function. Some experts suggest that this may also occur in human beings.

Allergic reaction. According to the *Merck Manual,* pork is one of the 12 foods most likely to trigger classic food allergy symptoms: hives, swelling of the lips and eyes, and upset stomach. The others are berries (blackberries, blueberries, raspberries, strawberries), chocolate, corn, eggs, fish, legumes (green peas, lima beans, peanuts, soybeans), milk, nuts, peaches, shellfish, and wheat.

Food/Drug Interactions

Tetracycline antibiotics (demeclocycline [Declomycin]), doxycycline [Vibtamycin], methacycline [Rondomycin], minocycline [Minocin], oxytetracycline [Terramycin], tetracycline [Achromycin V, Panmycin, Sumycin]). Because meat contains iron, which binds tetracyclines into compounds the body cannot absorb, it is best to avoid meat for two hours before and after taking one of these antibiotics.

Potatoes

See also Sweet potatoes.

Nutritional Profile

Energy value (calories per serving): *Moderate*
Protein: *Moderate*
Fat: *Low*
Saturated fat: *Low*
Cholesterol: *None*
Carbohydrates: *High*
Fiber: *High (with skin)*
Sodium: *Low*
Major vitamin contribution: *Folate, Vitamin C*
Major mineral contribution: *Potassium*

About the Nutrients in This Food

Potatoes are high-carbohydrate foods, rich in starch and dietary fiber, including insoluble cellulose and lignin in the skin and soluble pectins in the flesh. When potatoes are stored, their starches slowly turn to sugar. The longer a potato is stored, the sweeter and less tasty it will be.

The proteins in potatoes are limited in the essential amino acids methionine and cystine. Potatoes are a good source of the B vitamin folate and vitamin C. Fresh potatoes have more vitamin C than stored potatoes; after three months' storage, the potato has lost about one-third of its vitamin C; after six to seven months, about two-thirds.

One six-ounce baked potato with its skin has four grams dietary fiber, four grams protein, 0.2 g total fat, 48 mcg folate (12 percent of the RDA), and 16 mg vitamin C (21 percent of the RDA for a woman, 13 percent of the RDA for a man).

One ounce of regular (not low-fat) potato chips has 1.4 g dietary fiber, two grams protein, 9.8 g total fat, 13 mcg folate (3 percent of the RDA), and 8.8 mg vitamin C (12 percent of the RDA for a woman, 10 percent of the RDA for a man).

Potatoes are members of the nightshade family, Solanaceae, which includes eggplant, peppers, tomatoes, and some mushrooms. These plants produce neurotoxins (nerve poisons) called glycoalkaloids. The glycoalkaloid in potatoes is solanine, a chemical that interferes with acetylcholinesterase, a neurotransmitter that enables cells to transmit impulses.

Solanine is made in the green parts of the plant, the leaves, the stem, and any green spots on the skin. Potatoes exposed to light produce solanine more quickly and in higher amounts than potatoes stored in the dark, but *all* potatoes produce some solanine *all* the time. Solanine does not dissolve in water, nor is it destroyed by heat; any solanine present in a raw potato will still be there after you cook it. It is estimated than an adult might have to eat about three pounds of potatoes or 2.4 pounds of potato skins at one sitting to experience the first gastrointestinal or neurological signs of solanine poisoning. A child will react to smaller amounts, 1.5 pounds potatoes, 1.4 pounds potato skins. The U.S. government does not permit the sale of potatoes containing more than 200 ppm (*parts per million*) solanine. The potatoes we buy usually contain only 100 ppm, but the safest course is to discard *all* sprouting potatoes or potatoes with green spots on the skin.

Diets That May Exclude or Restrict This Food

Low-carbohydrate diet
Low-salt diet (canned potatoes, potato chips, potato sticks, and the like)

The Most Nutritious Way to Serve This Food

As fresh as possible, with meat, milk, or grains to complete the potato's proteins.
　　With the skin, which is a valuable source of food fiber.

Buying This Food

Look for: Firm potatoes with unscarred, unblemished skin. Different varieties of potatoes have skins of different thickness. This has no effect at all on the nutritional value of the potato.

Avoid: Potatoes with peeling skin (an immature vegetable that won't store well); potatoes with wrinkled or blemished skin (there may be decay inside); potatoes with green spots or sprouts growing out of the eyes (higher than normal levels of solanine); or moldy potatoes (potentially hazardous toxins).

Storing This Food

Store potatoes in a dark, dry cabinet or root cellar to prevent sprouting and protect them from mold. The temperature should be cool, but not cold, since temperatures below 50°F encourage the conversion of the potato's starches to sugar. If the potatoes are frozen, they will develop black rings inside.
　　Use potatoes as quickly as possible. Vitamin C is sensitive to oxygen, so the longer potatoes are stored, the less vitamin C they will have.

Do not wash potatoes before you store them nor store them in the refrigerator; dampness encourages the growth of molds.

Preparing This Food

Discard potatoes with green spots, sprouting eyes, or patches of mold on the skin, and scrub the rest with a stiff vegetable brush under cool running water. When you peel and slice potatoes, throw out any that have rot or mold inside.

Don't peel or slice potatoes until you are ready to use them. When you cut into a potato and tear its cell walls you release polyphenoloxidase, an enzyme that hastens the oxidation of phenols in the potato, creating the brownish compounds that darken a fresh-cut potato. You can slow this reaction (but not stop it completely) by soaking the peeled sliced fresh potatoes in ice water, but many of the vitamins in the potatoes will leach out into the soaking water. Another alternative is to dip the sliced potatoes in an acid solution (lemon juice and water, vinegar and water), but this will alter the taste.

What Happens When You Cook This Food

Starch consists of granules packed with the molecules of amylose and amylopectin. When you cook a potato, its starch granules absorb water molecules that cling to the amylose and amylopectin molecules, making the granules swell. If the granules absorb enough water, they will rupture, releasing the nutrients inside. If you are cooking potatoes in a stew or soup, the amylose and amylopectin molecules that escape from the ruptured starch granule will attract and hold water molecules in the liquid, thickening the dish.

However you prepare them, cooked potatoes have more nutrients available than raw potatoes do. They may also be a different color. Like onions and cauliflower, potatoes contain pale anthoxanthin pigments that react with metal ions to form blue, green, or brown compounds. That's why potatoes may turn yellowish if you cook them in an aluminum or iron pot or slice them with a carbon-steel knife. To keep potatoes pale, cook them in a glass or enameled pot.

See *Adverse Effects Associated with This Food.*

How Other Kinds of Processing Affect This Food

Freezing. A potato's cells are like a box whose stiff walls are held rigidly in place by the water inside the cell. When you freeze a cooked potato, the water in its cells forms ice crystals that can tear the cell walls, allowing liquid to leak out when the potatoes are defrosted, which is why defrosted potatoes taste mushy. Commercial processors get around this by partially dehydrating potatoes before they are frozen or by freezing potatoes in a sauce that gives an interesting flavor to take your mind off the texture.

Dehydrating. Potato "flakes" and "granules" have fewer vitamins and minerals than fresh potatoes; potato chips and sticks are usually much higher in salt.

Potato salad. Commercially prepared potato salads may be treated with a sulfite such as sulfur dioxide to inactivate polyphenoloxidase and keep the potatoes from darkening. People who are sensitive to sulfites may suffer serious allergic reactions, including potentially fatal anaphylactic shock if they eat potato salads treated with these chemicals.

Medical Uses and/or Benefits

To soothe a skin rash. Potato starch, like corn starch, may be used as a dusting powder or added to a lukewarm bath to soothe a wet, "weepy" skin rash. The starch, which is very drying, should never be used on a dry rash or without a doctor's advice.

As an antiscorbutic. Raw potatoes, which are high in vitamin C, were once used as an antiscorbutic, a substance that prevents or cures the vitamin C–deficiency disease scurvy. Today we have much more effective means of preventing scurvy.

Adverse Effects Associated with This Food

Allergic reactions to sulfite. See *How other forms of processing affect this food,* above.

Solanine poisoning. See *About the nutrients in this food,* above.

Potential carcinogenicity. A 2004 study from Stockholm University (Sweden) shows that exposing high-carbohydrate foods such as potatoes and grains to very high cooking temps triggers the production of odorless white crystals of acrylamide, a chemical the U.S. Environmental Protection Agency calls a "probable human carcinogen" in food. Currently, there is no evidence that the amount of acrylamide in potato chips and bread poses a serious threat to human health. However, in 2008, a report in the *Journal of the Science of Food and Agriculture* explained that (1) washing raw potatoes, or (2) soaking them in water for 30 minutes, or (3) soaking them in water for two hours reduced the formation of acrylamide by 23 percent, 38 percent, and 48 percent respectively, so long as the potatoes were then fried only to a light gold.

Food/Drug Interactions

* * *

Poultry

(Chicken, duck, goose, turkey)

Nutritional Profile*

Energy value (calories per serving): *Moderate*
Protein: *High*
Fat: *Low to high*
Saturated fat: *High*
Cholesterol: *Moderate (chicken, turkey)*
                High (duck, goose)
Carbohydrates: *None*
Fiber: *None*
Sodium: *Moderate*
Major vitamin contribution: *B vitamins*
Major mineral contribution: *Zinc, magnesium*

About the Nutrients in This Food

Like meat, fish, eggs, and dairy foods, poultry has high-quality proteins with adequate amounts of all the essential amino acids). Poultry fat is usually lower in saturated fats than that of red meat. Most poultry (especially white meat) has less fat than an equal-size serving of most beef, lamb, pork, or veal. A serving of white meat chicken or turkey has about the same amount of cholesterol as a four-ounce serving of lean beef; dark meat from chicken or turkey has about the same amount of cholesterol as pork and lamb; duck and goose have more. Like other foods from animals, poultry is a good source of heme iron, the form of iron most easily absorbed by your body.

Fat and Cholesterol Content of Roast Poultry, Meat Only (100 g/3.5 oz.)

Poultry	Total fat (g)	Saturated fat (g)	Cholesterol (mg)
Chicken			
light meat	4.51	1.2	85
dark meat	9.73	2.6	93
Duck	11.20	4.2	89

---

* Values are for roasted mixed dark and white meat.

Fat and Cholesterol Content of Roast Poultry, Meat Only (100 g/3.5 oz.)
(Continued)

Poultry	Total fat (g)	Saturated fat (g)	Cholesterol (mg)
Turkey			
light meat	3.3	1	69
dark meat	7.2	2.4	85
Beef			
eye, round, lean only	3.9	1.3	52

Source: USDA Nutrient Data Laboratory. National Nutrient Database for Standard Reference. Available online. URL: http://nal.usda.gov/fnic/foodcomp/search/.

The Most Nutritious Way to Serve This Food

Broiled or roasted, with the skin removed to reduce the fat. Soups and stews should be skimmed.

Diets That May Restrict or Exclude This Food

Controlled-fat, low cholesterol diet (duck, goose)
Low-protein diet

Buying This Food

Look for: Poultry with fresh, unblemished skin and clear unblemished meat. If you buy whole fresh chickens that have not been prepacked, try to bend the breastbone—the more flexible it is, the younger the bird and the more lean and tender the flesh.

Choose the bird that fits your needs. Young birds (broiler, fryer, capon, rock cornish hen, duckling, young turkey, young hen, and young tom) are good for broiling, frying, and roasting. Older birds (hen, stewing chicken, fowl, mature duck) have tougher muscle fiber, which requires long stewing or steaming to tenderize the meat.

Avoid: Poultry whose skin is dry or discolored.

Storing This Food

Refrigerate fresh poultry immediately. Refrigeration prolongs freshness by slowing the natural multiplication of bacteria on the surface of the chicken, turkey, duck, or goose. Left unchecked, these bacteria will convert proteins and other substances on the surface of the poultry to mucopolysaccharides, a slimy film. They will also convert the sulfur-containing amino acids methionine and cystine into smelly sulfur compounds called mercaptans, which give spoiled poultry a characteristic unpleasant odor. The bacteria multiply most on poultry wrapped in plastic, which is why it often smells bad when you unwrap it at home. Never use, store or freeze any poultry that does not smell absolutely fresh. Throw it out or return it to the store.

Cover fresh poultry and refrigerate it in a dish that keeps it from dripping and contaminating other foods or the refrigerator. Properly wrapped fresh poultry will keep for one or two days at 40°F. For longer storage, freeze the poultry.

Preparing This Food

Wash the poultry under cool running water to flush off the bacteria on its surface. There are more bacteria on an animal's skin than in its flesh. Since we buy poultry with the skin on, it has a much higher population of bacteria (including the ones that cause *Salmonella* food poisoning) than beef, veal, pork, and lamb. Beef and pork may have a few hundred bacteria per square centimeter; chicken will have several thousand.

Discard any poultry that feels slimy to the touch. If you are preparing duck or goose, pull as much fat out of the abdominal cavity as possible. To cut down on the fat in chicken, remove the skin before cooking.

To prevent poultry-borne illness:

1. Keep raw chicken cold, frozen chicken frozen solid, and leftover cooked chicken in the refrigerator. Use fresh chicken within one or two days.
2. Keep cutting boards and utensils clean by washing in hot soapy water to prevent any cross contamination between raw poultry (or its juices) and other foods.
3. Cook poultry thoroughly to an internal temperature of 180°F (no guessing— use a meat thermometer).

Fresh chicken stays fresh one to two days in the fridge; plain cooked chicken, three to four days; chicken in gravy, two days.

What Happens When You Cook This Food

Cooking changes the way poultry looks and tastes, alters its nutritional content, and makes it safer to eat.

Heat changes the structure of the poultry's proteins. It denatures the protein molecules so that they break apart into smaller fragments or change shape or clump together. These changes force moisture out of the tissues so that the poultry turns opaque as it cooks. As it loses water, the poultry also loses water-soluble B vitamins, which drip out into the pan. Since they are not destroyed by heat, they can be saved by using the skimmed pan drippings for gravy. Cooking also caramelizes proteins and the small amounts of sugar on the bird's surface, a "browning" reaction that gives the skin of the bird its characteristic sweet taste.

As moisture escapes from the skin, it turns crisp. At the same time, the heat liquifies the fat in the bird, which runs off into the pan, lowering the fat and cholesterol content.

Finally, cooking kills the *Salmonella* and other microorganisms on the skin and flesh of poultry. For maximum safety, poultry should be cooked to a uniform internal temperature of 180°F. If you are cooking your poultry in a microwave oven, check to be sure that the surface of the bird—which is cooled by evaporating moisture—is as hot as the inside, otherwise bacteria on the skin may remain alive.

How Other Kinds of Processing Affect This Food

Freezing.   When poultry is frozen, the water in its cells turns into ice crystals which rupture the cell walls. When you thaw the poultry, liquid escapes from the cells and the chicken, turkey, duck, or goose may taste dry and stringy.

The unsaturated fatty acids in poultry will continue to oxidize (and eventually turn rancid) while the bird is frozen. Poultry cut into pieces will spoil more quickly than a whole bird because it has more surfaces exposed to the air. Fresh whole chicken and turkey will keep for up to 12 months at 0°F; chicken pieces will keep for nine months; turkey pieces and whole duck and goose for six months.

Smoking.   Smoking (which means slowly roasting a bird in the smoke from an open fire) gives poultry a rich taste that varies according to the wood used in the fire. Birds smoked over an open fire may pick up carcinogenic chemicals from the smoke, including a-benzo-pyrene, the most prominent carcinogen in tobacco smoke. Artificial smoke flavoring is commercially treated to remove tar and a-benzopyrene. Smoked poultry has less moisture and proportionally more fat than fresh poultry.

Self-basting" turkeys.   To make these birds "self-basting," fat or oil is inserted under the skin of the breast before the bird is packed or frozen. As the bird cooks, the fat warms, melts, and oozes out, basting the turkey. "Self-basting" turkeys are higher in fat than other turkeys; depending on what kind of fat is inserted into the breast, they may also be higher in cholesterol.

Medical Uses and/or Benefits

To relieve the congestion of a cold.   Hot chicken soup, the quintessential folk remedy, does appear to relieve the congestion that comes with a head cold. Exactly why remains a mystery but some researchers have suggested that the hot steam from the soup helps liquify mucus and clear the nasal passages.

Adverse Effects Associated with This Food

Increased risk of cardiovascular disease.   Like other foods from animals, poultry is a significant source of cholesterol and saturated fats, which increase the amount of cholesterol circulating in your blood and raise your risk of heart disease. To reduce the risk of heart disease, the National Cholesterol Education Project recommends following the Step I and Step II diets.

The Step I diet provides no more than 30 percent of total daily calories from fat, no more than 10 percent of total daily calories from saturated fat, and no more than 300 mg of cholesterol per day. It is designed for healthy people whose cholesterol is in the range of 200–239 mg/dL.

The Step II diet provides 25–35 percent of total calories from fat, less than 7 percent of total calories from saturated fat, up to 10 percent of total calories from polyunsaturated fat, up to 20 percent of total calories from monounsaturated fat, and less than 300 mg cholesterol per day. This stricter regimen is designed for people who have one or more of the following conditions:

◆ Existing cardiovascular disease
◆ High levels of low-density lipoproteins (LDLs, or "bad" cholesterol) or low levels of high-density lipoproteins (HDLs, or "good" cholesterol)
◆ Obesity
◆ Type 1 diabetes (insulin-dependent diabetes, or diabetes mellitus)
◆ Metabolic syndrome, a.k.a. insulin resistance syndrome, a cluster of risk factors that includes type 2 diabetes (non-insulin-dependent diabetes)

Food/Drug Interactions

* * *

Prunes

(Dried plums)

See also Plums.

Nutritional Profile*

Energy value (calories per serving): *Moderate*

Protein: *Low*

Fat: *Low*

Saturated fat: *Low*

Cholesterol: *None*

Carbohydrates: *High*

Fiber: *Very high*

Sodium: *Low (fresh or dried fruit)*

       High (dried fruit treated with sodium sulfur compounds)

Major vitamin contribution: *Vitamin A, folate, vitamin C*

Major mineral contribution: *Iron, Potassium*

About the Nutrients in This Food

Prunes are a high-carbohydrate food, rich in sugars (sucrose and fructose) and very high in dietary fiber: insoluble cellulose and lignin in the skin and soluble pectins in the flesh. Prunes are a good source of vitamin A, with moderate amounts of vitamin C and nonheme iron, the form of iron found in plants.

    One serving (five uncooked pitted prunes) has 3.5 g dietary fiber, 370 IU vitamin A (16 percent of the RDA for a woman, 12.5 percent of the RDA for a man), and 0.5 mg iron (3 percent of the RDA for a woman, 6 percent of the RDA for a man).

The Most Nutritious Way to Serve This Food

With meat or a food rich in vitamin C to increase the absorption of iron from the prunes. Meat makes the stomach more acid (iron is absorbed better in an acid medium), while vitamin C changes the iron from ferric iron to ferrous iron, a more easily absorbed form.

---

* Values are for dried, uncooked prunes

Diets That May Restrict or Exclude This Food

Antiflatulence diet
Low-fiber diet
Low-residue diet
Low-potassium diet
Low-sodium diet (prunes treated with sodium bisulfite, sodium metabisulfite, sodium sulfite)

Buying This Food

Look for: Tightly sealed boxes or bags of fruit that are protected from air, moisture, and insects. Prunes come in different sizes, but size has no bearing on taste or quality. Pitted prunes are more convenient but also more expensive than prunes with their pits still in place.

Storing This Food

Store prunes in a tightly closed container at room temperature, where they may stay fresh for up to six months. Check periodically to be sure that there is no insect infestation and no mold.

Preparing This Food

Do not soak prunes before you cook them. The sugars that make prunes so distinctively sweet are soluble and will leach out into the soaking water.

What Happens When You Cook This Food

When you stew dried prunes, their water-soluble pectins and hemicellulose dissolve and their cells absorb water. Uncooked dried "nugget"-type prunes are 2.5 percent water; when stewed, they are 50.7 percent water. Uncooked "softened" dried prunes are 28 percent water; when stewed, they are 66.4 percent water. Since the water displaces nutrients, ounce for ounce stewed prunes (of either type) may have only one-third as much vitamin C and B vitamins, vitamin A, iron, and fiber as uncooked prunes.

How Other Kinds of Processing Affect This Food

* * *

Medical Uses and/or Benefits

To relieve or prevent constipation. Prunes are a high-fiber food that helps relieve constipation. However, since prune juice, which has only a trace of fiber, is also a laxative, some food chemists suggest that what makes the prune such an effective laxative is not its fiber but another constituent, an unidentified derivative of the organic chemical isatin, which is related to another natural substance, biscodyl, the active ingredient in some over-the-counter laxative tablets and suppositories. Biscodyl is a contact laxative that induces the secretion of fluid in the bowel and stimulates contractions of the intestines that push waste through the colon more quickly and efficiently.

Protection against the risk of some forms of cancer. According to the American Cancer Society, foods high in fiber and vitamin A may offer some protection against cancers of the gastrointestinal and respiratory tracts as well as cancers induced by chemicals.

Adverse Effects Associated with This Food

Allergic reactions to sulfite. When they are dried, prune plums may be treated with sulfites (sulfur dioxide, sodium bisulfite, and the like) to inactivate polyphenoloxidase, an enzyme that hastens the oxidation of phenols in the prunes, forming brownish compounds that darken the fruit. People who are sensitive to sulfite may suffer serious allergic reactions, including potentially fatal anaphylactic shock, if they eat prunes treated with sulfites. Also, prunes treated with sulfite compounds are high in sodium.

Diarrhea. Very large amounts of prunes, alone or with other high-fiber foods, may cause diarrhea.

Food/Drug Interactions

* * *

Pumpkin

See also Winter squash.

Nutritional Profile

Energy value (calories per serving): *Low*
Protein: *Moderate*
Fat: *Low*
Saturated fat: *Low*
Cholesterol: *None*
Carbohydrates: *High*
Fiber: *Very high*
Sodium: *Low*
Major vitamin contribution: *Vitamin A, B vitamins*
Major mineral contribution: *Potassium, iron (seeds)*

About the Nutrients in This Food

Pumpkins are very high in dietary fiber (soluble pectins), with moderate amounts of sugar, a little protein, some vitamin C, and a truly extraordinary supply of vitamin A derived from the deep yellow carotenes (including beta-carotene) in the golden pumpkin flesh.

Pumpkin seeds are an excellent source of dietary fiber and are particularly high in insoluble cellulose and lignin (in the seed covering). They are high in fat (primarily unsaturated fatty acids rich in vitamin E). Their proteins are plentiful but limited in the essential amino acid lysine. They are a good source of the B vitamin folate and nonheme iron, the form of iron in plants.

One-half cup boiled pumpkin has 1.3 g dietary fiber, 6,115 IU vitamin A (2.6 times the RDA for a woman, 2.1 times the RDA for a man), and 5.8 mg vitamin C (8 percent of the RDA for a woman, 6 percent of the RDA for a man).

One ounce dried pumpkin (or squash) seeds has 1.1 g dietary fiber, 13 g total fat (2.5 g saturated fat, 4 g monounsaturated fat, 5.9 g polyunsaturated fat), seven grams protein, 16 mcg folate (4 percent of the RDA for a woman, 53 percent of the RDA for a man).

The Most Nutritious Way to Serve This Food

Pumpkin. Baked. Boiled pumpkin absorbs water, so ounce for ounce, baked pumpkin has more nutrients than boiled pumpkin.

Pumpkin seeds. Dried, with beans (peanuts)—to complete the proteins in the seeds.

Diets That May Restrict or Exclude This Food

Low-fat (the seeds)
Low-fiber (particularly the seeds)

Buying This Food

Look for: A pumpkin with a bright orange, blemish-free rind. The pumpkin should feel heavy for its size.

Look for: Seeds in sealed packages to protect them from air and moisture.

Storing This Food

Store pumpkins in a cool, dry place and use within a month. Vitamin A is vulnerable to oxygen; the longer the pumpkin is stored, the less vitamin A it will have.

Preparing This Food

Wash the pumpkin under cold running water, then cut it in half or in quarters or in smaller portions, as you wish. Pull off the stringy parts and collect and set aside the seeds. Leave the rind on if you plan to bake large pieces of the pumpkin; peel it off for boiling. If the pumpkin is small enough and/or your oven is large enough, you can simply scoop out the strings and seeds and bake the pumpkin whole, as you would a large acorn squash.

What Happens When You Cook This Food

Pumpkin. When you bake a pumpkin, the soluble food fibers in its cell walls dissolve and the pumpkin gets softer. If you bake it too long, the moisture inside the cells will begin to evaporate and the pumpkin will shrink. When you boil pumpkin, it's just the opposite. The cell walls still soften, but its cells absorb water and the vegetable swells. (Boil it too long, though, and the cells will rupture, moisture will escape, and the pumpkin once again will shrink).

Baking also caramelizes sugars on the cut surface of the pumpkin, browning the vegetable. Since the pumpkin is not extraordinarily high in sugars, we help this along by dusting it with brown sugar before baking. Either way, the pumpkin will retain its color and its vitamin A since its carotenoids are impervious to the normal heat of cooking.

Pumpkin seeds. When you toast pumpkin seeds, their moisture evaporates and they turn crisp and brown. Commercially toasted pumpkin seeds are usually salted and must be considered high-sodium food. To toast pumpkin seeds at home, remove the outer cover of the seeds and toss the seeds on an ungreased skillet on top of the stove or on a cookie sheet in a 350°F oven. Stir often to keep the seeds from burning. They are done when golden.

How Other Kinds of Processing Affect This Food

Canning. According to the USDA, canned "pumpkin" may be a mixture of pumpkin and other yellow orange winter squash, all of which are similar in nutritional value.

Medical Uses and/or Benefits

Lower risk of some cancers. According to the American Cancer Society, foods rich in beta-carotene may lower the risk of cancers of the larynx, esophagus, and lungs. There is no similar benefit from beta-carotene supplements; indeed, one controversial study actually showed a higher rate of lung cancer among smokers taking the supplement.

Adverse Effects Associated with This Food

* * *

Food/Drug Interactions

* * *

Quinces

Nutritional Profile

Energy value (calories per serving): *Moderate*
Protein: *Low*
Fat: *Low*
Saturated fat: *Low*
Cholesterol: *None*
Carbohydrates: *High*
Fiber: *Moderate*
Sodium: *Low*
Major vitamin contribution: *Vitamin C*
Major mineral contribution: *Potassium*

About the Nutrients in This Food

Quinces look like pears, and, like pears, they are members of the apple family. They are high in sugar, with moderate amounts of dietary fiber (insoluble pectins). Fresh quinces are a good source of vitamin C.

One raw 3.3-ounce quince has 1.7 g dietary fiber and 13.8 mg vitamin C (18 percent of the RDA for a woman, 15 percent of the RDA for a man).

The seeds of the quince, like apple seeds, pear seeds, and apricot, cherry, peach, and plum pits, contain amygdalin, a natural cyanide/sugar compound that breaks down into hydrogen cyanide in your stomach (see APPLES).

The Most Nutritious Way to Serve This Food

Baked without sugar to save calories.

Diets That May Restrict or Exclude This Food

* * *

Buying This Food

Look for: Firm, round, or pear-shape fruit with a pale yellow, fuzzy skin.

Avoid: Small, knobby fruit or fruit with bruised skin.

Storing This Food

Store quinces in the refrigerator and use them within two weeks.

Preparing This Food

Wash the quince under cold running water, wipe off the fuzz, cut off the stem and the blossom ends, core the fruit, and bake or stew it.

What Happens When You Cook This Food

When you cook a quince, heat and the acids in the fruit convert the quince's colorless leucoanthocyanin pigments to red anthocyanins, turning its flesh from pale yellow to pink or red. Cooking also transforms the raw quince's strong, unpleasant, astringent taste to a more mellow flavor, halfway between apple and a pear.

How Other Kinds of Processing Affect This Food

* * *

Medical Uses and/or Benefits

Lower levels of cholesterol. Foods high in soluble gums and pectins appear to lower the amount of cholesterol in the blood and offer some protection against heart disease. The exact mechanism by which this occurs is still unknown, but one theory is that the pectins in the apple form a gel in your stomach that sops up fats and cholesterol, carrying them out of your body.

Adverse Effects Associated with This Food

* * *

Food/Drug Interactions

* * *

Radishes

(Daikon, horseradish)

Nutritional Profile

Energy value (calories per serving): *Low*
Protein: *High*
Fat: *Low*
Saturated fat: *Low*
Cholesterol: *None*
Carbohydrates: *High*
Fiber: *Moderate*
Sodium: *Low*
Major vitamin contribution: *Vitamin C*
Major mineral contribution: *Iron, potassium*

About the Nutrients in This Food

Radishes are cruciferous vegetables, members of the same family as broccoli, brussels sprouts, cabbage, and cauliflower. They have small amounts of dietary fiber (insoluble cellulose and lignin) and vitamin C. One serving of ten small fresh red radishes has 0.3 g dietary fiber and 3 mg vitamin C (4 percent of the RDA for a woman, 3 percent of the RDA for a man).

The Most Nutritious Way to Serve This Food

Fresh, crisp red or daikon radishes; freshly grated fresh horseradish or recently opened prepared horseradish.

Diets That May Restrict or Exclude This Food

Antiflatulence diet

Buying This Food

Look for: Firm, well-shaped radishes. The skin should be clear, clean, and free of blemishes. If there are green tops on the radish, they should be crisp and fresh. If you are buying radishes in plastic bags, check them carefully through the plastic to see that they are free of mold.

Avoid: Misshapen radishes, spongy radishes, radishes with soft spots (which suggest decay or discoloration underneath), and withered or dry radishes (they have lost vitamin C, which is sensitive to oxygen).

Storing This Food

Cut off any green tops and refrigerate fresh radishes in plastic bags to keep them from drying out.

Preparing This Food

Scrub the radishes under cold running water. Cut off the tops and the roots. Don't slice or grate radishes until you are ready to use them. When you cut into a radish, you tear its cells, releasing moisture that converts an otherwise mild chemical called sinigrin into an irritant mustard oil that gives radishes their hot taste.

What Happens When You Cook This Food

* * *

How Other Kinds of Processing Affect This Food

Prepared horseradish. Prepared horseradish should be used within a few weeks after you open the bottle. The longer it is exposed to air, the more bitter (rather than spicy) its mustard oils will be.

Medical Uses and/or Benefits

Lower risk of some kinds of cancer. Indoles, isothiocyanates, glucosinolates, dithiolethiones, and phenols, naturally occurring in radishes, broccoli, Brussels sprouts, cabbage, cauliflower, and other cruciferous vegetables, appear to reduce the risk of some cancers, perhaps by preventing the formation of carcinogens in your body or by blocking cancer-causing substances from reaching or reacting with sensitive body tissues or by inhibiting the transformation of healthy cells to malignant ones.

Brussels sprouts, broccoli, cauliflower, and other cruciferous vegetables all contain sulforaphane, a member of a family of chemicals known as isothiocyanates. In experiments with laboratory rats, sulforaphane appears to increase the body's production of phase-2 enzymes, naturally occurring substances that inactivate and help eliminate carcinogens. At the Johns Hopkins University in Baltimore (MD), 69 percent of the rats injected with a chemical known to cause mammary cancer developed tumors vs. only 26 percent of the rats given the carcinogenic chemical plus sulforaphane.

In 1997, Johns Hopkins researchers discovered that broccoli seeds and three-day-old broccoli sprouts contain a compound converted to sulforaphane when the seed and sprout cells are crushed. Five grams of three-day-old broccoli sprouts contain as much sulforaphane as 150 grams of mature broccoli. The sulforaphane levels in other cruciferous vegetables have not been calculated.

Adverse Effects Associated with This Food

Enlarged thyroid gland (goiter). Cruciferous vegetables, including radishes, contain goitrin, thiocyanate, and isothiocyanate. These chemicals, known collectively as goitrogens, inhibit the formation of thyroid hormones and cause the thyroid to enlarge in an attempt to produce more. Goitrogens are not hazardous for healthy people who eat moderate amounts of cruciferous vegetables, but they may pose problems for people who have a thyroid disorder.

Food/Drug Interactions

False-positive test for occult blood in the stool. The active ingredient in the guaiac slide test for hidden blood in feces, alphaguaiaconic acid, a chemical that turns blue in the presence of blood. Alphaguaiaconic acid also turns blue in the presence of peroxidase, a chemical that occurs naturally in radishes. Eating radishes in the 72 hours before taking the guaiac test may produce a false-positive result in people who do not actually have any blood in their stool.

Raisins

(Currants)

See also Grapes.

Nutritional Profile

Energy value (calories per serving): *High*
Protein: *Low*
Fat: *Low*
Saturated fat: *Low*
Cholesterol: *None*
Carbohydrates: *High*
Fiber: *Very high*
Sodium: *Low (fresh or dried fruit)*
       High (dried fruit treated with sodium sulfur compounds)
Major vitamin contribution: *B vitamins*
Major mineral contribution: *Iron, potassium*

About the Nutrients in this Food

Raisins are dried grapes. Raisins with seeds big enough to see or feel with your tongue are dried Muscat grapes. Raisins whose seeds are barely perceptible are dried Thompson grapes. Raisins with no seeds at all are dried sultana grapes. "Currants" are dried, dark-skinned black Corinth grapes.

All raisins are high-carbohydrate food, rich in sugars, with moderate amounts of dietary fiber (insoluble cellulose and lignin in the skin; soluble pectins in the fruit) and small amounts of vitamin C and nonheme iron, the inorganic form of iron found in plant foods.

One 1.5-ounce serving of seedless raisins has 1.6 g dietary fiber, 1 mg vitamin C (less than 1 percent of the RDA for either a woman or a man), and 0.8 mg iron (4 percent of the RDA for a woman, 10 percent of the RDA for a man).

The Most Nutritious Way to Serve This Food

With meat or with a food rich in vitamin C. Nonheme iron is five times less available to the body than heme iron, the organic form of iron found in meat, fish, poultry, milk, and eggs. Eating raisins with meat or vitamin C increases the amount you absorb because meat increase the secretion of stomach acid (iron is more easily absorbed in an acid environment), while vitamin C may change iron from ferric iron (which is hard for your body to absorb) to ferrous iron (which your body absorbs more easily).

Diets That May Restrict or Exclude This Food

Low-fiber diet
Low-carbohydrate diet

Buying This Food

Look for: Tightly sealed packages that protect the raisins from air (which will make them dry and hard) and insects.

Storing This Food

Store sealed packages of raisins in a cool, dark cabinet, where they may stay fresh for as long as a year. Once the package is opened, the raisins should be stored in an air- and moisture-proof container at room temperature and used within a few months. Check periodically for mold or insect infestation.

Preparing This Food

To use raisins in a bread or cake, "plump" them first by soaking them in water (or wine, rum, or brandy for a fruit cake) for about 15 minutes. Otherwise the raisins will be hard and dry when the cake or bread is baked.

What Happens When You Cook This Food

If you cook raisins in water, their pectins and gum will dissolve and the raisins will soften. They will also absorb liquids and swell up. Cook them long enough and the water will leak out again, allowing the raisins to collapse.

How Other Kinds of Processing Affect This Food

* * *

Medical Uses and/or Benefits

Iron supplementation. See *About the nutrients in this food,* above.

Adverse Reactions Associated with This Food

Sulfite allergies. To keep light grapes from drying to a dark brown color the grapes are treated with sulfites such as sulfur dioxide. People who are sensitive to sulfite may experience serious allergic reactions, including potentially fatal anaphylactic shock, if they eat raisins treated with sulfites.

Food/Drug Interactions

MAO inhibitors. Monoamine oxidase (MAO) inhibitors are drugs used an antidepressants or antihypertensives. They inhibit the action of natural enzymes that break down tyramine so that it can be eliminated from the body. Tyramine is a pressor amine, a chemical that constricts blood vessels and raises blood pressure. Tyramine, a natural by-product of protein metabolism, occurs naturally in many foods, particularly fermented or aged foods. If you eat a food rich in tyramine while you are taking an MAO inhibitor, the pressor amines cannot be efficiently eliminated from your body and the result may be a hypertensive crisis (sustained elevated blood pressure). There has been one report of an adverse side effect (severe headache) in a patient who ate two small packages of dark raisins while using an MAO inhibitor.

Raspberries

Nutritional Profile

Energy value (calories per serving): *Low*
Protein: *Low*
Fat: *Low*
Saturated fat: *Low*
Cholesterol: *None*
Carbohydrates: *High*
Fiber: *High*
Sodium: *Low*
Major vitamin contribution: *Vitamin C, folate*
Major mineral contribution: *Potassium, iron*

About the Nutrients in This Food

Raspberries are a high-fiber food with insoluble cellulose in the skin and soluble pectins in the fruit. They are a good source of vitamin C.

One-half cup fresh raspberries has four grams dietary fiber and 16 mg vitamin C (21 percent of the RDA for a woman, 18 percent of the RDA for a man).

The Most Nutritious Way to Serve This Food

Fresh or thawed, with cereal for even more fiber.

Diets That May Restrict or Exclude This Food

* * *

Buying This Food

Look for: Plump, shiny berries.

Avoid: Packages with juice stains or leaks suggesting crushed—and possibly moldy—berries inside.

Storing This Food

Refrigerate fresh berries. Do not wash or handle before storing. Washing increases the possibility of mold; handling damages cells, releasing enzymes that inactivate vitamins and make the berries less nutritious.

Preparing This Food

Rinse the berries under cool running water, then drain and pick over carefully to remove all debris.

What Happens When You Cook This Food

Heat dissolves the pectins in berry cells, making the berries softer. It also destroys some of the vitamin C.

How Other Kinds of Processing Affect This Food

Freezing. When you thaw frozen berries, some liquid leaks out, which means there is less water and more berry flesh per serving. However, freezing destroys some vitamins. A cup of frozen raspberries has twice the fiber, but less folate and vitamin C, than fresh berries.

Medical Uses and/or Benefits

Antiscorbutics. Foods high in vitamin C cure or prevent the vitamin C deficiency disease scurvy, characterized by bleeding gums and slow healing of wounds.

Adverse Effects Associated with This Food

Allergic reaction. Many people are sensitive to berries including raspberries. In fact, according to the *Merck Manual,* berries are one of the 12 foods most likely to trigger classic food allergy symptoms: hives, swelling of the lips and eyes, and upset stomach. The others are chocolate, corn, eggs, fish, legumes (peas, lima beans, peanuts, soybeans), milk, nuts, peaches, pork, shellfish, and wheat (see WHEAT CEREALS).

Food-borne illness. Small fruits such as berries appear to be a growing source of contamination by disease-causing organisms such as *E. coli* O157:H7 and salmonella. Common methods of decontamination such as vigorously washing the fruit are impractical with berries because they damage the fruit. In 2007, researchers from the University of Pennsylvania delivered a report at the annual meeting of the American Society of Agricultural and Biological Engineers, describing the use of pulsed ultraviolet light to decontaminate raspberries and strawberries with no observable damage to the fruit, which would give growers and food distributors a way to make their products safer before shipping.

Food/Drug Interactions

* * *

Rhubarb

Nutritional Profile

Energy value (calories per serving): *Low*
Protein: *Low*
Fat: *Low*
Saturated fat: *Low*
Cholesterol: *None*
Carbohydrates: *High*
Fiber: *Low*
Sodium: *Low*
Major vitamin contribution: *Vitamin A, vitamin C*
Major mineral contribution: *Potassium*

About the Nutrients in This Food

Despite its crunchy stringiness, rhubarb provides only small amounts of fiber, including the insoluble cellulose and lignin in the stiff cells of its stalk and "strings" and the soluble pectins in the flesh. Rhubarb has some sugar, no starch, and only a trace of protein and fat.

Rhubarb is a relatively good source of dietary fiber and vitamin C. One-half cup cooked rhubarb has 2.4 g dietary fiber including insoluble cellulose and lignin in the "strings" and soluble pectins in the flesh. One-half cup cooked rhubarb has 2.4 g dietary fiber and 4 mg vitamin C (5 percent of the RDA for a woman, 4 percent of the RDA for a man).

Rhubarb also has some calcium (174 mg per serving), but oxalic acid (one of the naturally occurring chemicals that give rhubarb its astringent flavor) binds the calcium into calcium oxalate, an insoluble compound the body cannot absorb. The other astringent chemicals in rhubarb are tannins (also found in tea, red wines, and some unripe fruits) and phenols. Tannins and phenols coagulate proteins on the surface of the mucous membrane lining of the mouth, making the mouth "pucker" when eating rhubarb.

The Most Nutritious Way to Serve This Food

Cooked. Only the stalks of the rhubarb are used as food; *THE LEAVES ARE POISONOUS, WHETHER RAW OR COOKED.*

Diets That May Restrict or Exclude This Food

Low-oxalate diet (for people who form calcium oxalate kidney stones)

Buying This Food

Look for: Crisp, bright, fresh stalks of rhubarb. Although color is not necessarily a guide to quality, the deeper the red, the more flavorful the stalks are likely to be. The medium-size stalks are generally more tender than large ones, which, like large stalks of celery, may be stringy.

Storing This Food

Wrap rhubarb in plastic and store it in the refrigerator to keep cool and humid. Rhubarb is fairly perishable; use it within a few days after you buy it.

Preparing This Food

Remove and discard all leaves on the rhubarb stalk. *RHUBARB LEAVES ARE NOT EDIBLE; THEY ARE POISONOUS, RAW OR COOKED.*

Wash the rhubarb under cool running water. Trim the end and cut off any discolored parts. If the stalks are tough, peel them to get rid of hard "strings." (Most of the rhubarb we buy is grown in hothouses and bred to have a thin skin that doesn't have to be peeled.)

What Happens When You Cook This Food

Rhubarb is colored with red anthocyanin pigments that turn redder in acid and turn bluish in bases (alkalis) and brownish if you cook them with sugar at very high heat. If you cook rhubarb in an aluminum or iron pot, metal ions flaking off the pot will interact with acids in the fruit to form brown compounds that darken both the pot and the rhubarb.

How Other Kinds of Processing Affect This Food

* * *

Medical Uses and/or Benefits

* * *

Adverse Effects Associated with This Food

Kidney stones. More than 50 percent of all kidney stones are composed of calcium oxalate or calcium oxalate plus phosphate. People with a metabolic disorder that leads them to excrete large amounts of oxalates in their urine or who have had ileal disease or who eat large amounts of foods high in oxalic acid are the ones most likely to form these stones. Rhubarb, like beets, cocoa, nuts, parsley, spinach, and tea, is high in oxalic acid.

Food/Drug Interactions

* * *

Rice

(Wild rice)

See also Wheat cereals.

Nutritional Profile

Energy value (calories per serving): *Moderate*
Protein: *Moderate*
Fat: *Low*
Saturated fat: *Low*
Cholesterol: *None*
Carbohydrates: *High*
Fiber: *Low to high*
Sodium: *Low**
Major vitamin contribution: *B vitamins*
Major mineral contribution: *Iron, calcium*

About the Nutrients in This Food

All rice is a high-carbohydrate food, rich in starch, with moderate amounts of dietary fiber. Brown rice, which has the bran (outer seed covering), is high in fiber.

Rice's proteins are plentiful but limited in the essential amino acids lysine and isoleucine. All rice is low in fat, but brown rice, with its fatty germ (the center of the seed), has about twice as much fat as white rice.

Brown rice is higher in vitamins and minerals than plain milled white rice. Enriched white rice is equivalent to plain brown rice. All rice is a source of B vitamins, including folates. In 1998, FDA ordered food manufacturers to add folates—which protect against birth defects of the spinal cord and against heart disease—to flour, rice, and other grain products. One year later, data from the Framingham Heart Study, which has followed heart health among residents of a Boston suburb for nearly half a century, showed a dramatic increase in blood levels of folic acid. Before the fortification of foods, 22 percent of the study participants had a folic acid deficiency; after, the number fell to 2 percent. Rice is also a source of calcium and nonheme iron, the form of iron found in plant foods.

---

* Dry uncooked rice is low in sodium. Cooked rice has absorbed liquid; its sodium content depends on the sodium content of the liquid in which it's cooked.

Fiber, B Vitamins, and Iron in Cooked Rice (¹/₂ cup)

Rice	Fiber (g)	Folate (mcg)	Thiamin (mg)	Niacin (mg)	Iron (mg)
Brown	1.8	4	0.1	1.3	0.5
White, long-grain, enriched	0.7	64	0.2	1.8	1.4
White, long-grain, instant, enriched	0.5	58	0.1	1.4	1.5
White, glutinous ("sticky"), unenriched	0.9	1	0.02	0.3	0.1

Source: USDA Nutrient Data Laboratory. National Nutrient Database for Standard Reference. Available online. URL: http://nal.usda.gov/fnic/foodcomp/search/.

The Most Nutritious Way to Serve This Food

With legumes (beans, peas). The proteins in rice are deficient in the essential amino acids lysine and isoleucine and rich in the essential amino acids tryptophan, methionine, and cystine. The proteins in legumes are exactly the opposite. Combining the two foods in one dish "complements" or "completes" their proteins.

With meat or a food rich in vitamin C (tomatoes, peppers). Both will increase the availability of the iron in the rice. Meat increases the secretion of stomach acids (iron is absorbed better in an acid environment); vitamin C changes the iron in the rice from ferric iron (which is hard to absorb) to ferous iron (which is easier to absorb).

Diets That May Restrict or Exclude This Food

Low-calcium diet (brown rice, wild rice)
Low-fiber diet

Buying This Food

Look for: Tightly sealed packages that protect the rice from air and moisture, which can oxidize the fats in the rice and turn them rancid.

Choose the rice that meets your needs. *Long-grain rice,* which has less starch than *short-grain* ("Oriental") rice, will be fluffier and less sticky when cooked. *Brown rice* has a distinctive nutty taste that can overwhelm delicate foods or "fight" with other strong flavors.

Avoid: Stained boxes of rice, even if they are still sealed. Whatever spilled on the box may have seeped through the cardboard onto the rice inside.

Storing This Food

Store rice in air- and moistureproof containers in a cool, dark cabinet to keep it dry and protect its fats from oxygen. White rice may stay fresh for as long as a year. Brown rice, which retains its bran and germ and thus has more fats than white rice, may stay fresh for only a few months before its fats (inevitably) oxidize. All rice spoils more quickly in hot, humid weather. Aging or rancid rice usually has a distinctive stale and musty odor.

Preparing This Food

Should you wash rice before you cook it? Yes, if you are preparing imported rice or rice purchased in bulk. No, if you are preparing prepacked white or brown rice.

You wash all varieties of bulk rices to flush away debris and/or insects. You wash imported rices to rinse off the cereal or corn-syrup coating. You should pick over brown and white rices to catch the occasional pebble or stone, but washing is either worthless or detrimental.

Washing brown rice has no effect one way or the other. Since the grains are protected by their bran, the water will not flush away either starches or nutrients. Washing long-grain white rices, however, will rinse away some of the starch on the surface, which can be a plus if you want the rice to be as fluffy as possible. The downside is that washing the rice will also rinse away any nutrients remaining on plain milled rice and dissolve the starch/nutrient coating on enriched rices. Washing the starches off short-grain, Oriental rices will make the rice uncharacteristically dry rather than sticky.

What Happens When You Cook This Food

Starch consists of molecules of the complex carbohydrates amylose and amylopectin packed into a starch granule. When you cook rice, the starch granules absorb water molecules. When the temperature of the water reaches approximately 140°F, the amylose and amylopectin molecules inside the starch granules relax and unfold, breaking some of their internal bonds (bonds between atoms on the same molecule) and forming new bonds between atoms on different molecules. The result is a starch network of starch molecules that traps and holds water molecules, making the starch granules even more bulky. In fact, rice holds so much water that it will double or even triple in bulk when cooked.[*]

If you continue to cook the rice, the starch granules will eventually break open, the liquid inside will leak out, the walls of the granules will collapse, and the rice will turn soft and mushy. At the same time, amylose and amylopectin molecules escaping from the granules will make the outside of the rice sticky—the reason why overcooked rice clumps together.

There are several ways to keep rice from clumping when you cook it. First, you can cook the rice in so much water that the grains have room to boil without bumping into each other, but you will lose B vitamins when you drain the excess water from the rice. Second, you can sauté the rice before you boil it or add a little fat to the boiling liquid. Theoretically, this

---

[*] Cooking rice in liquids other than water (tomato juice, bouillon, wine) keeps the rice firmer, since the grains will absorb solids along with water.

should make the outside of the grains slick enough to slide off each other. But this method raises the fat content of the rice—with no guarantee that it will really keep the rice from clumping. The best method is to cook the rice in just as much water as it can absorb without rupturing its starch granules and remove the rice from the heat as soon as the water is almost all absorbed. Fluff the cooked rice with a fork as it is cooling, to separate the grains.

How Other Kinds of Processing Affect This Food

"Converted" rice.   "Converted" rice is rice that is parboiled under pressure before it is milled. This process drives the vitamins and minerals into the grain and loosens the bran so that it slips off easily when the rice is milled. Converted rice retains more vitamins and minerals than conventionally milled white rice.

"Quick-cooking" rice.   This is rice that has been cooked and dehydrated. Its hard, starchy outer covering and its starch granules have already been broken so it will reabsorb water almost instantly when you cook it.

Medical Uses and/or Benefits

To soothe irritated skin.   Like corn starch or potato starch, powdered rice used as a dusting powder or stirred into the bath water may soothe and dry a "wet" skin rash. It is so drying, however, that it should *never* be used on a dry skin rash or on any rash without a doctor's advice.

As a substitute for wheat flour in a gluten-free diet.   People with celiac disease have an inherited metabolic disorder which makes it impossible for them to digest gluten and gliadin, proteins found in wheat and some other grains. Rice and rice flour, which are free of gluten and gliadin, may be a useful substitute in some recipes.

Adverse Effects Associated with This Food

Beri-beri: Beri-beri is the thiamin (vitamin B_1)-deficiency disease. Beri-beri, which is rare today, occurs among people for whom milled white rice, stripped of its B vitamins, is a dietary mainstay. Enriching the rice prevents beri-beri.

Mold toxins.   Rice, like other grains, may support the growth of toxic molds, including *Aspergillus flavus,* which produces carcinogenic aflatoxins. Other toxins found on moldy rice include citrinin, a penicillium mold too toxic to be used as an antibiotic; rubratoxins, mold products known to cause hemorrhages in animals who eat the moldy rice; and nivalenol, a mold toxin that suppresses DNA and protein synthesis in cells. Because mold may turn the rice yellow, moldy rice is also known as yellow rice.

Food/Drug Interactions

* * *

Shellfish

(Abalone, clams, conch, crabs, crayfish, lobster, mussels, oysters, prawns, scallops, shrimp, snails)

Nutritional Profile*

Energy value (calories per serving): *Moderate*

Protein: *High*

Fat: *Low*

Saturated fat: *Low*

Cholesterol: *Moderate to high*

Carbohydrates: *Trace*

Fiber: *None*

Sodium: *Moderate to high*

Major vitamin contribution: *B vitamins*

Major mineral contribution: *Iron (clams), iodine, copper, zinc (oysters), arsenic*

About the Nutrients in This Food

Like meat, fish, poultry, and eggs, shellfish are an excellent source of high-quality proteins with sufficient amounts of all the essential amino acids required by human beings.

Mollusks (abalone, clams, oysters, scallops, snails) are comparable in total fat content to meat and poultry. Crustaceans (crabs, lobster, shrimp) are lower in total fat content. Both types of shellfish have less saturated fat than meat does. They do have comparable amounts of cholesterol, but this is offset by the fact that like other seafood, shellfish provide omega-3 fatty acids, the class of heart-protective fats that includes linolenic acid, eicosapentaenoic acid (EPA), and docosahexaenoic acid (DHA).

Like other foods from animals, all shellfish are good sources of B vitamins, heme iron (the organic form of iron most easily absorbed by the body), and zinc. As an added bonus, they—like other fish—are rich in iodine, the mineral that protects against goiter (swelling of the thyroid gland).

All shellfish provide B vitamins. The crustaceans—crabs, lobsters, shrimp—also have vitamin A produced by their diet of carotenoid-rich green vegetation. A four-ounce serving of cooked Dungeness crab has 350 IU vitamin A (9 percent of the RDA for a healthy woman, 7 percent of the RDA for a healthy man).

---

*   Values are for raw or steamed shellfish.

Cholesterol Content of Shellfish

Shellfish	Serving	Cholesterol (mg)
Clams, raw	4 oz.	39
Crab, blue fresh		
cooked	4 oz.	113
canned	4 oz.	101
Crab, Dungeness	4 oz.	86
Lobster	1 cup	104
Oyster, raw	1 cup	124–131
Scallops, steamed	1/2 cup	57
Shrimp, boiled	6 large	167
Beef, lean sirloin	4 oz.	101

Source: USDA Nutrient Database: www.nal.usda.gov/fnic/cgi-bin/nut_search.pl., *Nutritive Value of Foods,* Home and Gardens Bulletin, No. 72 (USDA, 1989).

Shellfish also have heme iron, the organic form of iron found in meat, fish, poultry, milk and eggs, as well as the trace minerals copper and iodine. Oysters are a good source of zinc, a mineral which helps ensure the proper functioning of the male reproductive system.

The Most Nutritious Way to Serve This Food

Thoroughly cooked, to prevent food poisoning.

Diets That May Restrict or Exclude This Food

Controlled-fat, low-cholesterol diet
Low-protein diet
Low-sodium diet

Buying This Food

Look for: Clams, mussels, and oysters, shucked or live in the shell. Live clams, mussels, and oysters should be tightly shut or close with a snap when you touch them. Shucked clams, mussels, and oysters should be plump and shiny and smell absolutely fresh. There should be very little liquid in the container.

Choose live crabs that are actively moving their legs around. Lump crabmeat should be pink and white (not tan or yellowed), and it should smell absolutely fresh, as should cooked crabs.

Choose live lobsters and crayfish that look fresh, smell good, and are moving about actively. American lobsters come in four sizes: chicken ($^3/_4$–1 lb.), quarter (1.25 lb.), large

(1.5–2.25 lbs.), and jumbo (over 2.5 lbs.). Cooked lobsters should have a bright-red shell and a fresh aroma. If the tail curls back when you pull it down, the lobster was alive when cooked. Female lobsters, which have fluffy fins ("swimmerettes") at the juncture of tail and body, may contain roe or coral that turns red when you cook the lobster.

Choose dry, creamy, sweet-smelling scallops; unlike clams, oysters, and mussels, they can't be kept alive out of the water. Sea scallops, the large ones, may be sold fresh or frozen; bay scallops, the smaller shellfish, are usually only sold fresh.

Choose fresh shrimp and prawns that look dry and firm in the shell.

Choose tightly sealed cans of snails.

In 1998, the FDA National Center for Toxicological Research released for testing an inexpensive indicator called "Fresh Tag." The indicator, to be packed with seafood, changes color if the product spoils.

NOTE: Because of the possibility of industrial and microbial contamination of waters, live shellfish should be gathered only in waters certified by local health authorities.

Storing This Food

Refrigerate all shellfish and use as quickly as possible. Like other seafood shellfish are extremely perishable once they are no longer alive, and their fats, which are higher in unsaturated than saturated fatty acids, will oxidize and turn rancid fairly quickly. As a general rule, live clams in the shell may keep for up to two weeks, oysters in the shell for five days, shelled scallops for a day or two, and mussels should be used the day you buy them. Regardless of these estimates, *check the shellfish frequently to see that it is still alive and unspoiled.*

Cook live crabs and lobsters before storing to prolong their storage time. Shrimps and prawns will also stay fresh longer if you cook them before storing them. Use within a day. If you wait longer, check frequently to see that the crustaceans still look and smell fresh.

Preparing This Food

WHEN YOU ARE READY TO PREPARE SHELLFISH, SNIFF THEM FIRST. IF THEY DON'T SMELL ABSOLUTELY FRESH, THROW THEM OUT.

Abalone. Tenderize the abalone meat by pounding, then trim off any dark part, and slice the fish against the grain.*

Clams. All clams are sandy when you bring them home. To get rid of the grit, wash the closed clams thoroughly under cold running water. Then either immerse them in a salty solution (about 1/3 cup salt to a gallon of water or sprinkle them with cornmeal and cover them with water. Refrigerate the clams. They will take in the salt water (or cornmeal) and disgorge sand Clams covered with salt water will be clean in about half an hour, clams covered with cornmeal in about three hours. Before serving or cooking, discard any clams that are open or do not close immediately when you touch them or remain closed or float in the water.

---

* Some abalone are all black. Check with your fish market.

Conch.　Steam the conch or crack its shell. Open the shell and pull out the meat. Cut away and discard the stomach (it's right in the middle) and the dark tail. Peel off the skin, slice the meat thin, and pound it to tenderize the meat. Rinse, pat dry, and cook.

Crabs.　To clean *hard-shell crabs,* cook them first. Then plunge the hot crabs into cold water to firm up the meat. Remove the tail, snap off the claws, and pull off the shell. Cut away the gills and the digestive organs in the middle of the body and pull the meat away from the skeleton. *Soft-shell crabs* should be washed in cold water. They are ready to cook when you buy them.

Lobsters and crayfish (live).　If you plan to boil the lobsters, you can cook them just as they come from the store. If you plan to broil a lobster, kill it first by inserting a knife into the space between the head and the body and slicing through the crustacean's spinal cord. Then split the lobster and remove the internal organs. Live crayfish that have been stored in fresh running water do not have to be eviscerated before you boil them. If you wish to eviscerate the crayfish, grasp the middle fin on the tail, twist, and pull hard to pull out the stomach and intestine.

Mussels.　In the shell, mussels, like clams, are apt to be sandy. To get rid of the grit, scrub the mussels under cold running water, then put them in a pot of cold water and let them stand for an hour or two. Discard any that float to the top. Rinse the rest once more under cold running water, trim the "beard" with scissors, and prepare as your recipe directs.

Oysters.　Unlike clams and mussels, oysters in the shell are free of sand when you buy them. To prepare them, just wash the oysters thoroughly under cold running water. Discard any that don't close tight when you touch them or that float in water. Cook them in the shell or pry open the shell, strain the liquid for any stray grit, and use the oysters with or without the shell, as you recipe directs.

Scallops.　Shelled scallops in bulk should be relatively free of liquid. Rinse them in cold running water and use as your recipe directs.

Shrimp and prawns.　Wash the shrimp or prawns in cold running water. Then cook them in the shell to enhance the flavor of a soup or stew, or peel off the shell and remove the black "vein" (actually the digestive tract) running down the back, and prepare the shellfish as your recipe directs. (The orange line sometimes found running alongside the "vein" is edible roe.)

Snails (canned).　Prepare as your recipe directs.

　　When you are done, clean all utensils thoroughly with soap and hot water. Wash your cutting board, wood or plastic, with hot water, soap, and a bleach-and-water solution. For ultimate safety in preventing the transfer of microorganisms from the shellfish to other foods, keep one cutting board exclusively for fish, meat, or poultry, and a second one for everything else.

What Happens When You Cook This Food

When you cook shellfish, heat changes the structure of its proteins. The protein molecules are "denatured," which means they may break apart into smaller fragments, change shape, or clump together. All these changes force moisture out of protein tissues, making the shellfish opaque. The loss of moisture also changes the texture of the shellfish; the longer they are cooked, the more rubbery they will become. Shellfish should be cooked long enough to turn the flesh opaque and destroy any microorganisms living on the food.

How Other Kinds of Processing Affect This Food

Freezing.   When you freeze shellfish, the water in their cells forms ice crystals that can tear the cell membranes so the liquids inside leak out when the shellfish is defrosted—which is the reason defrosted shellfish tastes tougher and has less B vitamins than fresh shellfish. Defrosting the shellfish slowly in the refrigerator, lessens the loss of moisture and B vitamins. Frozen shrimp and prawns can be boiled whole, in the shells, without defrosting.

Canning.   Virtually all canned shellfish is higher in sodium than fresh shellfish. To reduce the sodium content, rinse the shellfish in cold water before you use it.

Medical Uses and/or Benefits

As a source of calcium.   Ground oyster shells, which are rich in calcium carbonate, are the calcium source in many over-the-counter supplements. Calcium carbonate is an efficient source of the mineral, but it is also likely to cause constipation.

Protective effects of omega-3 fatty acids.   Shellfish have small amounts of omega-3 fatty acids, a family of fatty acids which includes the essential fatty acid linolenic acid. Two other omega-3s, eicosapentaenoic acid (EPA) and docosahexaenoic acid (DHA), most abundant in fish living in cold waters, are the primary unsaturated fatty acids in oils from fish (anchovy, herring, mackerel, menhaden, salmon, sardines, trout, tuna) and shellfish, as well as human breast milk.

The omega-3s appear to reduce the risk of heart attack and "sudden death." A 20-year project at the University of Leyden in the Netherlands, comparing the eating habits of more than 800 men at risk of heart disease, found that men who ate more than an ounce of fish a day had a 50 percent lower rate of heart attacks. Since then, a lengthening list of studies has shown similar protection among men who eat fish at least two or three times a week. Possible explanations for this effect are the omega-3s ability to lower the levels of tryglicerides in your blood (high triglycerides are a risk factor for heart disease) and the fact that your body converts omega-3s to a compound similar to prostacyclin, a naturally occurring chemical that inhibits the formation of blood clots.

In the United States, about 250,000 people die each year from sudden cardiac failure caused by ventricular fibrillation, an unexpectedly irregular heartbeat. Those most at risk are people with blocked arteries (atherosclerosis), congestive heart failure, or abnormal thickening of the heart muscle. In a 1995 study from the Australian Commonwealth Scientific and Industrial Research Organization (Adelaide), laboratory monkeys fed omega-3 oils from fish had a steady heartbeat when exposed to electrical current twice as powerful as that which caused ventricular fibrillation in animals that did not get the fish oils. However, the heart benefits of the small amounts of omega-3s in shellfish such as shrimp may be offset by the high cholesterol content. (See below.)

Omega-3s also inhibit the production of leuketrienes, naturally occurring chemicals that trigger inflammation. This may be beneficial to people with rheumatoid arthritis. In 1995, the Arthritis Foundation published the results of a study by Piet Geusens at the Catholic University in Pellenberg (Belgium) suggesting that patients who take omega-3 fatty acid supplements along with their regular arthritis medications have improved pain relief. Previous studies had demonstrated the omega-3s ability to reduce inflammation, joint stiffness and swelling.

Finally, omega-3s may protect bone density. A 1997 study at Purdue University (Indiana) demonstrated that animals fed increased amounts of the omega-3 fatty acids formed new bone faster than animals fed a regular diet. This result has also shown up in studies with SOYBEANS.

Adverse Effects Associated with This Food

Allergic reaction. According to the *Merck Manual,* shellfish are one of the 12 foods most likely to trigger classic food allergy symptoms: hives, swelling of the lips and eyes, and upset stomach. The others are berries (blackberries, blueberries, raspberries, strawberries), chocolate, corn, eggs, fish, legumes (green peas, lima beans, peanuts, soybeans), milk, nuts, peaches, pork, and wheat (see WHEAT CEREALS). NOTE: Shrimp treated with sulfur compounds to prevent their darkening can cause serious allergic reactions in people sensitive to sulfites.

Food-borne infectious diseases. In the past two decades, food scientists have identified an increasing number of bacteria and viruses, including the cholera organism, the hepatitis virus, and *Vibrio vulnificus,* in live shellfish. According to the Food and Drug Administration, *Vibrio cholera* organisms introduced when wastes are thrown into the ocean are now permanent residents along some parts of the Atlantic and Gulf coasts, found all the way from Maine to Texas. Cholera-contaminated shrimp and crabs have been found in Louisiana, contaminated blue crabs in Galveston, (Texas), and contaminated oysters in Florida. Shellfish from infected water may carry the hepatitis B virus; *Vibrio vulnificus,* another organism carried in shellfish, causes fever, chills, and shock.

While it is true that cooking kills these organisms, the Centers for Disease Control—which advises cooking ALL shellfish—warns that viruses can survive quick steaming. The CDC further warns that raw shellfish are particularly hazardous for people with a weakened immune system: the very young, the very old, those who are HIV-positive or undergoing cancer chemotherapy or have liver disease, diabetes, or chronic gastrointestinal disease.

"Red Tide" poisoning. "Red tide" is a blanket of reddish organisms called dinoflagellates that float on the surface of the coastal waters of the Pacific and New England coasts between July and October. The dinoflagellates produce a neurological toxin that can be carried by any shellfish (clams, mussels, oysters) that eat the plankton. The toxin, which cannot be destroyed by cooking, can cause nausea, vomiting, and abdominal cramps, followed by muscle weakness and paralysis. Death may occur due to respiratory failure. These symptoms

generally begin to appear within a half-hour after you eat the contaminated shellfish. Other plankton ingested by shellfish may contain a diarrheic poison that causes gastric symptoms once thought to be caused by bacterial or viral food poisoning.

Worms or parasites.   Raw shellfish, like raw meat, may be host to worms, parasites, or their eggs and cysts. These organisms are killed by cooking the shellfish until the flesh is completely opaque.

Production of uric acid.   Purines are the natural metabolic by-products of protein metabolism in the body. They eventually break down into uric acid, which may form sharp crystals that may cause gout if they collect in your joints or kidney stones if they collect in urine. Shrimp are a source of purines; eating them raises the concentration of purines in your body. Although controlling the amount of purine-producing foods in the diet may not significantly affect the course of gout (which is treated with medication such as allopurinol, which inhibits the formation of uric acid), limiting these foods is still part of many gout regimens.

Food/Drug Interactions

* * *

Soybeans

See also Beans, Bean sprouts.

Nutritional Profile

Energy value (calories per serving): *Moderate*
Protein: *High*
Fat: *Moderate*
Saturated fat: *Moderate*
Cholesterol: *None*
Carbohydrates: *Moderate*
Fiber: *High*
Sodium: *Low*
Major vitamin contribution: *B vitamins, folate*
Major mineral contribution: *Iron, potassium*

About the Nutrients in This Food

Like other beans, soybeans are very high in fiber. Unlike other beans, they are also high in fat, and their proteins are high-quality, complete with sufficient amounts of all the essential amino acids.

Soybeans have insoluble dietary fiber (cellulose and lignin) in the bean covering and soluble pectins and gums in the bean. Their highly unsaturated fat (soybean oil) includes omega-3 fatty acids—the essential fatty acid linolenic acid, plus eicosapentaenoic acid (EPA) and docosahexaenoic acid [DHA], the two most plentiful unsaturated fatty acids in fish oils.

Soybeans are a good source of B vitamins, including folate and iron. They are the most abundant food source of isoflavones (genistein and daidzein), naturally occurring estrogenic compounds in plants.

One-half cup boiled mature soybeans has three grams dietary fiber, eight grams total fat (1.1 g saturated fat, 1.7 g monounsaturated fat, 4.4 g polyunsaturated fat), 14 g protein, 46 mcg folate (12 percent of the RDA), and 4.4 mg iron (24 percent of the RDA for a woman, 55 percent of the RDA for a man).

One-half cup dry roasted soybeans has seven grams dietary fiber, 18.6 g total fat (2.7 g saturated fat, 4.1 g monounsaturated fat, 10.5 g polyunsaturated fat), 34 g protein, 176 mcg folate (44 percent of the RDA), and 3.4 mg iron (19 percent of the RDA for a woman, 43 percent of the RDA for a man).

Soybeans are a good source of B vitamins, particularly vitamin B_6. They are rich in nonheme iron (the inorganic iron found in plant foods) but, like grains, beans contain phytic acid which binds their iron into insoluble compounds your body cannot absorb. As a result, nonheme iron is five to six times less available to the body than heme iron, the organic form of iron in meat, fish, and poultry.

Raw soybeans contain a number of antinutrients, including enzyme inhibitors (chemicals that interfere with the enzymes that make it possible for us to digest proteins); hemagglutinens (chemicals that make red blood cells clump together); and goitrogens (chemicals that make it hard for the thyroid to absorb iodine, which makes the gland swell in an effort to absorb more iodine; we call the swelling goiter). These chemicals are inactivated by cooking the soybeans.

The Most Nutritious Way to Serve This Food

With meat or a food rich in vitamin C to increase the amount of iron you can absorb from the soybeans. Meat makes your stomach more acid (iron is absorbed more easily in an acid environment); vitamin C may convert the iron in soybeans from ferric iron (which is hard to absorb) to ferrous iron (which is easier to absorb).

Diets That May Restrict or Exclude This Food

Low-calcium diet
Low-fiber diet
Low-protein diet
Low-purine (antigout) diet

Buying This Food

Look for: Tightly sealed packages that protect the beans from air and moisture. The beans should be smooth-skinned, uniformly sized, evenly colored, and free of stones and debris. It is easy to check beans sold in plastic bags, but the transparent material lets in light that may destroy pyridoxine and pyridoxal, the natural forms of vitamin B_{12}.

Storing This Food

Store beans in air- and moistureproof containers in a cool, dark cabinet where they are protected from heat, light, and insects.

Preparing This Food

Wash the beans and pick them over carefully, discarding damaged beans, withered beans, or beans that float. (The only beans light enough to float in water are those that have withered away inside.)

Soak "fresh" dried soybeans as directed on the package and then discard the water. If you use canned beans, discard the liquid in the can and rinse the beans in cool running water. In discarding this liquid you are getting rid of some of the soluble indigestible sugars that may cause intestinal gas when you eat beans.

What Happens When You Cook This Food

When soybeans are cooked in liquid, their cells absorb water, swell, and eventually rupture, releasing pectins, gums, and the nutrients inside the cell. In addition, cooking destroys antinutrients in beans, making them safe to eat.

How Other Kinds of Processing Affect This Food

Tofu. Tofu is a bland white cheeselike food made of liquid squeezed from soybeans and stiffened with a firming agent such as gluconolactone, calcium chloride, or calcium sulfate.

Heating tofu evaporates moisture and further coagulates proteins, making the tofu firmer and more dense. Tofu can be frozen; defrosted tofu is caramel-colored rather than creamy white with a spongy texture that soaks up sauce and flavorings.

Tofu is a useful cholesterol-free vegetarian substitute for meat, fish, or poultry. One 3-ounce serving of tofu equals one meat serving on the USDA/Health and Human Services Food Guide Pyramid. One four-ounce serving of regular tofu has one gram dietary fiber, six grams fat (0.9 g saturated fat), 10 g protein, 130 mg calcium, and 70 mg isoflavones.

Soy milk. Soy milk is a blend of soy flour (ground soybeans) and water. It is not a natural source of calcium, but most commercial soy milks are calcium-fortified, a useful alternative for people who cannot eat dairy foods. One cup calcium-fortified soy milk may have as much as 300 mg calcium.

Soy sauce. Soy sauce is made by adding salt to cooked soybeans and setting the mixture aside to ferment. Soy sauce is high in sodium, and it may interact with monoamine oxidase (MAO) inhibitors, antidepressant drugs that inactivate naturally occurring enzymes in your body that metabolize tyramine, a substance found in many fermented foods such as soy sauces. Tyramine is a pressor amine; it constricts blood vessels and increases blood pressure. If you eat a food containing tyramine while you are taking an MAO inhibitor, you cannot effectively eliminate the tyramine from your body, and the result may be a hypertensive crisis.

Milling. Soy flour is a powder made from soybeans. It is high in protein (37–47 percent). It can be used as a substitute for up to 20 percent of the wheat flour in any recipe. Unlike wheat flour, it has no gluten or gliadin, which makes it useful for people who have celiac disease, a metabolic disorder that makes it impossible for them to digest these wheat proteins (see FLOUR).

Canning. The heat of canning destroys some of the B vitamins in soybeans. Since the B vitamins are water-soluble, you could save them by using the liquid in the can. But the liquid also contains the indigestible sugars that cause intestinal gas when you eat beans.

Preprocessing. Preprocessed dried soybeans have already been soaked. They take less time to cook, but they are lower in B vitamins.

Medical Uses and/or Benefits

Lower risk of some birth defects. Up to two of every 1,000 babies born in the United States each year may have cleft palate or a neural tube (spinal cord) defect due to their mothers' not having gotten adequate amounts of folate during pregnancy. The current RDA for folate is 180 mcg for a woman and 200 mcg for a man, but the FDA now recommends 400 mcg for a woman who is or may become pregnant. Taking a folate supplement before becoming pregnant and continuing through the first two months of pregnancy reduces the risk of cleft palate; taking folate through the entire pregnancy reduces the risk of neural tube defects.

Possible lower risk of heart attack. In the spring of 1998, an analysis of data from the records for more than 80,000 women enrolled in the long-running Nurses' Health Study at Harvard School of Public Health/Brigham and Women's Hospital, in Boston, demonstrated that a diet providing more than 400 mcg folate and 3 mg vitamin B6 daily, either from food or supplements, might reduce a woman's risk of heart attack by almost 50 percent. Although men were not included in the study, the results were assumed to apply to them as well.

However, data from a meta-analysis published in the *Journal of the American Medical Association* in December 2006 called this theory into question. Researchers at Tulane University examined the results of 12 controlled studies in which 16,958 patients with preexisting cardiovascular disease were given either folic acid supplements or placebos ("look-alike" pills with no folic acid) for at least six months. The scientists, who found no reduction in the risk of further heart disease or overall death rates among those taking folic acid, concluded that further studies will be required to ascertain whether taking folic acid supplements reduces the risk of cardiovascular disease.

Lower cholesterol levels. A 1997 meta-analysis of 38 studies with more than 730 volunteers by James Anderson of the Metabolic Research Group at the Veterans Administration Medical Center and the University of Kentucky in Lexington demonstrates that substituting soy protein for animal proteins can lead to an average 9.3 percent decline in total cholesterol, a 12.3 percent decline in levels of low-density lipoproteins (the fat and protein particles that carry cholesterol into your arteries), and a 2.4 percent rise in HDL levels. People whose original cholesterol readings are "high" (250–289 mg/dl) are likely to see a greater decrease, as much as 24 percent lower total cholesterol.

There are currently two theories to explain how beans reduce cholesterol levels. The first theory is that the pectins in the beans may form a gel in your stomach that sops up fats and keeps them from being absorbed by your body. The second is that bacteria in the gut may feed on the bean fiber, producing short-chain fatty acids that inhibit the production of cholesterol in your liver. Whether soy's isoflavones affect cholesterol levels remains unanswered.

Lower levels of homocysteine. Homocysteine is an amino acid produced during the digestion of proteins. In 1998, the American Heart Association announced that high levels of homocysteine may be an independent risk factor for heart disease because homocysteine may damage smooth muscle cells in the lining of your arteries or make them grow faster (which could lead to arterial blockage) or may cause blood clots. Substituting soybeans for high-protein foods from animals lowers homocysteine production.

Protective effects of omega-3 fatty acids. Omega-3s appear to reduce the risk of heart attack. A 20-year project at the University of Leyden in the Netherlands, comparing the eating habits of more than 800 men at risk of heart disease, found that men who ate more than an ounce of fish a day had a 50 percent lower rate of heart attacks. Since then, a lengthening list of studies has shown similar protection among men who eat fish at least two or three times a week. One possible explanation is that omega-3s reduce triglyceride levels. Another is that your body converts omega-3s to a compound similar to prostacyclin, a naturally occurring chemical that inhibits the formation of blood clots.

Omega-3s also reduce the risk of "sudden death" heart attack. In the United States, about 250,000 people die each year from sudden cardiac failure caused by ventricular fibrillation, an unexpectedly irregular heartbeat. A 1995 study from the Australian Commonwealth Scientific and Industrial Research Organization (Adelaide), showed that laboratory monkeys fed omega-3 oils from fish had a steady heartbeat when exposed to electrical current twice as powerful as that which caused ventricular fibrillation in animals that did not get the fish oils.

Omega-3s inhibit the production of leuketrienes, naturally occurring chemicals that trigger inflammation. This may be beneficial to people with rheumatoid arthritis. In 1995, the Arthritis Foundation published the results of a study by Piet Geusens at the Catholic University in Pellenberg (Belgium) suggesting that patients who take omega-3 fatty acid supplements along with their regular arthritis medications have improved pain relief. Previous studies had demonstrated the omega-3s ability to reduce inflammation, joint stiffness and swelling.

Like isoflavones (see below), omega-3s may protect bone density. One 1997 study at Purdue University (Indiana) demonstrated that animals fed increased amounts of the omega-3 fatty acids formed new bone faster than animals fed a regular diet.

Potential protective effects of isoflavones. Soybeans are the most prominent source of isoflavones, plant compounds that mimic the effect of estrogen. The isoflavones in soybeans, genistein and daidzein, appear to protect bone density, and in the January 2008 issue of *Menopause* researchers at Beth Israel Deaconess Medical Center (Boston) report that a daidzein supplement may reduce the severity of menopausal hot flashes. However, earlier claims that consuming soy isoflavones might protect against breast, ovarian, and uterine cancers have not been proven.

As a source of carbohydrates for people with diabetes. Beans are digested very slowly, producing only a gradual rise in blood-sugar levels. As a result, the body needs less insulin to control blood sugar after eating beans than after eating some other high-carbohydrate foods (bread or potato). In studies at the University of Kentucky, a bean, whole-grain, vegetable, and fruit-rich diet developed at the University of Toronto and recommended by the American Diabetes Association enabled patients with type 1 diabetes (who do not produce any insulin themselves) to cut their daily insulin intake by 38 percent. For patients with type 2 diabetes (who can produce some insulin) the bean diet reduced the need for injected insulin by 98 percent. This diet is in line with the nutritional guidelines of the American Diabetes Association, but people with diabetes should always consult their doctor and/or dietitian before altering their diet.

As a diet aid. Although beans are high in calories, they are also high in fiber; even a small serving can make you feel full. And, because they are insulin-sparing, they put off the rise in insulin levels that makes us feel hungry again soon after eating. Research at the University of Toronto suggests the insulin-sparing effect may last for several hours after you eat the beans, perhaps until after your next meal.

Adverse Effects Associated with This Food

Allergic reaction. According to the *Merck Manual,* legumes, including soybeans, are one of the 12 foods most likely to trigger classic food allergy symptoms: hives, swelling of the lips and eyes, and upset stomach. The others are berries (blackberries, blueberries, raspberries, strawberries), chocolate, corn, eggs, fish, milk, nuts, peaches, pork, shellfish, and wheat (see WHEAT CEREALS).

Intestinal gas. Soybeans contain raffinose and stachyose, complex sugars that human beings cannot digest. The sugars sit in the gut, where they are fermented by intestinal bacteria, which then produce gas that distends the intestines and makes us uncomfortable. You can lessen this effect by covering the beans with boiling water and soaking them for four to six hours before you cook them so that the indigestible sugars leach out into the soaking water, which can be discarded. Or you may soak the beans for four hours in nine cups of water for every cup of beans, discard the soaking water, and add new water as your recipe directs. Then cook the beans and drain them before serving.

Production of uric acid. Purines are the natural metabolic by-products of protein metabolism in the body. They eventually break down into uric acid, which forms sharp crystals that may concentrate in joints, a condition known as gout. If uric acid crystals collect in the urine, the result may be kidney stones. Eating dried beans, which are rich in proteins, may raise the concentration of purines in your body. Although controlling the amount of purines in the diet does not significantly affect the course of gout (which is treated with allopurinol, a drug that prevents the formation of uric acid crystals), limiting these foods is still part of many gout regimens.

Food/Drug Interactions

* * *

Spinach

See also Greens, Lettuce.

Nutritional Profile

Energy value (calories per serving): *Low*
Protein: *High*
Fat: *Low*
Saturated fat: *Low*
Cholesterol: *None*
Carbohydrates: *Moderate*
Fiber: *Low*
Sodium: *Moderate*
Major vitamin contribution: *Vitamin A, folate, vitamin C*
Major mineral contribution: *Potassium*

About the Nutrients in This Food

Spinach has some sugar, a trace of starch; a moderate amount of proteins considered "incomplete" because they are deficient in the essential amino acids tryptophan, methionine, and cystine; very little fat; and no cholesterol. It has moderate amounts of cellulose, and the noncarbohydrate food fiber lignin, which is found in roots, seed coverings, stems, and the ribs of leaves. Spinach is a good source of vitamin A and vitamin C. It is also rich in iron, but oxalic acid (a naturally-occurring chemical in spinach leaves) binds the iron into an insoluble compound the body cannot absorb. Only 2 to 5 percent of the iron in spinach is actually available for absorption.

One cup of chopped fresh spinach leaves has 0.7 g dietary fiber, 2,813 IU vitamin A (1.2 times the RDA for a woman, 95 percent of the RDA for a man), 58 mcg folate (15 percent of the RDA), 84 mg vitamin C (1.1 times the RDA for a woman, 93 percent of the RDA for a man), and 0.8 mg iron (4 percent of the RDA for a woman, 10 percent of the RDA for a man).

The Most Nutritious Way to Serve This Food

Fresh, lightly steamed, to protect its vitamin C.

With a cream sauce. The sauce, which can be made of low-fat milk, provides the essential amino acids needed to complete the proteins in the spinach.

Diets That May Restrict or Exclude This Food

Low-calcium, low-oxalate diet (for people who form calcium-oxalate kidney stones)
Low-sodium diet

Buying This Food

Look for: Fresh, crisp dark-green leaves that are free of dirt and debris.

Avoid: Yellowed leaves. These are aging leaves whose chlorophyll pigments have faded, allowing the carotenoids underneath to show through. Wilted leaves or leaves that are limp and brownish have lost vitamin C.

Storing This Food

Refrigerate loose leaves in a roomy plastic bag. If you bought the spinach already wrapped in plastic, unwrap it and divide it up into smaller packages so the leaves are not crowded or bent, then refrigerate.

Preparing This Food

Wash the spinach thoroughly under cool running water to remove all sand and debris. Discard damaged or yellowed leaves. Trim the ribs and stems but don't remove them entirely; they are rich in food fiber. If you plan to use the spinach in a salad, refrigerate the damp leaves to make them crisp.

What Happens When You Cook This Food

Chlorophyll, the pigment that makes green vegetables green, is sensitive to acids. When you heat spinach, the chlorophyll in its leaves will react with acids in the vegetable or in the cooking water, forming pheophytin, which is brown. The pheophytin turns cooked spinach olive-drab or, if the spinach leaves contain a lot of yellow carotenes, bronze.

To keep cooked spinach green, you have to keep the chlorophyll from reacting with acids. One way to do this is to cook the spinach in a lot of water (which dilutes the acids), but this increases the loss of vitamin C. Another alternative is to cook the spinach with the lid off the pot so the volatile acids can float off into the air. Or you can steam the spinach quickly in very little water so that it retains its vitamin C and cooks before there is time for the chlorophyll/acid reaction to occur.

Spinach also contains astringent tannins that react with metals to create dark pigments. If you cook the leaves in an aluminum or iron pot, these pigments will discolor the pots and the spinach. To keep the spinach from darkening, cook in an enameled or glass pot.

How Other Kinds of Processing Affect This Food

Canning and freezing.   Canned spinach, which is processed at high heat, is olive or bronze rather than green. Like cooked spinach, canned spinach and frozen spinach have only 50 percent of the vitamin C in fresh spinach.

Medical Uses and/or Benefits

Reduced risk of cardiovascular disease, cancer, decline of brain function, and other diseases of aging.   Antioxidants prevent free radicals, fragments of molecules, from hooking up with other fragments to produce compounds that damage body cells, thus lowering your risk of heart disease, cancer, memory loss, and other conditions associated with aging or damaged cells. In 1996, researchers at the USDA Jean Mayer Human Nutrition Research Center on Aging at Tufts University (Boston) showed that, ounce for ounce, strawberries, blueberries, and spinach were the most potentially potent antioxidants of 40 foods tested. While blueberries scored number one in the Tufts study, antioxidant ranking of these foods may vary depending on growing conditions, season, and other variables.

Lower risk of some birth defects.   As many as two of every 1,000 babies born in the United States each year may have cleft palate or a neural tube (spinal cord) defect due to their mother's not having gotten adequate amounts of folate during pregnancy. The current RDA for folate is 180 mcg for a woman and 200 mcg for a man, but the FDA now recommends 400 mcg for a woman who is or may become pregnant. Taking folate supplements before becoming pregnant and continuing through the first two months of pregnancy reduces the risk of cleft palate; taking folate through the entire pregnancy reduces the risk of neural tube defects.

Possible lower risk of heart attack.   In the spring of 1998, an analysis of data from the records for more than 80,000 women enrolled in the long-running Nurses' Health Study at Harvard School of Public Health/Brigham and Women's Hospital, in Boston, demonstrated that a diet providing more than 400 mcg folate and 3 mg vitamin B_6 daily, either from food or supplements, might reduce a woman's risk of heart attack by almost 50 percent. Although men were not included in the study, the results were assumed to apply to them as well.

However, data from a meta-analysis published in the *Journal of the American Medical Association* in December 2006 called this theory into question. Researchers at Tulane University examined the results of 12 controlled studies in which 16,958 patients with preexisting cardiovascular disease were given either folic acid supplements or placebos ("look-alike" pills with no folic acid) for at least six months. The scientists, who found no reduction in the risk of further heart disease or overall death rates among those taking folic acid, concluded that further studies will be required to ascertain whether taking folic acid supplements reduces the risk of cardiovascular disease.

Lower risk of stroke.   Various nutrition studies have attested to the power of adequate potassium to keep blood pressure within safe levels. For example, in the 1990s, data from the long-running Harvard School of Public Health/Health Professionals Follow-Up Study of male doctors showed that a diet rich in high-potassium foods such as bananas, oranges, and plantain may reduce the risk of stroke. In the study, the men who ate the higher number of potassium-rich foods (an average of nine servings a day) had a risk of stroke 38 percent lower than that of men who consumed fewer than four servings a day. In 2008, a similar survey at the Queen's Medical Center (Honolulu) showed a similar protective effect among men and women using diuretic drugs (medicines that increase urination and thus the loss of potassium).

Adverse Effects Associated with This Food

Nitrate/nitrite poisoning. Spinach, like beets, celery, eggplant, lettuce, radish, and collard and turnip greens, contains nitrates that convert naturally into nitrites in your stomach and then react with the amino acids in proteins to form nitrosamines. Although some nitrosamines are known or suspected carcinogens, this natural chemical conversion presents no known problems for a healthy adult. However, when these nitrate-rich vegetables are cooked and left to stand at room temperature, bacterial enzyme action (and perhaps some enzymes in the plants) converts the nitrates to nitrites at a much faster rate than normal. These higher-nitrite foods may be hazardous for infants; several cases of "spinach poisoning" been reported among children who ate cooked spinach that had been left standing at room temperature.

Food/Drug Interactions

Anticoagulants Spinach is rich in vitamin K, the blood-clotting vitamin produced naturally by bacteria in the intestines. Consuming large quantities of this food may reduce the effectiveness of anticoagulants (blood thinners) such as warfarin (Coumadin). One cup of drained canned spinach contains 988 mcg vitamin K, 16 times the RDA for a healthy adult; one cup of shredded raw spinach contains 144 mcg vitamin K, nearly three times the RDA for a healthy adult.

MAO inhibitors. Monoamine oxidase (MAO) inhibitors are drugs used as antidepressants or antihypertensives. They interfere with the action of enzymes that break down tyramine, a chemical produced when long-chain protein molecules are broken into smaller pieces. Tyramine is a pressor amine, a chemical that constricts blood vessels and raises blood pressure. If you eat a food rich in tyramine while you are taking an MAO inhibitor, the pressor amine cannot be eliminated from your body and the result may be a hypertensive crisis (sustained elevated blood pressure). There has been at least one report of such an interaction in a patient who consumed New Zealand prickly spinach while using an MAO inhibitor.

Squid (Calamari)

(Octopus)

Nutritional Profile:

Energy value (calories per serving): *Moderate*
Protein: *High*
Fat: *Low*
Saturated fat: *Low*
Cholesterol: *High*
Carbohydrates: *Low*
Fiber: *None*
Sodium: *Moderate*
Major vitamin contribution: *B vitamins*
Major mineral contribution: *Iron*

About the Nutrients in This Food

Like meat, fish, and poultry, squid and octopus provide high-quality proteins with sufficient amounts of all the essential amino acids. Both have less saturated fat than meat and small amounts of omega-3 fatty acids, a group that includes the essential fatty acid linolenic acid, plus eicosapentaenoic acid (EPA) and docosahexaenoic acid (DHA), the primary unsaturated fatty acids in oils from fish. However, like shellfish, squid and octopus may be a significant source of cholesterol. The cholesterol content of squid and octopus can vary from animal to animal; there is no reliable guide to choosing the one that is lower in cholesterol. As a general rule, the mantle (body) generally has less cholesterol than the tentacles. Four ounces of raw squid has 1.6 g total fat (0.4 g saturated fat, 0.1 g monounsaturated fat, 0.7 g polyunsaturated fat), 264 mg cholesterol, and 17.7 g protein. Four ounces of raw octopus has 3.5 g total fat (0.7 g saturated fat, 0.6 g monounsaturated fat, and 0.8 g polyunsaturated fat), 163 mg cholesterol, and 17 g protein. According to the National Marine Fisheries Service Northeast Fisheries Laboratories, squid and octopus have approximately 86 mg omega-3s per ounce.

The Most Nutritious Way to Serve This Food

Prepared with little or no added fat, to preserve the seafood's status as a low-fat food.

Diets That May Restrict or Exclude This Food

Low-cholesterol diet
Low-protein diet
Low-sodium diet (frozen squid or octopus)

Buying This Food

Look for: Fresh whole squid with clear, smooth skin. The squid should smell absolutely fresh. Squid larger than 8 inches may be tough.

Choose fresh, whole baby octopus or octopus meat that looks and smells absolutely fresh. Octopus larger than two to 2.5 pounds may be tough.

Storing This Food

Refrigerate fresh, cleaned octopus or squid immediately and use it within a day or two. Frozen squid or octopus will keep for one month in a 0°F freezer.

Preparing This Food

NOTE: Handle live squid or octopus with care. They bite.

Squid. Whole squid are usually sold cleaned, like any other seafood. If you are cleaning the squid yourself, your goal is to throw out everything but the empty saclike body and the tentacles. Start by removing the beak. Then reach into the body cavity and pull out all the innards, including the cartilage. (If you tear or puncture the ink sac and spill the ink, just wash it off your hands.) Cut the innards away from the body and throw them out. Peel off the skin. Squeeze the thick end of the tentacles and discard the small yellowish piece of meat that pops out. Rinse the squid meat thoroughly, inside and out, under cool running water. Stuff the sac whole for baking or cut it into rings and stew it along with chunks of the tentacles.

Octopus. Cleaned, dressed octopus needs only be rinsed thoroughly under cold running water. To prepare a small whole octopus, remove the beak, eyes, anal area, and ink sac. Cut off the tough ends of the tentacles, slice the tentacles into rounds or chunks, rinse them thoroughly under cold running water to remove all the gelatinous cartilage, and pound the meat to tenderize.

When you are done, clean all utensils thoroughly with soap and hot water. Wash your cutting board, wood or plastic, with hot water, soap, and a bleach-and-water solution. For ultimate safety in preventing the transfer of microorganisms from the squid to other foods, keep one cutting board exclusively for raw fish, meats, or poultry, and a second one for everything else. Don't forget to wash your hands.

What Happens When You Cook This Food

Heat changes the structure of the proteins in the squid and octopus. The proteins are denatured, which means that they break into smaller fragments or change shape or clump together. These changes cause protein tissues to lose moisture and shrink, so that the sea-food becomes opaque as it cooks.

Squid cooks fairly quickly. Its thin-walled body can be fried or sautéed in less than a minute and stewed in half an hour. Octopus, on the other hand, may need to be simmered for as long as three hours. But take care: the longer you cook the octopus, the more moisture you squeeze out of its protein tissues and the more rubbery it becomes.

How Other Kinds of Processing Affect This Food

Freezing. Commercially processed squid are soaked in brine before freezing, which makes them much higher in sodium than fresh squid.

Medical Uses and/or Benefits

Protective effects of omega-3 fatty acids. Omega-3s appear to reduce the risk of heart attack. A 20-year project at the University of Leyden in the Netherlands, comparing the eating habits of more than 800 men at risk of heart disease, found that men who ate more than an ounce of fish a day had a 50 percent lower rate of heart attacks. Since then, a lengthening list of studies has shown similar protection among men who eat fish at least two or three times a week. One possible explanation is that omega-3s reduce triglyceride levels. Another is that your body converts omega-3s to a compound similar to prostacyclin, a naturally occurring chemical that inhibits the formation of blood clots.

Omega-3s also reduce the risk of "sudden death" heart attack. In the United States, about 250,000 people die each year from sudden cardiac failure caused by ventricular fibrillation, an unexpectedly irregular heartbeat. A 1995 study from the Australian Commonwealth Scientific and Industrial Research Organization (Adelaide), showed that laboratory monkeys fed omega-3 oils from fish had a steady heartbeat when exposed to electrical current twice as powerful as that which caused ventricular fibrillation in animals that did not get the fish oils.

Omega-3s inhibit the production of leuketrienes, naturally occurring chemicals that trigger inflammation. This may be beneficial to people with rheumatoid arthritis. In 1995, the Arthritis Foundation published the results of a study by Piet Geusens at the Catholic University in Pellenberg (Belgium) suggesting that patients who take omega-3 fatty acid supplements along with their regular arthritis medications have improved pain relief.

Previous studies had demonstrated the omega-3s ability to reduce inflammation, joint stiffness, and swelling.

Finally, like isoflavones, omega-3s may protect bone density. One 1997 study at Purdue University (Indiana) demonstrated that animals fed increased amounts of the omega-3 fatty acids formed new bone faster than animals fed a regular diet.

Adverse Effects Associated with This Food

Allergic reaction.   Shellfish are one of the 12 foods most likely to cause the classic symptoms of food allergy, including upset stomach, hives, and angioedema (swelling of the lips and eyes). The others are berries (blackberries, blueberries, raspberries, strawberries), chocolate, corn, eggs, fish, legumes (peas, lima beans, peanuts, soybeans), milk, nuts, peaches, pork, and wheat (see WHEAT CEREALS).

Parasitical, viral, and bacterial infections and/or food poisoning.   Like raw meat, raw shellfish may carry various pathogens, including *Salmonella* bacteria. These organisms are destroyed by thorough cooking.

Elevated levels of serum cholesterol.   People whose blood-cholesterol levels are abnormally high are considered at risk for heart disease, but experts disagree as to the effects of dietary cholesterol on serum cholesterol. Patients with hypercholesteremia, a metabolic disorder that influences cholesterol production in the liver, may benefit from a diet low in dietary cholesterol, but there is no conclusive proof that lowering a healthy person's consumption of dietary cholesterol will significantly change the amount of cholesterol he or she produces. In 1986 the American Heart Association issued new guidelines suggesting that healthy adults reduce their consumption of fat to 30 percent of total calories and limit cholesterol intake to 300 mg per day or 100 mg per 1000 calories, whichever is less (3.5 ounces of squid or octopus have 300 mg cholesterol).

Food/Drug Interactions

* * *

Strawberries

Nutritional Profile

Energy value (calories per serving): *Low*
Protein: *Moderate*
Fat: *Low*
Saturated fat: *Low*
Cholesterol: *None*
Carbohydrates: *High*
Fiber: *Moderate*
Sodium: *Low*
Major vitamin contribution: *Folate, vitamin C*
Major mineral contribution: *Potassium*

About the Nutrients in This Food

Strawberries are high in dietary fiber: insoluble lignin in the tiny seeds that dot the surface of the berry and soluble pectins in the fruit itself. Strawberries are also a good source of the B vitamin folate and high in vitamin C.

One-half cup sliced fresh strawberries has 1.7 g dietary fiber, 20 mcg folate (5 percent of the RDA), and 49 mg vitamin C (65 percent of the RDA for a woman, 54 percent of the RDA for a man).

The Most Nutritious Way to Serve This Food

Fresh and ripe, to preserve the vitamin C.

Diets That May Restrict or Exclude This Food

Low-fiber diet

Buying This Food

Look for: Bright red berries with fresh green caps. Pale berries are immature; berries with dark, red wet spots are overmature; berries whose caps have browned are aging. Small berries are generally more flavorful than large ones.

Storing This Food

Refrigerate strawberries with their caps on. When you remove the caps you tear cells in the berries, activating ascorbic acid oxidase, an enzyme that destroys vitamin C. Keeping strawberries cool also helps keep them bright red; the anthocyanin pigments that make strawberries red turn brown faster at high temperatures.

Preparing This Food

When you are ready to use the berries, rinse them thoroughly under cool running water. Then remove the caps. (If you hull the berries before you rinse them, water may run into the berry and dilute the flavor.)

Don't slice the berries until you are ready to use them. When you slice a strawberry, you tear cell walls, releasing ascorbic acid oxidase, the enzyme that breaks down vitamin C. This reduces the nutritional value of the strawberries. It may also be linked to the degradation of the pigments that make strawberries red. Acids retard the color loss; sprinkling the sliced berries with lemon juice helps preserve color.

You can soften and sweeten strawberries by dusting them with sugar and letting them sit for a while. The sugar dissolves in moisture on the surface of the berry, producing a solution that is more dense than the liquid inside the strawberry's cells. Then the liquid inside the cells will flow across the cell walls to the denser sugar-water solution (a phenomenon known as osmosis); the cell walls that were held apart by the water will collapse inward and the strawberry will be softer.

What Happens When You Cook This Food

The red anthocyanin pigments in strawberries are heat-sensitive; they break apart and turn brown when you heat them. Adding sugar speeds up the process even further because some of the chemicals produced when sugars are heated also break down anthocyanins. That's why strawberries cooked in boiling, sugared water turn brown faster than strawberries steamed quickly without sugar.

Red anthocyanins also change color in acids and bases (alkalis). They are bright red in acids such as lemon juice and bluish or purple in bases such as baking soda. If you cook strawberries in an aluminum or iron pot, their acids will react with metal ions from the surface of the pot to create dark brown compounds that darken either the pot or the fruit.

Strawberries also lose heat-sensitive vitamin C when you cook them.

How Other Forms of Processing Affect This Food

Heat processing (canning: making jams, jellies, and preserves). As noted above, strawberries turn brown when you heat them with sugar. Lemon juice added to jams, jellies, and preserves makes the taste tart and helps preserve the color.

Medical Uses and/or Benefits

Lower risk of some birth defects. Up to two of every 1,000 babies born in the United States each year may have cleft palate or a neural tube (spinal cord) defect due to their mothers' not having gotten adequate amounts of folate during pregnancy. The current RDA for folate is 180 mcg for a woman and 200 mcg for a man, but FDA now recommends 400 mcg for a woman who is or may become pregnant. Taking a folate supplement before becoming pregnant and continuing through the first two months of pregnancy reduces the risk of cleft palate; taking folate through the entire pregnancy reduces the risk of neural tube defects.

Possible lower risk of heart attack. In the spring of 1998, an analysis of data from the records for more than 80,000 women enrolled in the long-running Nurses' Health Study at Harvard School of Public Health/Brigham and Women's Hospital, in Boston, demonstrated that a diet providing more than 400 mcg folate and 3 mg vitamin B_6 daily, either from food or supplements, might reduce a woman's risk of heart attack by almost 50 percent. Although men were not included in the study, the results were assumed to apply to them as well.

However, data from a meta-analysis published in the *Journal of the American Medical Association* in December 2006 called this theory into question. Researchers at Tulane University examined the results of 12 controlled studies in which 16,958 patients with preexisting cardiovascular disease were given either folic acid supplements or placebos ("look-alike" pills with no folic acid) for at least six months. The scientists, who found no reduction in the risk of further heart disease or overall death rates among those taking folic acid, concluded that further studies will be required to ascertain whether taking folic acid supplements reduces the risk of cardiovascular disease.

As an antiscorbutic. Strawberries, which (ounce for ounce) have more vitamin C than citrus fruits, help protect against scurvy, the vitamin C–deficiency disease.

Adverse Effects Associated with This Food

Allergic reaction. According to the *Merck Manual,* strawberries and other berries are one of 12 foods most likely to trigger classic food-allergy symptoms: upset stomach, hives, angioedema (swelling of the face, lips, and eyes), and a hay-feverlike reaction. The others are chocolate, corn, eggs, fish, legumes (peas, lima beans, peanuts, soybeans), milk, nuts, peaches, pork, shellfish, and wheat (see WHEAT CEREALS).

Food-borne illness. Small fruits such as berries appear to be a growing source of contamination by disease-causing organisms such as *E. coli* O157:H7 and salmonella. Common methods of decontamination such as vigorously washing the fruit are impractical with berries because they damage the fruit. In 2007, researchers from the University of Pennsylvania delivered a report at the annual meeting of the American Society of Agricultural and Biological Engineers, describing the use of pulsed ultraviolet light to decontaminate raspberries and strawberries with no observable damage to the fruit, offering growers and food distributors a way to make their products safer before shipping.

Food/Drug Interactions

* * *

Sugar

(Corn syrup, fructose, maple sugar, maple syrup, molasses)

See also Honey.

Nutritional Profile

Energy value (calories per serving): *High*

Protein: *None*

Fat: *None*

Saturated fat: *None*

Cholesterol: *None*

Carbohydrates: *High*

Fiber: *None*

Sodium: *None*

Major vitamin contribution: *B vitamins (molasses)*

Major mineral contribution: *Iron (molasses)*

About the Nutrients in This Food

The sugars we use in cooking—table sugar ("white sugar"), brown sugar, molasses, corn syrup, maple sugar—are all disaccharides ("double sugars") made from units of fructose ("fruit sugar") and glucose.

    Table sugar (also known as *granulated sugar, white sugar, refined sugar,* or simply *sugar*) is crystallized from sugar cane. *Confectioner's sugar* is table sugar mixed with corn starch. *Molasses* and *blackstrap molasses* are by-products of table sugar production. *Brown sugar* is table sugar with added molasses; the darker the sugar, the more molasses. *Raw sugar* (a.k.a. *turbinado sugar*) is cane sugar with some of the natural molasses left in. Because of its impurities, true raw sugar cannot be sold legally in the United States; "raw sugar" at the supermarket is usually plain white sugar colored with molasses. *Maple sugar* is concentrated from the sap of the maple tree. *Corn syrup* is glucose extracted from corn starch, with sucrose or fructose added to make it sweeter. (Glucose is only half as sweet as sucrose.)

    With the exception of molasses, which has about 0.9 mg iron per tablespoon (5 percent of the RDA for a woman, 11 percent of the RDA for a man), no sugar has an appreciable amount of any nutrient other than calories.

The Most Nutritious Way to Serve This Food

In moderation.

Diets That May Restrict or Exclude This Food

Low-calorie diet
Low-carbohydrate diet
Sucrose-free diet

Buying This Food

Look for: Tightly sealed boxes or sacks of dry sugars. Avoid stained packages; whatever stained the outside may have seeped through into the sugar.

Choose tightly sealed bottles or liquid sugars. The liquid inside should be clear; tiny bubbles and a gray scum on the surface of the sugar suggest that it has fermented.

Storing This Food

Store solid sugars in air- and moistureproof containers in a cool, dry cabinet.
Sugars are hydrophilic, which means that they will absorb moisture. If sugars get wet (or pick up excess moisture from hot, humid air), they will harden or cake.

Store tightly sealed, unopened containers of liquid sugars such as corn syrup, maple syrup, and molasses at room temperature. Once the container is opened, you can store the sugar in the refrigerator to protect it from molds and keep the sugars from fermenting.

Preparing This Food

Because they contain different amounts of water and have different levels of sweetness, sugars cannot simply be substituted equally for each other. As a general rule, one cup of white table sugar = one cup of firmly packed brown sugar = 1.75 cup confectioner's sugar (which cannot be substituted in baking) = two cups corn syrup (with a reduction of liquid in baking and substitution of corn syrup for only half the sugar) = 1.3 cups molasses (with reduced liquid and no more than substitution for half the sugar in baking).

To measure granulated white sugar, pour into a cup and use a knife to level. To measure brown sugar, pack tightly into a cup. Powdered (confectioner's) sugar can be sifted or not, as the recipe dictates.

What Happens When You Cook This Food

When you heat sugar its molecules separate. The sugar liquifies, then turns brown. The browning is called caramelization. When you heat sugar in water it attracts molecules of water and forms a syrup that can be thickened by heating the solution long enough to evaporate some of the water.

How Other Kinds of Processing Affect This Food

* * *

Medical Uses and/or Benefits

* * *

Adverse Effects Associated with This Food

Tooth decay. Fermentable carbohydrates, including sugars, may cling to the teeth and nourish the bacteria that cause cavities. Regular flossing and brushing remove the sugars mechanically; fluoridated water hardens the surface of the teeth so that they are more resistant to bacterial action.

Inability to metabolize sucrose. People with diabetes do not produce enough insulin to metabolize sugar properly to glucose (the form of sugar circulating in our blood). When they eat sugar, excess glucose builds up in urine and blood. Some people have precisely the opposite problem, reactive hypoglycemia, an excess secretion of insulin that can trigger trembling, anxiety, headache, fast heartbeat, and difficulty in thinking clearly. If untreated, the results of both insulin insufficiency and insulin over-secretion may be life-threatening.

Heart disease. In some people, a high-carbohydrate diet may cause an increase in the level of triglycerides (fatty acids) in the blood, but this rise is only temporary in people whose weight is normal. People who are overweight tend, as a rule, to have levels of triglycerides that are consistently higher than normal. When they lose weight the levels of triglycerides fall. The theory that sugar causes heart disease, first proposed by British researchers in the 1960s, has been successfully refuted by long-term studies from several countries that show no correlation at all between sugar intake and the incidence of coronary heart disease.

Possible hyperactivity in children. The popular belief that sugared foods causes hyperactivity in children remains controversial. In the 1990s, the National Institutes of Health (NIH) conducted studies in which children were given drinks sweetened with glucose, sucrose, or saccharin without the children or the testers knowing which child got what drink. The results showed no correlation between sugared drinks and hyperactivity. In fact, the children were generally quieter after drinking sugared beverages, an observation that is consistent with the accepted observation that consuming carbohydrates, including sugars, facilitates the brain's ability to produce the calming neurotransmitter serotonin. However, the NIH note that because refined sugars enter the bloodstream more quickly than complex carbohydrates such as starches (e.g., bread), they do produce fluctuation in blood glucose levels that might trigger the release of the "fight-or-flight" energizing hormone adrenaline, making a child more active for the moment.

Hypoglycemia.   Reactive hypoglycemia, an oversecretion of insulin in response to eating sugar, is a rare condition that causes trembling, anxiety, headache, fast heartbeat, and difficulty in thinking clearly. Hypoglycemia may also be caused by the presence of a pancreatic tumor or an overdose of insulin. This is a more serious condition that, uncorrected, may lead to coma or death.

Food/Drug Interactions

* * *

Summer Squash

(Yellow crookneck, yellow straightneck, zucchini)

Nutritional Profile

Energy value (calories per serving): *Low*
Protein: *High*
Fat: *Low*
Saturated fat: *Low*
Cholesterol: *None*
Carbohydrates: *High*
Fiber: *Moderate*
Sodium: *Low*
Major vitamin contribution: *Vitamin A, vitamin C*
Major mineral contribution: *Potassium*

About the Nutrients in This Food

Zucchini and the yellow summer squashes are high in dietary fiber: insoluble cellulose and lignin in the seeds and peel and soluble pectins in the vegetable itself.

Green and yellow summer squashes have small to moderate amounts of vitamin A derived from yellow carotenes (including beta-carotene) in the skin. Zucchini and the yellow crookneck and straightneck squashes also have some vitamin C.

One half-cup (four ounces) boiled zucchini slices has 1.2 g dietary fiber, 1,005 IU vitamin A (44 percent of the RDA for a woman, 34 percent of the RDA for a man), 18 mcg folate (5 percent of the RDA), and 4 mg vitamin C (5 percent of the RDA for a woman, 4 percent of the RDA for a man). A similar serving of yellow crookneck or straightneck squash has 1.3 g dietary fiber, 147 IU vitamin A (6 percent of the RDA for a woman, 5 percent of the RDA for a man), 15 mcg folate (4 percent of the RDA), and 5 mg vitamin C (7 percent of the RDA for a woman, 6 percent of the RDA for a man).

The Most Nutritious Way to Serve This Food

Steamed quickly in very little water, to preserve the vitamin C.

Diets That May Restrict or Exclude This Food

Low-fiber diet

Buying This Food

Look for: Dark green slender zucchini with pale yellow or white striping. Yellow crookneck squash should be brightly colored with lightly pebbled skin. Yellow straightneck squash may have either smooth or pebbled skin.

Choose smaller (and therefore more tender) squash. The best zucchini are four to nine inches long; the best crooknecks and straightnecks are four to six inches long.

Avoid: Limp squash. They have lost moisture and vitamins. Avoid squash whose skin is bruised or cut; handle squash gently to avoid bruising them yourself. Bruising tears cells, activating ascorbic acid oxidase, an enzyme that destroys vitamin C. Avoid squash with a hard rind; the harder the rind, the older the squash and the larger and harder the seeds inside.

Storing This Food

Refrigerate summer squash, which are perishable and should be used within a few days.

Preparing This Food

Scrub the squash with a vegetable brush and cut off each round end. Peel older, larger squash, then slice them in half and remove the hard seeds. Younger, more tender squash can be cooked with the peel and seeds.

What Happens When You Cook This Food

As the squash cooks, its cells absorb water, the pectins in the cell walls dissolve, and the vegetable gets softer. The seeds, stiffened with insoluble cellulose and lignin, will remain firm.

Chlorophyll, the pigment that makes green vegetables green, is sensitive to acids. When you heat zucchini, its chlorophyll reacts with acids in the vegetable or in the cooking water to form pheophytin, which is brown. The pheophytin makes cooked zucchini look olive-drab. To keep the cooked zucchini green, you have to keep the chlorophyll from reacting with the acids. One way to do this is to cook the zucchini in a large quantity of water (which will dilute the acids), but this increases the loss of vitamin C. A second alternative is to leave the top off the pot so that the volatile acids can float off into the air. Or you can stir-fry the zucchini or steam it in very little water so the vegetable cooks before the chlorophyll/acid reaction can occur.

Yellow squash stays bright yellow no matter how long you cook it; its carotene pigments are impervious to the normal heat of cooking.

How Other Kinds of Processing Affect This Food

Canning. Canned zucchini has about as much vitamin C as fresh-cooked zucchini.

Medical Uses and/or Benefits

Lowering the risk of some cancers. According to the American Cancer Society, foods rich in beta-carotene may lower the risk of cancers of the larynx, esophagus, and lungs. There is no similar benefit from beta-carotene supplements; indeed, one controversial study actually showed a higher rate of lung cancer among smokers taking the supplement.

Adverse Effects Associated with This Food

* * *

Food/Drug Interactions

* * *

Sweet Potatoes

(Yams)

See also Potatoes.

Nutritional Profile

Energy value (calories per serving): *Moderate*
Protein: *Moderate*
Fat: *Low*
Saturated fat: *Low*
Cholesterol: *None*
Carbohydrates: *High*
Fiber: *High*
Sodium: *Low*
Major vitamin contribution: *Vitamin A, folate, vitamin C*
Major mineral contribution: *Potassium*

About the Nutrients in This Food

Sweet potatoes are high-carbohydrate foods, rich in starch and high in dietary fiber (soluble pectins in the flesh). *Alpha amylase,* an enzyme in sweet potatoes, converts starches to sugars as the potato matures or when it is stored or while it is cooking, so older sweet potatoes are sweeter than young ones.

Sweet potatoes are an extraordinary source of vitamin A derived from the carotene pigments that make the potato orange yellow. The deeper the color, the higher the vitamin A content. Sweet potatoes are also a good source of the B vitamin folate, vitamin C, and potassium.

One baked 5" × 2" sweet potato has 3.8 g dietary fiber, 21,907 IU vitamin A (nearly 10 times the RDA for a woman, seven times the RDA for a man), 22.3 mg vitamin C (30 percent of the RDA for a woman, 25 percent of the RDA for a man), and 542 mg potassium, nearly twice as much as one-half cup (four ounces) fresh orange juice.

Raw sweet potatoes, like raw lima beans, contain cyanogenic glycosides, natural chemicals that break down into hydrogen cyanide in your stomach or when the potato is heated. If you pierce the potato while it is baking or leave the lid off the pot while it is boiling, the hydrogen cyanide (a gas) will float off harmlessly into the air.

The Most Nutritious Way to Serve This Food

Baked or boiled.

Diets That May Restrict or Exclude This Food

* * *

Buying This Food

Look for: Solid, well-shaped sweet potatoes, thick in the center and tapering toward the ends. The potatoes should feel heavy for their size and the skin should be evenly colored and free of blemishes, bruises, and mold. Moldy sweet potatoes may be contaminated with a number of toxins including the liver toxin ipomeamarone and a toxic derivative, ipomeamaronol. These toxins cannot be destroyed by normal boiling or baking.

Storing This Food

Handle sweet potatoes gently to avoid bruising. When you bruise a sweet potato you tear some of its cells, releasing polyphenoloxidase, an enzyme that hastens the oxidation of phenols in the potato, creating brown compounds that darken the potato.

Store sweet potatoes in a cool (55–60°F), dark cabinet, not in the refrigerator. Like bruising, very cold temperature damage the potato's cells, releasing polyphenoloxidase and darkening the potato.

Store home-grown sweet potatoes at 85°F for four to six days right after harvesting to sweeten them by increasing the natural conversion of starches to sugars.

Preparing This Food

Scrub sweet potatoes under cool running water. Boiling the potatoes in their skin will save more vitamins since you will be able to peel them more closely after they are cooked. If you plan to bake the sweet potatoes, pierce the skin with a cake tester to let the steam escape as the potato cooks, and insert an aluminum "potato nail" to carry heat evenly through as it bakes.

What Happens When You Cook This Food

Cooking sweetens the potato by converting some of its starches to sugars. Cooking also changes the potato's texture. When you bake a sweet potato, the water inside its cells dissolves some of the pectins in its cell walls, so the potato gets softer. As it continues to bake, moisture begins to evaporate from the cells and the potato shrinks. When you boil sweet potatoes, the initial reaction is just the opposite: at first, the starch granules in the potato absorb moisture and swell so that the potato looks bigger. If you continue to boil the potato, however, its starch granules will absorb so much water that they rupture. The water inside will leak out and the potato, once again, will shrink.

How Other Kinds of Processing Affect This Food

Canning. Sweet potatoes canned in water have the same nutrients as cooked fresh sweet potatoes. Sweet potatoes canned in sugar syrups have more carbohydrates and more calories.

Medical Uses and/or Benefits

Lower risk of stroke. Various nutrition studies have attested to the power of adequate potassium to keep blood pressure within safe levels. For example, in the 1990s, data from the long-running Harvard School of Public Health/Health Professionals Follow-Up Study of male doctors showed that a diet rich in high-potassium foods such as bananas, oranges, and plantain may reduce the risk of stroke. In the study, the men who ate the higher number of potassium-rich foods (an average of nine servings a day) had a risk of stroke 38 percent lower than that of men who consumed fewer than four servings a day. In 2008, a similar survey at the Queen's Medical Center (Honolulu) showed a similar protective effect among men and women using diuretic drugs (medicines that increase urination and thus the loss of potassium).

Adverse Effects Associated with This Food

* * *

Food/Drug Interactions

* * *

Tangerines

(Clementine, tangelo)

Nutritional Profile

Energy value (calories per serving): *Low*
Protein: *Moderate*
Fat: *Low*
Saturated fat: *Low*
Cholesterol: *None*
Carbohydrates: *High*
Fiber: *Moderate*
Sodium: *Low*
Major vitamin contribution: *Vitamin C*
Major mineral contribution: *Potassium*

About the Nutrients in This Food

Tangerines are also known as "mandarin oranges." Clementines are small Algerian tangerines. Tangelos are a cross between the grapefruit and the tangerine. All there are high in sugar with moderate amounts of dietary fiber (soluble pectins), good sources of vitamin A and vitamin C.

One peeled tangerine, 2.5 inches in diameter, has 1.6 g dietary fiber, 599 IU vitamin A (26 percent of the RDA for a woman, 20 percent of the RDA for a man), and 24 mg vitamin C (32 percent of the RDA for a woman, 27 percent of the RDA for a man).

The Most Nutritious Way to Serve This Food

Freshly peeled.

Diets That May Restrict or Exclude This Food

Low-fiber diet

Buying This Food

Look for: Tangerines that are heavy for their size (which means they will be juicy). The skin should be deep orange, almost red, and naturally puffy and easy to peel.

Choose firm, heavy tangelos, with a thin, light-orange skin that is less puffy than the tangerine's.

Choose small-to-medium clementines with bright orange skin. They should be heavy for their size.

Storing This Food

Refrigerate tangerines and clementines. Tangerines are very perishable; use them within a day or two. Store tangelos at room temperature for a few days. Refrigerate them for longer storage.

Preparing This Food

Wash the fruit under cold running water. Don't peel it until you are ready to use it; peeling tears cells and activates ascorbic acid oxidase, an enzyme that destroys vitamin C.

Although many people prefer citrus fruits very cold, bringing the tangerines, clementines, and tangelos to room temperature before you serve them liberates the aromatic molecules that make the fruit smell and taste good, intensifying the flavor and aroma.

What Happens When You Cook This Food

* * *

How Other Kinds of Processing Affect This Food

Canning.   Before they are canned, Mandarin oranges are blanched briefly in steam to inactivate ascorbic acid oxidase, an enzyme that would otherwise destroy the fruit's vitamin C. Canned Mandarin oranges contain approximately as much vitamin C as fresh ones.

Medical Uses and/or Benefits

Antiscorbutics.   Like other citrus fruits, tangerines, tangelos, and clementines are useful in preventing or curing the vitamin C–deficiency disease scurvy.

Adverse Effects Associated with This Food

Contact dermatitis.   The oils in the peel of the tangerine, tangelo, or clementine may be irritating to sensitive individuals.

Aphthous ulcers. Eating citrus fruit, including tangerines, tangelos, and clementines, may trigger an attack of apthous ulcers (canker sores) in sensitive people, but eliminating these foods from your diet will neither cure nor prevent an attack.

Food/Drug Interactions

Aspirin and other nonsteroidal anti-inflammatory drugs (NSAIDs: ibuprofen, naproxen, etc.). Taking aspirin or NSAIDs with acidic foods such as grapefruit intensifies the drugs' ability to irritate your stomach and cause gastric bleeding.

Tea

Nutritional Profile

Energy value (calories per serving): *Low*
Protein: *None*
Fat: *None*
Saturated fat: *None*
Cholesterol: *None*
Carbohydrates: *Low*
Fiber: *None*
Sodium: *None*
Major vitamin contribution: *Folate*
Major mineral contribution: *Fluoride, magnesium*

About the Nutrients in This Food

White tea, green tea, black tea, and oolong tea all come from the same plant, *Camellia Sinensis*. What differentiates one tea from another is the way the tea leaves are processed. White tea (which actually brews up slightly pinkish) is made from tea buds and very young leaves which are steamed or "fired" (heated) and then dried. Green teas are brewed from slightly more mature leaves, which are allowed to wither before they are steamed or dried. Oolong teas are made from teas allowed to dry in the air for a longer time than white or green teas (but for less time than black teas) before being steamed or fired. Leaves meant for black teas are rolled and broken up to allow full drying before they are processed. During fermentation polyphenoloxidase, an enzyme in the leaves, hastens the oxidation of phenols in the leaves, creating brown pigments that darken the leaves and intensify their flavor.* (*Souchong, pekoe,* and *orange pekoe* are terms used to describe grades of black-tea leaves. Souchong leaves are round; orange pekoe leaves are thin and wiry; pekoe leaves are shorter and rounder than orange pekoe.)

The tea plant is a good source of the B vitamin folate, and it is high in fluorides. It is not uncommon to find a tea plant with a fluoride concentration of 100 ppm (parts per million). By comparison, fluoridated water is

---

* Polyphenoloxidase is the enzyme that turns fruits and vegetables brown when you slice or peel them. (See, for example, APPLES OR POTATOES.)

generally 1 ppm fluoride. The USDA estimates that a six-ounce cup of tea prepared with tap water may provide 663 mcg fluoride.

Like coffee and chocolate, tea contains the methylxanthine stimulants, caffeine, theophylline, and theobromine. (Coffee has more caffeine; tea has more theophylline; and chocolate has more theobromine.) The amount of caffeine in the tea depends on how it's made: Tea brewed from loose leaves almost always has more caffeine than tea made from tea bags or instant tea.

Caffeine and Fluoride Content of Brewed Teas

Tea	Caffeine (mg/8-oz. cup)	Fluoride (mg/8-oz. cup)
White	15	(na)
Green	20	0.3–0.4
Black	40	0.2–0.5
Oolong	30	0.1–0.2
Decaffeinated	2	(na)
Coffee (5-oz. cup)	40–170*	(na)

* Depends on brewing method

Sources: Stash Tea Company. "Caffeine Information on Tea." Available online. URL: www.stashtea.com/caffeine.htm. Linus Pauling Institute, Oregon State University. "Bioactive Compounds in Tea." Available online. URL: http://lpi.oregonstate.edu/infocenter/phytochemicals/tea/#components.

Tea leaves are also rich in flavonoids, naturally occurring chemical compounds credited with tea's ability to lower cholesterol, reduce the risk of some kinds of cancer, and protect the teeth from cavity-causing bacteria. Fresh tea leaves are rich in flavonoids called catechins, but processing the leaves to make black and green teas releases enzymes that enable individual catechins to join with others, forming new flavor and coloring agents called polyphenols (*poly* means *many*) that give flavor and color to black and green teas. The length of time tea leaves are left to dry before processing affects the rate at which their catechins are converted to polyphenols. For example, white teas have fewer polyphenols than green teas, which have fewer than oolong, which has fewer than black teas. As a result, nutrition researchers at the Linus Pauling Institute at Oregon State University report that the catechin content of white tea is three times that of green tea, with black tea a distant third. (See below, *Medical uses and/or benefits*.)

Finally, tea leaves also contain antinutrient enzymes that can split the thiamin (vitamin B_1) molecule so that it is no longer nutritionally useful. This is not generally considered a problem for healthy people who eat a balanced diet and consume normal amounts of tea, but it might trigger a thiamin deficiency if you drink a lot of tea and your diet is marginal in thiamin. The tannins in tea are also potential antinutrients that bind calcium and iron into insoluble compounds your body cannot absorb. According to the National Research Council of the National Academy of Sciences, an "inordinate" consumption of tea might substantially reduce the absorption of iron from foods. Tannins also interfere with the absorption of thiamin (vitamin B_1) and vitamin B_{12}. Finally, tea contains oxalates that can bind calcium and might contribute to the formation of calcium-oxalate kidney stones in people predisposed to form stones.

Catechin Content of Various Teas

Tea/8-oz. serving	Catechins
White tea	20.7 (estimate)*
Green tea	6.9 mg
Oolong	(na)
Black tea	3.5 mg

*Based on the theory that white tea has three times as much as green tea.

Sources: www.stashtea.com/caffeine.htm

The Most Nutritious Way to Serve This Food

With milk. Milk protein (casein) binds and inactivates tannins.

Diets That May Restrict or Exclude This Food

Bland diet
Low-oxalate diet (for people who form calcium-oxalate kidney stones)

Buying This Food

Look for: Tightly sealed packages. Tea loses flavor and freshness when it is exposed to air, moisture, or light.

Storing This Food

Store tea in a cool, dark cabinet in an air- and moistureproof container, preferably a glass jar.

Preparing This Food

When brewing tea, always start with an absolutely clean glass, china, or enamel pot and, if possible, soft, mineral-free water. The tannins in tea leaves react with metals and minerals to create the compounds that make up the film sometimes seen floating on top of a cup of tea.

What Happens When You Cook This Food

When tea leaves are immersed in water they begin to release flavoring agents plus bitter tannins, the astringent chemicals that coagulate proteins on the surface of the mucous membranes lining the mouth, making the tissues pucker. The best tea is brewed at the boiling point of water, a temperature that allows the tea leaves to release flavoring agents quickly without overloading the tea with bitter tannins. If the brewing water is below the boiling point, the leaves will release their flavoring agents so slowly that by the time enough flavor molecules have been released into the brew, the ratio of bitter tannins will be so high that the tea tastes bitter. Brewing tea in water that is too hot also makes a bitter drink. At temperatures above boiling, the tannins are released so fast that they turn tea bitter in a minute or two.

You cannot judge the flavor of brewed tea by its color. Brewed black teas turn reddish brown, brewed green teas are almost colorless, and brewed white teas may be pinkish, but they all have distinctive flavors.

How Other Kinds of Processing Affect This Food

Iced tea. Hot water can dissolve more pigments from tea leaves than cold water. When tea brewed in hot water is chilled, as for iced tea, the "extra" pigments will precipitate out and the tea will look cloudy.

Medical Uses and/or Benefits

As a stimulant and mood elevator. Caffeine is a stimulant. It increases alertness and concentration, intensifies muscle responses, quickens heartbeat, and elevates mood. Its effects derive from the fact that its molecular structure is similar to that of adenosine, a natural chemical by-product of normal cell activity. Adenosine is a regular chemical that keeps nerve cell activity within safe limits. When caffeine molecules hook up to sites in the brain where adenosine molecules normally dock, nerve cells continue to fire indiscriminately, producing the jangly feeling sometimes associated with drinking excess amounts of tea, coffee, and other caffeine products.

As a rule, it takes five to six hours to metabolize and excrete caffeine from the body. During that time, its effects may vary widely from person to person. Some find its stimulation pleasant, even relaxing; others experience restlessness, nervousness, hyperactivity, insomnia, flushing, and upset stomach after as little as one cup a day. It is possible to develop a tolerance for caffeine, so people who drink tea every day are likely to find it less immediately stimulating than those who drink it only once in a while.

NOTE: Theophylline, the primary stimulant in tea, relaxes the smooth muscles lining the bronchi (the small passages that carry air into the lungs). As a drug, theophylline is effective in relieving asthmatic spasms, but the relatively low concentrations in brewed tea are too small to produce therapeutic results.

Lower risk of some kinds of cancer. In 1991, a number of scientific teams at the Fourth Chemical Congress of North America announced the identification of chemicals in teas that show positive results in laboratory studies in which laboratory animals given green and black tea have lower rates of skin tumors, esophageal tumors, gastrointestinal tract tumors, and tumors of the lung, liver and pancreas. Eight years later, in January 1999, Purdue University researchers released a study showing that EGCg, a compound in green tea, inhibits an enzyme required for cancer cell growth, killing cancer cells in laboratory dishes without harming healthy cells. The Purdue findings suggest that drinking four cups of green tea a day may produce a lower overall risk of cancer. NOTE: People who drink tea when it is very hot (131°F to 153°F) have a higher risk of esophageal cancer than do people who drink tea at a temperature of 95°F to 117°F. The higher rate of cancer is almost certainly due to the tissues being injured repeatedly by the extremely hot liquid.

Lower risk of cardiovascular disease (heart attack and stroke). Numerous studies have suggested that consuming moderate amounts of tea (five cups per day) reduces both overall mortality (death from all causes) and the risk of death from cardiovascular disease. There are several possible explanations for this finding. For example, in 2008, a report from INSERM, France's national institute for medical research, found that women who drank three or more cups of tea a day were 11 percent less likely than non–tea drinkers to have cholesterol plaques (deposits) inside their arteries. In addition, drinking tea appears to increase the ability of blood vessels to expand, an important factor in protecting against blood clots that may block the vessel, leading to a heart attack or stroke. In a clinical trial, one group of patients with coronary artery disease and mildly elevated cholesterol levels were each given four to six cups of black tea a day for at least four weeks, while a second group got either a beverage with the equivalent amount of caffeine or plain hot water. The blood vessels of patients who drank tea daily dilated more effectively. Some researchers attribute this effect to the catechins in tea.

Many researchers do not consider these results conclusive either because many studies showing lower mortality were too small or because tea consumption in the general population was too low to allow reliable comparisons between tea drinkers and non–tea drinkers. As a result, while both black and green teas (and presumably white teas) appear to be protective, further research is needed to provide firm conclusions about tea and heart health.

Lower risk of some forms of cancer. Animal studies suggest that both green and black teas may reduce the risk of cancers of the skin, lung, mouth, esophagus, stomach, colon, pancreas, bladder, and prostate, while white tea and green tea reduce the incidence of intestinal polyps. Again, the effects are attributed to the flavonoids (catechins) in the teas. However, human studies have produced inconsistent results. For example, while some studies show a decreased risk of colon cancer among tea drinkers, others do not. In general, the assumption is that further evidence is required before linking tea consumption and cancer prevention.

Lower risk of dental cavities.   By observation, there appears to be a link between tea drinking and a lower risk of dental decay. In addition, one study of more than 6,000 14-year old children in the United Kingdom found that those who drank tea had significantly fewer dental caries than non–tea drinkers, regardless of whether they drank their tea plain or with sugar or milk and sugar. This result may be attributable to the natural presence of fluorides in tea leaves.

Methylxanthine (theophylline and caffeine) effects.   All methylxanthines are central-nervous-system stimulants, vasoactive compounds that dilate the skeletal blood vessels and constrict blood vessels in the brain. Theophylline, which effectively relaxes the smooth muscles in the bronchi—the small passages that carry air into the lungs—is used as an asthma medication, but the relatively low concentrations of theophylline in brewed tea are too small to produce therapeutic effects.

Adverse Effects Associated with This Food

Stimulation of the central nervous system.   Taken in excessive amounts, caffeine and theophylline may cause rapid heartbeat, restlessness, sleeplessness, and/or depression in sensitive individuals. Since different people can tolerate different amounts of caffeine and theophylline without suffering ill effects, exactly which dose produces problems varies from person to person.

Constipation.   The tannins in tea may be constipating.

Increased severity of premenstrual syndrome (PMS).   Beta-estradiol and progesterone, two hormones that rise and fall during the monthly menstrual cycle, directly affect brain levels of adenosine (see above). Beta-estradiol (an estrogen), which rises just before ovulation, keeps adenosine from slowing down nerve cell activity, which may be why many women feel pleasantly energized at mid-cycle. Progesterone encourages adenosine; it's a soothing hormone. That may be why many women feel tense and irritable when progesterone levels fall just before menstrual bleeding begins. Because caffeine alters adenosine activity in the brain, drinking tea may make beta-estradiol's "highs" higher and progesterone's "lows" lower. Because tea contains less caffeine than coffee, its effects would be much weaker.

Food/Drug Interactions

Drugs that make it harder to metabolize caffeine.   Some medical drugs slow the body's metabolism of caffeine, thus increasing its stimulating effect. The list of such drugs includes cimetidine (Tagamet), disulfiram (Antabuse), estrogens, fluoroquinolone antibiotics (e.g., ciprofloxacin, enoxacin, norfloxacin), fluconazole (Diflucan), fluvoxamine (Luvox), mexiletine (Mexitil), riluzole (Rilutek), terbinafine (Lamisil), and verapamil (Calan). If you are taking one of these medicines, check with your doctor regarding your consumption of caffeinated beverages.

Drugs whose adverse effects increase due to consumption of large amounts of caffeine.   This list includes such drugs as clozapine (Clozaril), ephedrine, epinephrine, metaproterenal (Alupent), monoamine oxidase inhibitors, phenylpropanolamine, and theophylline. In addition, suddenly decreasing your caffeine intake may increase blood levels of lithium, a drug used to control mood swings. If you are taking one of these medicines, check with your doctor regarding your consumption of caffeinated beverages.

Allopurinol. Tea and other beverages containing the methylxanthine stimulants (caffeine, theophylline, and theobromine) reduce the effectiveness of the xanthine inhibitor, antigout drug allopurinol.

Antibiotics. Drinking tea increases stomach acidity, which reduces the absorption of the antibiotics ampicillin, erythromycin, griseofulvin, penicillin, and tetracycline.

Anticoagulants. Green tea is high in vitamin K, the blood-clotting vitamin produced naturally by bacteria in our intestines. Using foods rich in vitamin K while you are taking an anticoagulant (warfarin, Coumadin, Panwarfin) may reduce the effectiveness of the anticoagulant, so larger doses are required.

Antiulcer medication. Drinking tea makes the stomach more acid and may reduce the effectiveness of normal doses of cimetidine and other antiulcer medication.

Iron supplements. Caffeine and tannic acid bind with iron to form insoluble compounds your body cannot absorb. Ideally, iron supplements and tea should be taken at least two hours apart.

Monoamine oxidase (MAO) inhibitors. Monoamine oxidase inhibitors are drugs used to treat depression. They inactivate naturally occurring enzymes in your body that metabolize tyramine, a substance found in many fermented or aged foods. Tyramine constricts blood vessels and increases blood pressure. Caffeine has some similarity to tyramine; if you consume excessive amounts of a caffeinated beverage such as tea while you are taking an MAO inhibitor, the result may be a hypertensive crisis.

Nonprescription drugs containing caffeine. The caffeine in brewed tea may add to the stimulant effects of the caffeine in some cold remedies, diuretics, pain relievers, stimulants, and weight-control products. Some over-the-counter cold pills contain 30 mg caffeine, some pain relievers 130 mg, and some weight-control products as much as 280 mg caffeine. There are 21 to 47 mg caffeine in a five-ounce cup of brewed tea.

Sedatives. The caffeine in tea may counteract the drowsiness caused by sedative drugs.

Theophylline. The theophylline and caffeine in brewed tea may intensify the effects and/or increase the risk of side effects from this antiasthmatic drug.

Tomatoes

Nutritional Profile

Energy value (calories per serving): *Low*
Protein: *Moderate*
Fat: *Low*
Saturated fat: *Low*
Cholesterol: *None*
Carbohydrates: *High*
Fiber: *High*
Sodium: *Low*
Major vitamin contribution: *Vitamin A, vitamin C*
Major mineral contribution: *Potassium*

About the Nutrients in This Food

Tomatoes are high in dietary fiber, insoluble cellulose and lignin in the skin and seeds. They have vitamin A, but not as much as you might think because red tomatoes get their color from lycopene, a carotenoid with very little vitamin A activity. Tomatoes are high in the B vitamin folate and an excellent source of vitamin C, found primarily in the jellylike substance around the seeds.

One medium ripe red tomato, 2.5 inches in diameter, has 1.5 g dietary fiber, 1,025 IU vitamin A (44 percent of the RDA for a woman, 35 percent of the RDA for a man), 18 mcg folate (5 percent of the RDA), 15.6 mg vitamin C (21 percent of the RDA for a woman, 17 percent of the RDA for a man), and 292 mg potassium, slightly more than half the potassium in

Average Vitamin C Content in One Medium Fresh Tomato

Tomato variety	Vitamin C (mg)
Green	28.8
Orange	17.8
Red	15.6
Yellow	19.1

Source: USDA Nutrient Data Laboratory. National Nutrient Database for Standard Reference. Available online. URL: http://nal.usda.gov/fnic/foodcomp/search/.

one 8-ounce cup of orange juice. NOTE: The amount of vitamin C in any one tomato depends on the variety and when the tomato is harvested. Those harvested from June through October in the northern hemisphere generally have more vitamin C per tomato than those harvested at other times during the year.

Tomatoes are members of the nightshade family, Solanacea. Other members of this family are eggplant, peppers, potatoes, and some mushrooms. These plants produce natural neurotoxins (nerve poisons) called glycoalkaloids. The glycoalkaloid in tomatoes is alpha-tomatine, found in the green parts of the plant. Ripe tomatoes have practically no alphatomatine, and it is estimated that an adult would have to eat 150 small green tomatoes to get a potentially lethal dose. But less than two ounces of tomato leaves is considered deadly for an adult.

The Most Nutritious Way to Serve This Food

Fresh and ripe.

With the seeds (for the most vitamin C). Cooked, with a bit of oil (for the most lycopene, see below *Medical uses and/or benefits*).

Diets That May Restrict or Exclude This Food

Low-fiber diet

Buying This Food

Look for: Smooth round or oval tomatoes. The tomatoes should feel heavy for their size; their flesh should be firm, not watery. If you plan to use the tomatoes right away, pick ripe ones whose skin is a deep orange red. If you plan to store the tomatoes for a few days, pick tomatoes whose skin is still slightly yellow.

Choose pear-shaped Italian plum tomatoes for sauce making. They have less water than ordinary tomatoes and more sugar.

Avoid: Bruised tomatoes or tomatoes with mold around the stem end. The damaged tomatoes may be rotten inside; the moldy ones may be contaminated with mycotoxins, poisons produced by molds.

Storing This Food

Store unripe tomatoes at room temperature until they turn fully orange red. Tomatoes picked before they have ripened on the vine will be at their most nutritious if you let them continue to ripen at a temperature between 60° and 75°F. Keep them out of direct sunlight, which can soften the tomato without ripening it and destroy vitamins A and C. At room temperature, yellow to light pink tomatoes should ripen in three to five days.

Refrigerate ripe tomatoes to inactivate enzymes that continue to soften the fruit by dissolving pectins in its cell walls. Fully ripe tomatoes should be used within two or three days.

Preparing This Food

Remove and discard all leaves and stalks. Wash the tomatoes under cool running water, then slice and serve. Or peel the tomatoes by plunging them into boiling water, then transferring them on a slotted spoon into a bowl of cold water. The change in temperature damages a layer of cells just under the skin so that the skin slips off easily.

To get rid of the seeds, cut the tomato in half across the middle and squeeze the halves gently, cut side down, over a bowl. The seeds should pop out easily.

What Happens When You Cook This Food

When a tomato is heated the soluble pectins in its cell walls dissolve and the flesh of the tomato turns mushy. But the seeds and peel, which are stiffened with insoluble cellulose and lignin, stay hard. This is useful if you are baking or broiling a tomato (the peel will act as a natural "cup") but not if you are making a soup or stew. If you add an unpeeled tomato to the dish the peel will split, separate from the tomato flesh, and curl up into hard little balls or strips.

Vitamin C is sensitive to heat. A cooked tomato has less vitamin C than a fresh one, but it has the same amount of vitamin A because carotenoid pigments are impervious to the heat of normal cooking.

How Other Kinds of Processing Affect This Food

Artificial ripening.   Tomatoes are available all year round. In the summer, when they can be picked close to the market and have less distance to travel, they are picked vine-ripened. In the winter, when they have to travel farther, they are picked while the skin is still a bit green so they will not spoil on the way to market. On the vine, in shipping, or in your kitchen, tomatoes produce ethylene, a natural ripening agent that triggers the change from green to red skin. In winter, if the tomatoes are still green when they reach the market, they are sprayed with ethylene—which turns them red. These tomatoes are called hard-ripened (as opposed to vine-ripened). You cannot soften hard-ripened tomatoes by storing them at room temperature. They should be refrigerated to keep them from rotting.

Juice.   Since 2000, following several deaths attributed to unpasteurized apple juice contaminated with *E. coli* O157:H7, the FDA has required that all juices sold in the United States be pasteurized to inactivate harmful organisms such as bacteria and mold.

Canning.   Most canned tomatoes are salted. Unless otherwise labeled, they should be considered high-sodium foods. NOTE: The *botulinum* organism whose toxin causes botulism thrives in an airless, nonacid environment like the inside of a vegetable can. Because tomatoes are an acid food, many people assume that canned tomatoes will not support the growth of the *botulinum* organism, but there have been reports of canned tomatoes contaminated with *botulinum* toxins. Tomatoes should therefore be treated like any other canned food. Cook them thoroughly before you use them. Throw out any unopened can that is bulging. And discard—*without tasting*—any canned tomatoes that look or smell suspicious.

Aseptic packaging. Tomatoes packed in aseptic boxes may taste fresher than canned tomatoes because they are cooked for a shorter time before processing.

Sun-drying. Sun-dried tomatoes will keep for several months in the refrigerator. If they are not packed in oil, they have to be "plumped" before you can use them. Plunge them in boiling water for a few minutes, then drain, soak, chop, and use within a day or so. Or cover them with olive oil and store them in the refrigerator.

Medical Uses and/or Benefits

Possible protection against some forms of cancer. Tomatoes contain the red carotenoid (pigment) lycopene, a strong antioxidant that may reduce the risk of some forms of cancer. Cooking the tomatoes and consuming tomato products with dietary fats such as olive oil makes the lycopene easier for the body to absorb. In November 2005, the FDA ruled that tomato and tomato-sauce products (including catsup) may carry labels with health claims regarding their ability to reduce the risk of prostate, gastric, ovarian, and pancreatic cancers, but that these claims must be described as "unlikely," "highly uncertain," and "highly unlikely." There is no evidence that pure lycopene, as in supplements, produces the effects of lycopene in tomato products.

Pale tomatoes, yellow tomatoes, green tomatoes, and tomatoes ripened after picking have less lycopene than deep-red tomatoes ripened on the vine.

Lower risk of stroke. Various nutrition studies have attested to the power of adequate potassium to keep blood pressure within safe levels. For example, in the 1990s, data from the long-running Harvard School of Public Health/Health Professionals Follow-Up Study of male doctors showed that a diet rich in high-potassium foods such as bananas, oranges, and plantain may reduce the risk of stroke. In the study, the men who ate the higher number of potassium-rich foods (an average of nine servings a day) had a risk of stroke 38 percent lower than that of men who consumed fewer than four servings a day. In 2008, a similar survey at the Queen's Medical Center (Honolulu) showed a similar protective effect among men and women using diuretic drugs (medicines that increase urination and thus the loss of potassium).

As an antiscorbutic. Fresh tomatoes, which are rich in vitamin C, help protect against scurvy, the vitamin C–deficiency disease.

Adverse Effects Associated with This Food

Orange skin. Lycopene, the red carotenoid pigment in tomatoes, can be stored in the fatty layer under your skin. If you eat excessive amounts of tomatoes (or tomatoes and carrots), the carotenoids may turn your palms, the soles of your feet, and even some of your other skin yellow orange. The color change is harmless and will disappear as soon as you cut back your consumption of these vegetables.

Latex-fruit syndrome.   Latex is a milky fluid obtained from the rubber tree and used to make medical and surgical products such as condoms and protective latex gloves, as well as rubber bands, balloons, and toys; elastic used in clothing; pacifiers and baby-bottle nipples; chewing gum; and various adhesives. Some of the proteins in latex are allergenic, known to cause reactions ranging from mild to potentially life-threatening. Some of the proteins found naturally in latex also occur naturally in foods from plants such as avocados, bananas, chestnuts, kiwi fruit, tomatoes, and food and diet sodas sweetened with aspartame. Persons sensitive to these foods are likely to be sensitive to latex as well. NOTE: The National Institute of Health Sciences, in Japan, also lists the following foods as suspect: Almonds, apples, apricots, bamboo shoots, bell peppers, buckwheat, cantaloupe, carrots, celery, cherries, chestnuts, coconut, figs, grapefruit, lettuce, loquat, mangoes, mushrooms, mustard, nectarines, oranges, passion fruit, papaya, peaches, peanuts, peppermint, pineapples, potatoes, soybeans, strawberries, walnuts, and watermelon.

Food/Drug Interactions

False-positive test for carcenoid tumors.   Carcenoid tumors, which may arise in tissues of the endocrine or gastrointestinal system, secrete serotonin, a natural chemical that makes blood vessels expand or contract. Because serotonin is excreted in urine, these tumors are diagnosed by measuring the levels of serotonin by products in the urine. Tomatoes contain large amounts of serotonin; eating them in the three days before a test for an endocrine tumor might produce a false-positive result, suggesting that you have the tumor when in fact you do not. (Other foods high in serotonin are avocados, bananas, eggplant, pineapple, plums, and walnuts.)

Turnips

(Rutabaga)

See also Greens.

Nutritional Profile

Energy value (calories per serving): *Low*
Protein: *Moderate*
Fat: *Low*
Saturated fat: *Low*
Cholesterol: *None*
Carbohydrates: *High*
Fiber: *High*
Sodium: *Moderate*
Major vitamin contribution: *Vitamin A, vitamin C*
Major mineral contribution: *Calcium*

About the Nutrients in This Food

White turnips and rutabagas (which are members of the same plant family) are taproots of plants belonging to the cabbage family (cruciferous vegetables). The white turnip is a creamy globe, tinged with rose at the top and capped with greens that may be used on their own as a rich source of calcium (see GREENS). The rutabaga is a large globe with bumpy tan skin and a yellow interior. The outside of the rutabaga is usually waxed to keep the vegetable from drying out on the way to market.

Both turnips and rutabagas are moderately good sources of fiber, pectin, and sugars. They have no starch, some protein, a trace of fat, and no cholesterol.

One-half cup mashed boiled turnips has two grams dietary fiber and 13 mg vitamin C (17 percent of the RDA for a woman, 14 percent of the RDA for a man). One-half cup mashed boiled rutabaga has 2.2 g dietary fiber and 22.6 mg vitamin C (30 percent of the RDA for a woman, 25 percent of the RDA for a man).

The Most Nutritious Way to Serve This Food

White turnips. Raw or steamed, to preserve the vitamin C. The peeled raw turnip may be grated into a salad or eaten like an apple.

Rutabagas. Steamed as quickly as possible, to protect the vitamin C.

398

Diets That May Restrict or Exclude This Food

Low-fiber diet
Low-sodium diet (white turnips)

Buying This Food

Look for: Firm, smooth, medium-sized white turnips with fresh green leaves on top. Choose smoothly waxed, medium-sized rutabagas with smooth, unscarred skin.

Avoid: White turnips with wilted greens or rutabagas with mold on the surface.

Storing This Food

Pull all the leaves off a white turnip, wash them, and store them separately in a plastic bag. (For information about preparing turnip greens, see GREENS.) Refrigerate the turnips in the vegetable crisper. Waxed rutabagas may be stored in a cool, dark cabinet.

Preparing This Food

White turnips. Wash the turnips under cool running water and peel to just under the line that separates the peel from the flesh.

Rutabagas. Cut the vegetables into quarters (or smaller pieces if necessary) and then cut away the waxed rind.

What Happens When You Cook This Food

When turnips and rutabagas are cooked, the pectins in their cells walls dissolve and the vegetable softens.

Like other cruciferous vegetables, turnips and rutabagas contain mustard oils bound to sugar molecules. These compounds are activated when you cook a turnip or rutabaga or cut into it, damaging its cell walls and releasing enzymes that separate the sugar and oil compounds into their smelly components (which include hydrogen sulfide, the chemical that makes rotten eggs smell rotten). Compared to the mustard oils in cabbage, brussels sprouts, and broccoli, the ones in turnips and rutabagas are very mild. They produce only a faint odor when these vegetables are cut or cooked, but the longer you cook a turnip or rutabaga, the more smelly chemicals you will produce and the stronger the taste and odor will be.

Cooking white turnips in an aluminum or iron pot will darken the turnips or discolor the pot. The turnips contain pale anthoxanthin pigments that interact with metal ions escaping from the surface of the pot to form brown or yellow compounds. Rutabagas, which get their color from carotenes that are impervious to the heat of normal cooking, stay bright yellow in any pot.

How Other Kinds of Processing Affect This Food

Freezing. Crisp fruit and vegetables like apples, carrots, potatoes, turnips, and rutabagas snap when you break or bite into them because their cells are so full of moisture that they pop when the cell walls are broken. When these vegetables are cooked and frozen, the water inside their cells turns into ice crystals that tear cell membranes so that the moisture inside leaks out when the vegetable is defrosted and the cells collapse inward, which is the reason defrosted turnips and rutabagas, like defrosted carrots and potatoes, have a mushy texture.

Medical Uses and/or Benefits

Lower risk of cancer. Naturally occurring chemicals (indoles, isothiocyanates, glucosinolates, dithiolethiones, and phenols) in cabbage, Brussels sprouts, broccoli, cauliflower, and other cruciferous vegetables appear to reduce the risk of some cancers, perhaps by preventing the formation of carcinogens in your body or by blocking cancer-causing substances from reaching or reacting with sensitive body tissues or by inhibiting the transformation of healthy cells to malignant ones.

All cruciferous vegetables contain sulforaphane, a member of a family of chemicals known as isothiocyanates. In experiments with laboratory rats, sulforaphane appears to increase the body's production of phase-2 enzymes, naturally occurring substances that inactivate and help eliminate carcinogens. At the Johns Hopkins University in Baltimore, Maryland, 69 percent of the rats injected with a chemical known to cause mammary cancer developed tumors vs. only 26 percent of the rats given the carcinogenic chemical plus sulforaphane.

In 1997, Johns Hopkins researchers discovered that broccoli seeds and three-day-old broccoli sprouts contain a compound converted to sulforaphane when the seed and sprout cells are crushed. Five grams of three-day-old broccoli sprouts contain as much sulforaphane as 150 grams of mature broccoli. The sulforaphane levels in other cruciferous vegetables have not yet been calculated.

Adverse Effects Associated with This Food

Enlarged thyroid gland (goiter). Cruciferous vegetables, including turnips, contain goitrogens, chemicals that inhibit the formation of thyroid hormones and cause the thyroid to enlarge in an attempt to produce more. Goitrogens are not hazardous for healthy people who eat moderate amounts of cruciferous vegetables, but they may pose problems for people who have thyroid disorder. The goitrogens in turnips are progoitrin and gluconasturtin.

Food/Drug Interactions

False-positive test for occult blood in the stool.   The active ingredient in the guaiac slide test for hidden blood in feces is alphaguaiaconic acid, a chemical that turns blue in the presence of blood. Alphaguaiaconic acid also turns blue in the presence of peroxidase, a chemical that occurs naturally in turnips. Eating turnips in the 72 hours before taking the guaiac test may produce a false-positive result in people who do not actually have any blood in their stool.

Variety Meats

(Brain, heart, sweetbreads, tripe, kidney, tongue)

See also Beef, Liver, Pork, Veal.

Nutritional Profile

Energy value (calories per serving): *Moderate*
Protein: *High*
Fat: *Moderate (muscle meats)*
    High (organ meats)
Saturated fat: *High*
Cholesterol: *High*
Carbohydrates: *None*
Fiber: *None*
Sodium: *Low to high*
Major vitamin contribution: *Vitamin A (kidneys), B vitamins*
Major mineral contribution: *Iron, copper*

About the Nutrients in This Food

Heart, tongue, and tripe (the muscular lining of the cow's stomach) are muscle meats. Brains, kidneys, and sweetbreads (the thymus gland) are organ meats. Like other foods of animal origin, both kinds of meats are rich sources of proteins considered "complete" because they have sufficient amounts of all the essential amino acids.

Organ meats have more fat than muscle meats. Their fat composition varies according to the animal from which they come. Ounce for ounce, beef fat has proportionally more saturated fatty acids than pork fat, slightly less cholesterol than chicken fat, and appreciably less than lamb fat.

Like fish, poultry, milk, and eggs, and other meat, variety meats are an excellent source of high-quality protein, with sufficient amounts of all the essential amino acids. They are an excellent source of B vitamins, including vitamin B_{12}, a nutrient found only in animal foods. Kidneys are high in natural vitamin A (retinol), the form of vitamin A also found in liver. All variety meats are high in heme iron, the form of iron most easily absorbed by your body.

Fat and Cholesterol Content of Beef Variety Meats (100-g/3.5-oz. serving)

Meat	Total Fat (g)	Saturated Fat (g)	Cholesterol (g)
Heart	4.7	1.4	212
Kidneys	4.7	1.1	716
Sweetbread (thymus gland)	25	8.6	294
Tongue	22	8.1	132
Tripe	4.1	1.4	157

Source: USDA Nutrient Data Laboratory. National Nutrient Database for Standard Reference. Available online. URL: http://nal.usda.gov/fnic/foodcomp/search/.

The Most Nutritious Way to Serve This Food

With a food rich in vitamin C. Vitamin C changes ferrous iron in foods into the more easily absorbed ferric iron.

Diets That May Restrict or Exclude This Food

Low-cholesterol, controlled-fat diet
Low-protein diet
Low-sodium diet

Buying This Food

Look for: Refrigerated meat that feels cold to the touch and looks and smells absolutely fresh. Frozen heart or tripe should be solid, with no give to the package and no drippings staining the outside.

Choose some variety meats by size. The smaller the tongue, for example, the more tender it will be. The most tender kidneys come from young animals. On the other hand, all brains and sweetbreads are by nature tender, while all heart, tongue, and tripe (the most solidly muscular of the variety meats) require long simmering to make them tender.

Storing This Food

Refrigerate variety meats immediately. All are highly perishable and should be used within 24 hours of purchase. Refrigeration prolongs the freshness of meat by slowing the natural multiplication of bacteria on the surface. Unchecked, these bacteria will digest the proteins on the surface of the meat, leaving a slimy film in their wake, and convert the meat's sulfur-containing amino acids (tryptophan, methionine, and cystine) into smelly chemicals called mercaptans. The combination of mercaptans with myoglobin, a pigment in blood that transfers oxygen hemoglobin to muscle tissues, creates the greenish pigment that makes rotten meat look so unpleasant.

Wrap fresh meat carefully before storing to keep the drippings from spilling and contaminating other food or the refrigerator/freezer shelves.

Preparing This Food

Brains. First wash the brains under cold running water and pull off the membranes. Then put the brains in a bowl of cold water and let them soak for a half hour. Change the water; let them soak for another half hour. Repeat the process one more time, for a total soaking time of an hour and a half. Now drain the water, put the brains in a saucepan, cover with water, add a tablespoon or two of acid (lemon juice or vinegar) to firm the brains, and cook them for 20 to 25 minutes over low heat without boiling. Drain and use as your recipe directs.

Kidneys. Pull off the white membrane and rinse the kidneys thoroughly under plenty of cold running water. Cut them in half, remove the inner core, and rinse once again. Slice them and use as your recipe directs. (Beef kidneys have a strong, distinctive flavor that can be toned down by soaking the kidneys for an hour in a solution of 1 teaspoon lemon juice to 1 cup of water before cooking.)

Heart. Cut out the blood vessels, rinse the heart thoroughly (inside and out) under cold running water, and prepare as your recipe directs.

Sweetbreads. Rinse the sweetbreads thoroughly under cold running water and soak in ice water for at least an hour, changing the water until it remains clear and free of blood. Then drain the sweetbreads and blanch them in water plus two teaspoons of acid (lemon juice or vinegar) to firm them. Drain the sweetbreads, cover them with ice water, and remove membranes and connective tissue. Then use as your recipe directs.

Tongue. Scrub the tongue with a vegetable brush under cold running water. Cover it with cold water, bring the water to a boil, and cook the tongue at a simmer for 30 minutes or soak and cook as directed on the package. Drain the tongue, peel off the skin, cut away the gristle and small bones, and prepare as your recipe directs. Some smoked tongues require long soaking, even overnight; check the directions on the package.

Tripe. Virtually all the tripe sold in markets today has been blanched and boiled until tender. All you have to do is wash it thoroughly under cold running water and use it as directed in your recipe. If you have to start from scratch with tripe, wash it in several changes of cold water, boil it for several hours until tender, then use as your recipe directs.

When you are done, clean all utensils thoroughly with soap and hot water. Wash your cutting board, wood or plastic, with hot water, soap, and a bleach-and-water solution. For ultimate safety in preventing the transfer of microorganisms from the meats to other foods, keep one cutting board exclusively for raw meat, fish, or poultry, and a second one for everything else. Don't forget to wash your hands.

What Happens When You Cook This Food

Heat changes the structure of proteins. It denatures protein molecules—they break apart into smaller fragments, change shape, or clump together. All these changes force moisture out of protein tissues. The longer you cook variety meats, the more moisture they will lose. The meat's pigments, also denatured by the heat, combine with oxygen and turn brown—the natural color of cooked meat.

As the meat cooks, its fats oxidize. Oxidized fats, whether formed in cooking or when the cooked meat is stored in the refrigerator, give cooked meat a characteristic warmed-over flavor the next day. Stewing and storing heart or kidneys under a blanket of antioxidants—catsup or a gravy made of tomatoes, peppers and other vitamin C–rich vegetables—reduces the oxidation of fats and the intensity of warmed-over flavor.

All variety meats must be cooked thoroughly.

How Other Kinds of Processing Affect This Food

Freezing. When meat is frozen, the water inside its cells freezes into sharp ice crystals that puncture cell membranes so that water (and B vitamins) leak out of the cells when the meat is thawed. Frozen heart, kidneys, and tripe are drier when thawed than they would have been fresh. They may also be lower in B vitamins. Freezing may also cause freezer burn, dry spots left when moisture evaporates from the surface of the meat. Waxed freezer paper is designed specifically to hold the moisture in frozen meat.

Medical Uses and/or Benefits

As a source of heme iron. Because the body stores excess iron in the heart, kidneys, and other organs, variety meats are an excellent source of heme iron.

Adverse Effects Associated with This Food

Increased risk of cardiovascular disease. Like other foods from animals, variety meats are a significant source of cholesterol and saturated fats, which increase the amount of cholesterol circulating in your blood and raise your risk of heart disease. To reduce the risk of heart disease, the National Cholesterol Education Project recommends following the Step I and Step II diets.

The Step I diet provides no more than 30 percent of total daily calories from fat, no more than 10 percent of total daily calories from saturated fat, and no more than 300 mg of cholesterol per day. It is designed for healthy people whose cholesterol is in the range of 200–239 mg/dL.

The Step II diet provides 25–35 percent of total calories from fat, less than 7 percent of total calories from saturated fat, up to 10 percent of total calories from polyunsaturated fat, up to 20 percent of total calories from monounsaturated fat, and less than 300 mg cholesterol per day. This stricter regimen is designed for people who have one or more of the following conditions:

◆ Existing cardiovascular disease
◆ High levels of low-density lipoproteins (LDLs, or "bad" cholesterol) or low levels of high-density lipoproteins (HDLs, or "good" cholesterol)
◆ Obesity
◆ Type 1 diabetes (insulin-dependent diabetes, or diabetes mellitus)
◆ Metabolic syndrome, a.k.a. insulin resistance syndrome, a cluster of risk factors that includes type 2 diabetes (non-insulin-dependent diabetes)

Production of uric acid. Purines are natural by-products of protein metabolism. Purines break down into uric acid, which form sharp crystals that can cause gout if they collect in your joints or kidney stones if they collect in urine. Sweetbreads and kidneys are a source of purines. Eating them raises the concentration of purines in your body. Although controlling the amount of purine-producing foods in the diet may not significantly affect the course of gout (treated with medication such as allopurinol, which inhibits the formation of uric acid), limiting these foods is still part of many gout treatment regimens.

Decline in kidney function. Proteins are nitrogen compounds. When metabolized by your body, they yield ammonia that is excreted through the kidneys. In laboratory animals, a sustained high-protein diet increases the flow of blood through the kidneys and may accelerate the natural decline in kidney function associated with aging. To date there is no proof that this also occurs in human beings.

Food/Drug Interactions

Tetracycline antibiotics (demeclocycline [Declomycin]), doxycycline [Vibtamycin], methacycline [Rondomycin], minocycline [Minocin], oxytetracycline [Terramycin], tetracycline [Achromycin V, Panmycin, Sumycin]). Because meat contains iron which binds tetracyclines into compounds the body cannot absorb, it is best to avoid meat for two hours before and after taking one of these antibiotics.

Monoamine oxidase (MAO) inhibitors. Monoamine oxidase inhibitors are drugs used to treat depression. They inactivate naturally occurring enzymes in your body that metabolize tyramine, a substance found in many fermented or aged foods. Tyramine constricts blood vessels and increases blood pressure. Pickling or preserving meat may produce tyramine. If you eat a food such as pickled tongue which is high in tyramine while you are taking an MAO inhibitor, your body cannot eliminate the tyramine and the result may be a hypertensive crisis.

Veal

Nutritional Profile*

Energy value (calories per serving): *Moderate*
Protein: *High*
Fat: *Moderate*
Saturated fat: *Low*
Cholesterol: *Moderate*
Carbohydrates: *None*
Fiber: *None*
Sodium: *Moderate*
Major vitamin contribution: *B vitamins*
Major mineral contribution: *Iron, zinc*

About the Nutrients in This Food

Veal is meat from cattle (usually) younger than three months and weighing less than 400 pounds, with proportionally more muscle and less fat than older animals.

Like fish, poultry, milk, eggs, and other meats, veal has high-quality protein with sufficient amounts of all the essential amino acids.

Veal is an excellent source of B vitamins, including niacin, vitamin B_6, and vitamin B_{12}, which is found only in animal foods. Veal is a good source of heme iron, the organic form of iron found in foods of animal origin. Heme iron is approximately five times more available to the body than nonheme iron, the inorganic form of iron found in plant foods.

One four-ounce serving of lean roast veal rib meat has 8.5 g total fat, 2.3 g saturated fat, 30 g protein, and 1.1 mg heme iron (6 percent of the RDA for a woman, 14 percent of the RDA for a man).

The Most Nutritious Way to Serve This Food

With a food rich in vitamin C. Ascorbic acid increases the absorption of iron from meat.

---

* Values are for lean roasted meat.

Diets That May Restrict or Exclude This Food

Controlled-fat, low-cholesterol diet
Low-protein diet (for some forms of kidney disease)

Buying This Food

Look for: The cut of veal that fits your recipe. Thick cuts, such as roasts, need long, slow cooking to gelatinize their connective tissue and keep the veal from drying out. A breast with bones, however, has more fat than a solid roast. Veal scallops and cutlets are the only kinds of veal that can be sauteed or broiled quickly.

Storing This Food

Refrigerate raw veal immediately, carefully wrapped to prevent its drippings from contaminating the refrigerator shelves or other foods. Refrigeration prolongs the freshness of veal by slowing the natural multiplication of bacteria on the surface of meat. Unchecked, these bacteria will convert proteins and other substances on the surface of the meat to a slimy film. Eventually, they will also convert the meat's sulfur-containing amino acids methionine and cystine into smelly chemicals called mercaptans that interact with myoglobin to create the greenish pigment that gives spoiled meat its characteristic unpleasant appearance.

Fresh veal will keep for three to five days in the refrigerator. As a general rule, large cuts of veal will keep a little longer than small ones. Ground veal, which has many surfaces where bacteria can live and work, should be used within 48 hours.

Preparing This Food

To lighten the color of veal, marinate the meat in lemon juice or milk overnight in the refrigerator. Or marinate it in lemon juice. Trim the meat carefully. By judiciously cutting away all visible fat you can significantly reduce the amount of fat and cholesterol in each serving.

Do not salt the veal before you cook it. The salt dissolves in water on the surface of the meat to form a liquid denser than the moisture inside the veal's cells. As a result the water inside the cells will flow out across the cell toward the denser solution, a phenomenon known as osmosis. The loss of moisture will make the veal less tender and stringy.

When you are done, clean all utensils thoroughly with soap and hot water. Wash your cutting board, wood or plastic, with hot water, soap, and a bleach-and-water solution. For ultimate safety in preventing the transfer of microorganisms from the meat to other foods, keep one cutting board exclusively for meat, fish, or poultry, and a second one for everything else.

What Happens When You Cook This Food

Cooking changes the way veal looks and tastes, alters its nutritional value, makes it safer, and extends its shelf life.

Browning meat before you cook it does not seal in the juices but does change the flavor by caramelizing proteins and sugars on the surface. Since meat has no sugars other than the small amounts of glycogen in its muscles, we usually add sugars in the form of marinades or basting liquids that may also contain acids (vinegar, lemon juice, wine) to break down muscle fibers and tenderize the meat. Browning has one minor nutritional drawback. It breaks amino acids on the surface of the meat into smaller compounds that are no longer useful proteins.

Heat changes the structure of proteins. It denatures the protein molecules, which means they break up into smaller fragments or change shape or clump together. All these changes force water out of protein tissues, which is why meat gets dryer the longer it is cooked. In addition, heat denatures the pigments in meat, which combine with oxygen and turn brown.

As the veal continues to cook, its fats oxidize. Oxidized fats, whether formed in cooking or when the cooked meat is stored in the refrigerator, give cooked the meat a characteristic warmed-over flavor. You can reduce the oxidation of fats and the warmed-over flavor by cooking and storing meat under a blanket of catsup or a gravy made of tomatoes, peppers, and other vitamin C–rich vegetables—all of which are natural antioxidants.

An obvious nutritional benefit of cooking is that it liquifies the fat in the meat so that it can run off. And, of course, cooking makes veal safer by killing *Salmonella* and other organisms.

How Other Kinds of Processing Affect This Food

Freezing. When you thaw frozen veal it may be less tender than fresh veal. It may also be lower in B vitamins. While the veal is frozen, the water inside its cells turn into sharp ice crystals that can puncture cell membranes. When the veal thaws, moisture (and some of the B vitamins) will leak out through these torn cell walls. The loss of moisture is irreversible.

Freezing can also cause freezer burn, the dry spots where moisture has evaporated from the surface of the meat. Waxed freezer paper is designed specifically to hold the moisture in meat.

Freezing slows the oxidation of fats and the multiplication of bacteria so that the veal stays usable longer than it would in a refrigerator. At 0°F fresh veal will keep for four to eight months. (Beef, which has fewer oxygen-sensitive unsaturated fatty acids than veal, will keep for up to a year.)

Medical Uses and/or Benefits

* * *

Adverse Effects Associated with This Food

Increased risk of cardiovascular disease. Like other foods from animals, veal is a source of cholesterol and saturated fats which increase the amount of cholesterol circulating in your blood and raise your risk of heart disease. To reduce the risk of heart disease, the National Cholesterol Education Project recommends following the Step I and Step II diets.

The Step I diet provides no more than 30 percent of total daily calories from fat, no more than 10 percent of total daily calories from saturated fat, and no more than 300 mg of cholesterol per day. It is designed for healthy people whose cholesterol is in the range of 200–239 mg/dL.

The Step II diet provides 25–35 percent of total calories from fat, less than 7 percent of total calories from saturated fat, up to 10 percent of total calories from polyunsaturated fat, up to 20 percent of total calories from monounsaturated fat, and less than 300 mg cholesterol per day. This stricter regimen is designed for people who have one or more of the following conditions:

◆ Existing cardiovascular disease
◆ High levels of low-density lipoproteins (LDLs, or "bad" cholesterol) or low levels of high-density lipoproteins (HDLs, or "good" cholesterol)
◆ Obesity
◆ Type 1 diabetes (insulin-dependent diabetes, or diabetes mellitus)
◆ Metabolic syndrome, a.k.a. insulin resistance syndrome, a cluster of risk factors that includes type 2 diabetes (non-insulin-dependent diabetes)

Antibiotic sensitivity. Cattle in this country are routinely given antibiotics to protect them from infection. By law, the antibiotic treatment must stop three days before the veal is slaughtered. Theoretically, the veal should then be free of antibiotic residues, but some people who are sensitive to penicillin or tetracycline may (rarely) have an allergic reaction to the meat.

Antibiotic-resistant Salmonella and toxoplasmosis. Veal treated with antibiotics may produce meat contaminated with antibiotic-resistant strains of *Salmonella,* and all raw beef may harbor *T. gondii,* the parasite that causes toxoplasmosis. Toxoplasmosis is particularly hazardous for pregnant women. It can be passed on to the fetus and may trigger a series of birth defects, including blindness and mental retardation. Both the drug-resistant *Salmonella* and *T. gondii* can be eliminated by cooking meat thoroughly and washing all utensils, cutting boards, and counters as well as your hands with hot soapy water before touching any other food.

Decline in kidney function. Proteins are nitrogen compounds. When metabolized, they yield ammonia that is excreted through the kidneys. In laboratory animals, a sustained high-protein diet increases the flow of blood through the kidneys and accelerates the natural decline in kidney function that comes with age. Some experts suggest that this may also occur in human beings, but this remains to be proven.

Food/Drug Interactions

Tetracycline antibiotics (demeclocycline [Declomycin]), doxycycline [Vibtamycin], methacycline [Rondomycin], minocycline [Minocin], oxytetracycline [Terramycin], tetracycline [Achromycin V, Panmycin, Sumycin]). Because meat contains iron which binds tetracyclines into compounds the body cannot absorb, it is best to avoid meat for two hours before and after taking one of these antibiotics.

Monoamine oxidase (MAO) inhibitors. Meat "tenderized" with papaya or a papain powder can interact with the class of antidepressant drugs known as monoamine oxidase inhibitors. Papain meat tenderizers work by breaking up the long chains of protein molecules. One by-product of this process is tyramine, a substance that constructs blood vessels and raises blood pressure. MAO inhibitors inactivate naturally occurring enzymes in your body that metabolize tyramine. If you eat a food such as papain-tenderized meat which is high in tyramine while you are taking an MAO inhibitor, you cannot effectively eliminate the tyramine from your body. The result may be a hypertensive crisis.

Vegetable Oils

(Coconut oil, corn oil, cottonseed oil, olive oil, peanut oil, safflower oil, sesame oil, soybean oil)

See also Butter, Nuts, Olives.

Nutritional Profile

Energy value (calories per serving): *High*
Protein: *None*
Fat: *High*
Saturated fat: *Moderate*
Cholesterol: *None*
Carbohydrates: *None*
Fiber: *None*
Sodium: *None*
Major vitamin contribution: *Vitamin E*
Major mineral contribution: *None*

About the Nutrients in This Food

Vegetable oils are low in saturated fat and high in monounsaturated and polyunsaturated fatty acids, including the essential fatty acid linoleic acid. The polyunsaturates are a good source of vitamin E, the collective name for a group of chemicals called tocopherols.[*] The tocopherol with the most vitamin E activity is alpha-tocopherol; the RDA for vitamin E is stated as milligrams of alpha-tocopherol equivalents (mg *a*-TE): 10 mg *a*-TE for a man, 8 mg *a*-TE for a woman.

---

[*] Vitamin E was first identified as a substance vital for reproduction in rats, hence the name *tocopherols* from the Greek words *tokos* (offspring) and *pherein* (to bear).

Fat and Vitamin E Content of Vegetables Oils (grams per tablespoon)*

Oil	Saturated (g)	Monounsaturated (g)	Polyunsaturated (g)	Vitamin E (a-TE) (mg)
Canola oil	1.0	8.2	4.1	2.93
Corn oil	1.8	3.4	8.2	2.94
Olive oil	1.9	10.3	1.2	0.7
Peanut oil	2.4	6.5	4.5	1.82
Safflower oil	1.3	1.7	10.4	5.46
Soybean oil	2.0	3.3	8.1	1.4
Sunflower oil	1.5	2.7	9.2	6.86
Butter	7.1	3.3	3.4	

* all oils have 14 grams total fat per tablespoon; butter has 11 grams total fat tablespoon

Sources: USDA Nutrient Database: www.nal.usda.gov/fnic/cgi-bin/nut_search.pl *Nutritive Value of Foods,* Home and Garden Bulletin No. 72 (USDA, 1989); Briggs, George M. and Doris Howes Callaway, *Nutrition and Physical Fitness,* 11th ed. (New York: Holt, Rinehart and Winston, 1984).

The Most Nutritious Way to Serve This Food

In moderation.

Diets That May Restrict or Exclude This Food

low-fat diet

Buying This Food

Look for: Tightly sealed bottles of vegetable oil, protected from light and heat.

Storing This Food

Store vegetable oils in a cool, dark cabinet to protect them from light, heat, and air. When exposed to air, fatty acids become rancid, which means that they combine with oxygen to form hydroperoxides, natural substances that taste bad, smell bad, and may destroy the vitamin E in the oil. The higher the proportion of polyunsaturated fatty acids in the oil, the more quickly it will turn rancid. Many salad and cooking oils contain antioxidant preservatives (BHT, BHA) to slow this reaction.

Preparing This Food

* * *

What Happens When You Cook This Food

Heat promotes the oxidation of fats, a chemical reaction accelerated by cooking fats in iron pots. Cooked fats are safe at normal temperatures, but when they are used over and over, they may break down into components known as free radicals—which are suspected carcinogens.

Most fats begin to decompose well below 500°F, and they may catch fire spontaneously with no warning without boiling first. The point at which they decompose and burn is called the smoking point. Vegetable shortening will burn at 375°F, vegetable oils at close to 450°F. Safflower, soybean, cotton-seed, and corn oils have higher smoking points than peanut and sesame oils.

How Other Kinds of Processing Affect This Food

Margarine and shortening. Margarine is made of hydrogenated vegetable oils (oils to which hydrogen atoms have been added). Adding hydrogen atoms hardens the oils into a semi-solid material than can be molded into bars or packed in tubs as margarine or shortening. Hydrogenation also changes the structure of some of the polyunsaturated fatty acids in the oils from a form known as "cis fatty acids" to a form known as "trans fatty acids." Questions have been raised as to the safety of trans fatty acids, but there is no proof so far that they are more likely than cis fatty acids to cause atherosclerosis. Margarines may also contain coloring agents (to make the margarine look like butter), emulsifiers, and milk or animal fats (including butter).

Margarine should be refrigerated, closely wrapped to keep it from picking up odors from other foods. It will keep for about two weeks in the refrigerator before its fatty acids oxidize to produce off odors and taste. Shortening can be stored, tightly covered, at room temperature.

Medical Uses and/or Benefits

Lower risk of cardiovascular disease. A diet high in cholesterol and saturated fats increases the amount of cholesterol circulating through your arteries and raises your risk of coronary artery disease (heart attack). To reduce the risk of heart disease, the National Cholesterol Education Project recommends following the Step I and Step II diets.

The Step I diet provides no more than 30 percent of total daily calories from fat, no more than 10 percent of total daily calories from saturated fat, and no more than 300 mg of cholesterol per day. It is designed for healthy people whose cholesterol is in the range of 200–239 mg/dL.

The Step II diet provides 25–35 percent of total calories from fat, less than 7 percent of total calories from saturated fat, up to 10 percent of total calories from polyunsaturated fat, up to 20 percent of total calories from monounsaturated fat, and less than 300 mg cholesterol per day. This stricter regimen is designed for people who have one or more of the following conditions:

◆ Existing cardiovascular disease
◆ High levels of low-density lipoproteins (LDLs, or "bad" cholesterol) or low levels of high-density lipoproteins (HDLs, or "good" cholesterol)
◆ Obesity
◆ Type 1 diabetes (insulin-dependent diabetes, or diabetes mellitus)
◆ Metabolic syndrome, a.k.a. insulin resistance syndrome, a cluster of risk factors that includes type 2 diabetes (non-insulin-dependent diabetes)

Adverse Effects Associated with This Food

* * *

Food/Drug Interactions

* * *

Water

Nutritional Profile

Energy value (calories per serving): *None*
Protein: *None*
Fat: *None*
Saturated fat: *None*
Cholesterol: *None*
Carbohydrates: *None*
Fiber: *None*
Sodium: *Low to high*
Major vitamin contribution: *None*
Major mineral contribution: *Sodium, calcium, magnesium, fluorides*

About the Nutrients in This Food

Water has no nutrients other than the minerals it picks up from the earth or the pipes through which it flows or that are added by a bottler to give the water a specific flavor. *Hard water* contains dissolved calcium and magnesium salts, usually in the form of bicarbonates, sulfates, and chlorides. *Soft* water has very little calcium and magnesium, but it may still contain sodium. Some bottled mineral waters may contain as much as 200 to 400 mg sodium in an eight-ounce glass.

The only absolutely pure water is *distilled water,* which has been vaporized, condensed, and collected free of any impurities. *Spring water* is water that flows up to the earth's surface on its own from an underground spring. *Well water* is water that must be reached through a hole drilled into the ground. *Naturally sparkling water* is spring water with naturally occurring carbon dioxide. *Sparkling water,* artificially carbonated with added carbon dioxide, is known as *seltzer. Club soda* is sparkling water flavored with salts, including sodium bicarbonate.

The purity of bottled water depends on the integrity of the bottler. In 1996, responding to questions about possible contaminants in some bottled waters, the FDA imposed limits on levels of contaminants in bottled water. In 1998, the FDA amended the rule to require bottlers to monitor water sources and finished products for contaminants once a year.

The Most Nutritious Way to Serve This Food

Filtered, if required, to remove impurities. (Bacteria may multiply on an ordinary faucet filter. Change the filter frequently to protect your drinking water.)

Diets That May Restrict or Exclude This Food

Low-sodium diets ("softened" water, some bottled waters)

Buying This Food

Look for: Tightly sealed bottles, preferably with a protective foil seal under the cap. If you are on a low-sodium diet, read the label on bottled waters carefully. Many bottled mineral waters contain sodium chloride or sodium bicarbonate.

Storing This Food

Store bottled water in a cool, dark cabinet. Water bottled in glass will keep longer than water bottled in plastic, which may begin to pick up the taste of the container after about two weeks.

Improve the taste of heavily chlorinated tap water by refrigerating it overnight in a glass bottle. The chlorine will evaporate and the water will taste fresh.

Preparing This Food

Let cold tap water run for a minute or two before you use it to pick up air, which will make it taste better.

What Happens When You Cook This Food

The molecules in a solid material are tightly packed together in an orderly crystal structure. The molecules in a gas have no particular order, which is why a gas will expand to fill the space available. A liquid is somewhere in between. The attractive forces that hold its molecules together are weaker than those between the molecules in a solid but stronger than those between the molecules in a gas. When you heat a liquid, you excite its molecules (increase their thermal energy) and disrupt the forces holding them together. As the molecules continue to absorb energy, they separate from each other and begin to escape from the liquid. When the concentration of the molecules escaping from the liquids equals the pressure of air above the surface, the liquid will boil and some of its molecules will vaporize to a gas that floats off the surface as the liquid evaporates.

At sea level, plain water boils at 212°F (100°C), the temperature at which its molecules have absorbed enough energy to begin to escape from the surface as steam. If you add salt to the water before it starts to boil, the water molecules will need to pick up extra energy in order to overcome the greater attractive forces between the salt and water molecules. Since the energy comes from heat, adding salt raises the boiling point of the water. Salted water boils at a higher temperature than plain water does. That is why pasta, rice, and other foods cook more quickly in boiling salted water than in plain boiling water.

How Other Kinds of Processing Affect This Food

Freezing.   Water is the only compound that expands when it freezes. A water molecule is shaped roughly like an open triangle, with an oxygen atom at the center and a hydrogen atom at the end of either arm. When water is frozen, its molecules move more slowly, and each hydrogen atom forms a temporary bond to the oxygen atom on a nearby water molecule. The phenomenon, known as hydrogen bonding, creates a rigid structure in which the molecules stretch out rather than pack closely together, as normally happens when a substance is cooled. An ounce of frozen water (ice) takes up more room than an ounce of liquid water.

"Softening."   Home water softeners that filter out "hard" calcium carbonate and replace it with sodium may increase the sodium content of tap water by as much as 100 mg per quart.

Medical Uses and/or Benefits

Maintaining body functions.   The body uses water in and around body cells and tissues to regulate body temperature; create blood, lymph, and body secretions; digest food; dissolve and circulate nutrients; eliminate waste; and lubricate joints.

Protection against dental cavities.   Fluoridated drinking water provides fluoride ions that are incorporated into the crystalline structure of dental enamel, hardening the tooth surface and making it more resistant to bacteria such as *Mutans streptococcus,* a type of bacteria that live in sticky dental plaque, digesting sugars and excreting acidic material that eats away at the tooth. To obtain the most protection, the American Dental Association says children should drink fluoridated water from birth through the eruption of their permanent teeth, around ages 12 to 13.

Relief from constipation.   Water bulks up stool and moves it more quickly and easily through your body; a glass of warm water first thing in the morning stimulates gastric juices and exerts a mild laxative effect.

Relief from stuffed nose caused by cold or seasonal (mold, pollen) allergy.   Warm beverages loosen mucous, making it easier to clear your nasal passages.

Prevention of heat-related illness. Heatstroke is a medical emergency caused by dehydration resulting from the failure to replace fluids lost through excess perspiration. Drinking adequate amounts of water while exercising or working in a hot environment reduces (but does not entirely eliminate) the risk of heatstroke. NOTE: Alcoholic beverages and caffeinated beverages are mild diuretics; drinking them increases your loss of water.

Antacid, diuretic, and laxative effects. Mineral waters are natural mild diuretics and, because they contain sodium bicarbonate, naturally antacid. Any kind of water, taken warm about a half hour before breakfast, appears to be mildly laxative, perhaps because it stimulates contractions of the muscles in the digestive tract.

Adverse Effects Associated with This Food

Contaminants. Drinking water may pick up a variety of chemical contaminants as it travels through the ground or through pipes. To date, more than 300 chemical contaminants, including arsenic, asbestos, nitrates and nitrites, pesticides, and lead, have been identified in the water systems of various American cities. Even chlorine, which is added to the water supply to eliminate potentially hazardous microorganisms, can be a problem. The free chlorine generated during the purification process may react with organic compounds in the water to produce trihalomethanes, such a chloroform, which are suspected carcinogens or mutagens (substances that alter the structure of DNA). To prevent this, the Environmental Protection Agency (EPA) monitors chlorinated water supplies to make sure that the level of trihalomethanes remains below 0.10 mg/liter (100 parts per billion), a level currently considered safe for human consumption.

Water overload. On an average day, a healthy adult may lose 2,500 ml (milliliters) water through breathing, perspiring, urinating, and defecating. An ounce is equal to 30 ml, so we can replace the fluid we lose with eight 10-ounce glasses of water or any equivalent combination of water plus other liquids and/or foods with a high water content. However, in 2008, an editorial in *The Journal of the American Society of Nephrology,* the professional publication of the association of doctors specializing in kidney diseases, questioned the validity of the "eight-glass-a-day" rule. They concluded that there is no clear evidence to support drinking large quantities of water and that it is more sensible for healthy people to drink when thirsty rather than to rely on a specific amount of water each day. Their reasoning was simple: If we take in much more water than we need to replace what we lose, the excess water will dilute the liquid inside our cells, lowering the normal concentration of electrolytes (sodium, potassium, chloride). Because a proper ratio of electrolytes is vital to the transmission of impulses from cell to cell, a continued excessive intake of fluid may cause water intoxication, a condition whose symptoms include lethargy, muscle spasms, convulsions, coma, and/or death. Healthy people whose kidneys are able to eliminate a temporary water overload are unlikely to suffer from water intoxication, but diets that require excessive water consumption may be hazardous for epileptics and others at risk of seizures.

Stained teeth. In some parts of the American Southwest, the groundwater is naturally fluoridated to concentrations as high as 10 ppm. Long-term consumption of water with fluoride concentrations higher than 2 ppm may discolor or stain your teeth.

Food/Drug Interactions

Diuretics. Diuretic drugs increase the loss of electrolytes through frequent urination. Check with your doctor for precise information regarding fluid requirements while you are taking these medications.

Wheat Cereals

See also Barley, Corn, Flour, Oats, Rice.

Nutritional Profile

Energy value (calories per serving): *Moderate*
Protein: *Moderate*
Fat: *Low*
Saturated fat: *Low*
Cholesterol: *None*
Carbohydrates: *High*
Fiber: *Low to very high*
Sodium: *Low*
Major vitamin contribution: *B vitamins*
Major mineral contribution: *Iron, zinc*

About the Nutrients in This Food

Wheat cereals such as bulgur wheat, farina, and kasha are grains that have been milled (ground) to remove the cellulose and lignin covering (bran) so that we can digest the nutrients inside.

When grain is milled, the bran may be mixed in with the cereal or discarded. Cereals with the bran are very high-fiber food. Cereals with the germ (the inner portion of the seed) are high in fat and may turn rancid more quickly than cereals without the germ.

The proteins in wheat cereals are limited in the essential amino acid lysine. Wheat cereals are naturally good sources of the B vitamins, including folate, plus iron and zinc. In 1998, the Food and Drug Administration ordered food manufactures to add folates—which protect against birth defects of the spinal cord and against heart disease—to flour, rice, and other grain products. One year later, data from the Framingham Heart Study, which has followed heart health among residents of a Boston suburb for nearly half a century, showed a dramatic increase in blood levels of folic acid. Before the fortification of foods, 22 percent of the study participants had a folic acid deficiency; after, the number fell to 2 percent.

One-half cup cooked bulgur wheat has 5.5 g dietary fiber, 16.5 mg folate (4 percent of the RDA), 0.87 mg iron (5 percent of the RDA for a woman, 11 percent of the RDA for a man), and .52 mg zinc (7 percent of the RDA for a woman, 5 percent of the RDA for a man).

One-half cup cooked farina has 0.7 g dietary fiber, 79 mg folate (20 percent of the RDA), 1.2 mg iron (7 percent of the RDA for a woman,

15 percent of the RDA for a man), and 0.2 mg zinc (3 percent of the RDA for a woman, 2 percent of the RDA for a man).

One-half cup cooked kasha (roasted buckwheat groats) has 4.5 g dietary fiber, 24 mg folate (6 percent of the RDA), 1.3 mg iron (7 percent of the RDA for a woman, 16 percent of the RDA for a man), and 1 mg iron (6 percent of the RDA for a woman, 17 percent of the RDA for a man).

The Most Nutritious Way to Serve This Food

With beans, milk, cheese, or meat, any of which will provide the essential amino acid lysine to "complete" the proteins in the grains.

Diets That May Restrict or Exclude This Food

Gluten-restricted, gliadin-free diet (farina, kasha)
Low-carbohydrate diet
Low-fiber, low-residue diet
Low-sodium diet (see *About the nutrients in this food,* above)

Buying This Food

Look for: Tightly sealed boxes or canisters.

Storing This Food

Keep cereals in air- and moisture-proof containers to protect them from potentially toxic fungi that grow on damp grains. Properly stored, degermed grains may keep for as long as a year. Whole-grain cereals, which contain the fatty germ, may become rancid and should be used as quickly as possible.

Preparing This Food

* * *

What Happens When You Cook This Food

Cereals are made of tightly folded molecules of the complex carbohydrates amylose and amylopectin packed into starch granules. As the granules are heated in liquid, they absorb water and swell. As the temperature of the liquid rises to approximately 140°F, amylose and amylopectin molecules inside the starch granules relax and unfold, breaking some of their internal bonds (bonds between atoms on the same molecule) and forming new bonds to other atoms on other molecules. This creates a network that traps and holds water molecules.*

Ounce for ounce, cereal has fewer vitamins and minerals after cooking simply because so much of the weight of the cooked cereal is water. Cereals are naturally sodium-free but absorb sodium from the soaking water.

How Other Kinds of Processing Affect This Food

* * *

Medical Uses and/or Benefits

As a source of carbohydrates for people with diabetes.   Plain cereals are digested very slowly, producing only a gradual rise in the level of sugar in the blood. As a result, the body needs less insulin to control blood sugar after eating unsugared cereals made from additive-free grain than after eating some other high-carbohydrate foods (such as bread or potato). In studies at the University of Kentucky, a whole-grain-, bean-, vegetable-, and fruit-rich diet developed at the University of Toronto and recommended by the American Diabetic Association enabled patients with type 1 diabetes (who do not produce any insulin themselves) to cut their daily insulin intake by 38 percent. For patients with type 2 diabetes (who can produce some insulin) the bean diet reduced the need for injected insulin by 98 percent. This diet is in line with the nutritional guidelines of the American Diabetes Association, although people with diabetes should always consult with their doctor and/or dietitian before altering their diets.

Lower risk of heart disease.   In 2007, researchers from the Harvard Medical School and Brigham and Women's Hospital, in Boston, released an analysis of data from the long-running 21,400-man Physicians Health Follow-Up Study showing that men who consume seven or more servings of whole-grain cereal a week are 21 percent less likely to suffer from heart failure than are men who do not consume whole grain cereals daily. The results held true regardless of how much the men weighed, whether they smoked or drank or took vitamin pills, or had a history of high blood pressure and high cholesterol. NOTE: In this study, "whole-grain cereals" are defined as those containing at least 25 percent whole grain or wheat bran by weight.

A lower risk of some kinds of cancer.   In 1998, scientists at Wayne State University in Detroit conducted a meta-analysis of data from more than 30 well-designed animal studies measuring the anti-cancer effects of wheat bran, the part of grain with highest amount of the

---

* When you use a little starch in a lot of liquid the amylose and amylopectin released when the starch granules rupture will thicken the liquid by attracting and immobilizing some of its water molecules. Amylose, a long unbranched spiral molecule, can form more bonds to water molecules than can amylopectin, a short branched molecule. Wheat flours, which have a higher ratio of amylose to amylopectin, are superior thickeners.

insoluble dietary fibers cellulose and lignin. They found a 32 percent reduction in the risk of colon cancer among animals fed wheat bran; now they plan to conduct a similar meta-analysis of human studies. Whole grain cereals are a good source of wheat bran. NOTE: The amount of fiber per serving listed on a food package label shows the total amount of fiber (insoluble and soluble).

However, early the following year, new data from the long-running Nurses' Health Study at Harvard School of Public Health and Brigham and Women's Hospital, in Boston, showed no difference in the risk of colon cancer between women who ate a high-fiber diet and those who did not. Nonetheless, many nutrition researchers remain wary of ruling out a protective effect for dietary fiber. They note that there are different kinds of dietary fiber which may have different effects, that most Americans do not consume a diet with the recommended amount of dietary fiber, and that gender, genetics, and various personal health issues may also affect the link between dietary fiber and the risk of colon cancer. NOTE: The current recommendations for dietary fiber consumption are 25 grams per day for women younger than 50, and 21 grams per day for women older than 50; 38 grams per day for men younger than 50, and 30 grams per day for men older than 50.

Adverse Effects Associated with This Food

Allergic reaction. According to the *Merck Manual,* wheat is one of the 12 foods most likely to trigger the classic food allergy symptoms: hives, swelling of the lips and eyes, and upset stomach. The others are berries (blackberries, blueberries, raspberries, strawberries), chocolate, corn, eggs, fish, legumes (green peas, lima beans, peanuts, soybeans), milk, nuts, peaches, pork, and shellfish.

Gluten intolerance. Celiac disease is an allergic intestinal disorder experienced by people sensitive to gliadin, a component of gluten, the sticky elastic protein that makes it possible for breads made with wheat and rye flour to rise. (All wheat cereals contain gluten.) People with celiac disease cannot digest the nutrients in these grains; if they eat foods such as farina or kasha that contain gluten, they may suffer anemia, weight loss, bone pain, swelling, and skin disorders.

Food/Drug Interactions

* * *

Wine

Nutritional Profile*

Energy value (calories per serving): *Moderate*
Protein: *Low*
Fat: *None*
Saturated fat: *None*
Cholesterol: *None*
Carbohydrates: *Low*
Fiber: *None*
Sodium: *Low*
Major vitamin contribution: *B vitamins*
Major mineral contribution: *Potassium*

About the Nutrients in This Food

Wine is a beverage produced by yeasts that digest the sugars in fruits and turn them into alcohol. Grapes are particularly well suited in winemaking because they are sweet enough to produce a beverage that is at least 10 percent alcohol and acid enough to encourage the growth of the friendly yeasts while discouraging the growth of potentially harmful bacteria.

Wines contain carbohydrates, a trace of protein, and small amounts of vitamins and minerals but no fats. Unlike food, which has to be metabolized before your body can use it for energy, the alcohol in wine can be absorbed into the bloodstream directly from the gastrointestinal tract. Ethyl alcohol (the alcohol in alcohol beverages) provides seven calories per gram.

Querceitin and querceitrin, the pale yellow pigments that make white wine "white," turn browner as they age. The darker the wine, the older it is. Red wine's ruby color comes from red anthocyanin pigments in red grape skins. As red wines age, their red pigments react with tannins in the wine and turn brown.

The USDA/Health and Human Services Dietary Guidelines for Americans defines one drink as 12 ounces of beer, five ounces of wine, or 1.25 ounces of distilled spirits. One five-ounce glass of wine has 106 calories, 96 of them (91 percent) from alcohol. But the beverage is more than empty

* Values are for table wines.

calories. Like beer, wine retains small amounts of some nutrients present in the food from which it was made. NOTE: *Table wines* are wines with an alcohol content lower than 15 percent.* *Dessert wines* are sweet wines whose alcohol content ranges between 15 and 24 percent. *Sherry, Madeira,* and *port* are *fortified wines,* wines to which brandy or spirits have been added. *Sparkling wines,* such as champagne, are bottled with a precisely measured yeast-and-sugar solution that ferments in the bottle to produce carbon dioxide bubbles.

The Nutrients in Red Table Wine (five-ounce glass)

Nutrients	Red	%RDA
Calcium	8 mg	0.8
Magnesium	13 mg	3.7–4.6*
Phosphorus	14 mg	0.8
Potassium	112 mg	n.a.
Zinc	0.09 mg	0.6–0.7*
Thiamin	0.005 mg	0.003–0.004*
Riboflavin	0.03 mg	1.8–2–2.3*
Vitamin B$_6$	0.03 mg	1.5
Folate	2 mcg	1

* The first figure is the %RDA for a man; the second, for a woman

Source: USDA Nutrients Database: www.nal.usda.gov/fnic/cgi-bin/nut_search.pl.

The Most Nutritious Way to Serve This Food

In moderation.

Diets That May Restrict or Exclude This Food

Bland diet
Lactose-free diet
Low-purine (antigout) diet
Low-sodium diet (cooking wines)

Buying This Food

Look for: Tightly sealed bottles stored away from direct sunlight, whose energy might disrupt the structure of molecules in the beverage and alter its flavor.

---

*   In the United States, "proof" is twice the alcohol content. A wine that is 15 percent alcohol by volume is 30 proof.

Choose wines sold only by licensed dealers. Products sold in these stores are manufactured under the strict supervision of the federal government.

Storing This Food

All wine should be stored in tightly sealed bottles in a cool, dry, dark place, protected from direct light—whose energy might disrupt the structure of the flavor molecules in the wine. (Most wine bottles are tinted amber or green to screen out ultraviolet light.)

After it is bottled, wine continues to react with the small amount of oxygen in the container, a phenomenon known as aging. Red wines improve ("mature") in the bottle; their taste is deeper and mellower after a year or two, and some continue to age for as long as 15 years. Keep the bottle on its side so that the wine flows down and keeps the cork wet. A wet cork expands to seal the bottle even more tightly and keep extra air from coming into the bottle and oxidizing the wine to vinegar. (Bottles with plastic corks or screw tops can be stored upright. Their seals are air-tight.)

Store leftover wine in a small bottle with a tight cap and as little air space as possible. Use leftover table wines as soon as possible (or let them oxidize to vinegar). Appetizer and dessert wines, which are higher in alcohol content than table wines, may taste good for as long as a month after the bottle is opened.

Preparing This Food

All wines contain volatile molecules that give the beverage its characteristic flavor and aroma. Warming the liquid excites these molecules and intensifies the flavor and aroma. While dry white or rosé wines are usually chilled before serving, sweet white wines and the more flavorful reds are best served at room temperature.

Stand a bottle of wine upright for a day before serving it, so that the sediment (dregs) will settle to the bottom. When you open a bottle of wine, handle it gently to avoid stirring up the sediment.

What Happens When You Cook This Food

When you heat wine, its alcohol evaporates but its flavor remains. Since evaporation concentrates the flavor, be sure the wine you're using tastes good enough to drink; cooking won't improve the flavor of a bad wine.

In cooking, when you add the wine depends on what you want it to do. As a tenderizer, add the wine when you start cooking; for flavor, near the end of the cooking process.

Alcohol is an acid. If you cook it in an aluminum or iron pot, it will react with metal ions to form dark compounds that discolor the pot and the food. Recipes made with wine should be prepared in an enameled, glass, or stainless steel pot.

How Other Kinds of Processing Affect This Food

* * *

Medical Uses and/or Benefits

Lower risk of stroke. In January 1999, the results of a 677-person study published by researchers at New York Presbyterian Hospital–Columbia University showed that moderate alcohol consumption reduces the risk of stroke due to a blood clot in the brain among older people (average age: 70). How the alcohol prevents stroke is still unknown, but it is clear that moderate use of alcohol is a key. Heavy drinkers (those who consume more than seven drinks a day) have a higher risk of stroke. People who once drank heavily, but cut their consumption to moderate levels, may also reduce their risk of stroke. Numerous later studies have confirmed these findings.

Reduced risk of heart attack. Data from the American Cancer Society's Cancer Prevention Study 1, an 12-year survey of more than 1 million Americans in 25 states, shows that men who take one drink a day have a 21 percent lower risk of heart attack and a 22 percent lower risk of stroke than men who do not drink at all. Women who have up to one drink a day also reduce their risk of heart attack. Numerous later studies have confirmed these findings.

Lower cholesterol levels. Beverage alcohol decreases the body's production and storage of low density lipoproteins (LDLs), the protein and fat particles that carry cholesterol into your arteries. As a result, people who drink moderately tend to have lower cholesterol levels and higher levels of high density lipoproteins (HDLs), the fat and protein particles that carry cholesterol out of the body.

Appetite stimulation. Alcohol beverages stimulate the production of saliva and gastric acids that cause the stomach contractions we call hunger pangs. Moderate amounts, which may help stimulate appetite, are often prescribed for geriatric patients, convalescents, and people who do not have ulcers or other chronic gastric problems.

Dilation of blood vessels. Alcohol dilates the tiny blood vessels just under the skin, bringing blood up to the surface. That's why moderate amounts of alcohol beverages (0.2–1 gram per kilogram of body weight—that is, 6.6 ounces of wine for a 150-pound adult) temporarily warms the drinker. But the warm blood that flows up to the surface of the skin will cool down there, making you even colder when it circulates back into the center of your body. Then an alcohol flush will make you perspire, so that you lose more heat. Excessive amounts of beverage alcohol may depress the mechanism that regulates body temperature.

Adverse Effects Associated with This Food

Increased risk of breast cancer. In 2008, scientists at the National Cancer Institute released data from a seven-year survey of more than 100,000 postmenopausal women showing that even moderate drinking (one to two drinks a day) may increase by 32 percent a woman's risk of developing estrogen-receptor positive (ER+) and progesterone-receptor positive (PR+) breast cancer, tumors whose growth is stimulated by hormones. No such link was found between consuming alcohol and the risk of developing ER-/PR- tumors (not fueled by hormones). The finding applies to all types of alcohol: beer, wine, and distilled spirits.

Increased risk of cancer of the colon and rectum.   In the mid-1990s, studies at the University of Oklahoma suggested that men who drink more than five beers a day are at increased risk of rectal cancer. Later studies suggested that men and women who are heavy beer or spirits drinkers (but not those who are heavy wine drinkers) have a higher risk of colorectal cancers. Further studies are required to confirm these findings.

Increased risk of oral cancer (cancer of the mouth and throat).   Numerous studies confirm the American Cancer Society's warning that men and women who consume more than two drinks a day are at higher risk of oral cancer than are nondrinkers or people who drink less. NOTE: *The Dietary Guidelines for Americans* describes one drink as 12 ounces of beer, five ounces of wine, or 1.5 ounces of distilled spirits.

Alcoholism.   Alcoholism is an addiction disease, the inability to control one's alcohol consumption. It is a potentially life-threatening condition, with a higher risk of death by accident, suicide, malnutrition, or acute alcohol poisoning, a toxic reaction that kills by paralyzing body organs, including the heart.

Malnutrition.   While moderate alcohol consumption stimulates appetite, alcohol abuse depresses it. In addition, an alcoholic may drink instead of eating. When an alcoholic does eat, excess alcohol in his/her body prevents absorption of nutrients and reduces the ability to synthesize new tissue.

Hangover.   Alcohol is absorbed from the stomach and small intestine and carried by the bloodstream to the liver, where it is oxidized to acetaldehyde by alcohol dehydrogenase (ADH), the enzyme our bodies use every day to metabolize the alcohol we produce when we digest carbohydrates. The acetaldehyde is converted to acetyl coenzyme A and either eliminated from the body or used in the synthesis of cholesterol, fatty acids, and body tissues. Although individuals vary widely in their capacity to metabolize alcohol, an adult of average size can metabolize the alcohol in 13 ounces (400 ml) of wine in approximately five to six hours. If he or she drinks more than that, the amount of alcohol in the body will exceed the available supply of ADH. The surplus, unmetabolized alcohol will pile up in the bloodstream, interfering with the liver's metabolic functions. Since alcohol decreases the reabsorption of water from the kidneys and may inhibit the secretion of an antidiuretic hormone, the drinker will begin to urinate copiously, losing magnesium, calcium, and zinc but retaining more irritating uric acid. The level of lactic acid in the body will increase, making him or her feel tired and out of sorts; the acid-base balance will be out of kilter; the blood vessels of the head will swell and throb and the stomach, its lining irritated by the alcohol, will ache. The ultimate result is a "hangover" whose symptoms will disappear only when enough time has passed to allow the body to marshal the ADH needed to metabolize the extra alcohol in the blood.

Changes in body temperature.   Alcohol dilates capillaries, tiny blood vessels just under the skin, producing a "flush" that temporarily warms the drinker. But drinking is not an effective way to stay warm in cold weather. Warm blood flowing up from the body core to the surface capillaries is quickly chilled, making you even colder when it circulates back into your organs. In addition, an alcohol flush triggers perspiration, further cooling your skin.

Finally, very large amounts of alcohol may actually depress the mechanism that regulates body temperature.

Sulfite allergy. Sulfur dioxide (a sulfite) is sometimes used as a preservative to control the growth of "wild" microorganisms that might turn wine to vinegar. People who are sensitive to sulfites may experience severe allergic reactions, including anaphylactic shock, if they drink these wines.

Migraine headaches. When grapes are fermented, their long protein molecules are broken into smaller fragments. One of these fragments, tyramine, inhibits PST, an enzyme that deactivates phenols (alcohols). The resulting build-up of phenols in your bloodstream may trigger a headache. All wines have some tyramine, but the most serious offenders appear to be red wines, particularly chianti.

Food/Drug Interactions

Acetaminophen (Tylenol, etc.). The FDA recommends that people who regularly have three or more drinks a day consult a doctor before using acetaminophen. The alcohol/acetaminophen combination may cause liver failure.

Anti-alcohol abuse drugs (disulfiram [Antabuse]). Taken concurrently with alcohol, the anti-alcoholism drug disulfiram can cause flushing, nausea, a drop in blood pressure, breathing difficulty, and confusion. The severity of the symptoms, which may vary among individuals, generally depends on the amount of alcohol consumed and the amount of disulfiram in the body.

Anticoagulants (blood thinners). Alcohol slows the body's metabolism of anticoagulants such as warfarin (Coumadin), intensifying the effect of the drugs and increasing the risk of side effects such as spontaneous nosebleeds.

Antidepressants. Alcohol may increase the sedative or other central nervous system effects of any antidepressant. Combining alcohol with monoamine oxidase (MAO) inhibitors is especially hazardous. MAO inhibitors inactivate naturally occurring enzymes in your body that metabolize tyramine, a substance found in many fermented or aged foods that constricts blood vessels and increases blood pressure. If you eat a food containing tyramine while you are taking an MAO inhibitor, you cannot effectively eliminate the tyramine from your body. The result may be a hypertensive crisis. Ordinarily, fermentation of beer and ale does not produce tyramine, but some patients have reported tyramine reactions after drinking some imported beers. Beer and ale are usually excluded from the diet when you are using MAO inhibitors.

Aspirin, ibuprofen, ketoprofen, naproxen and nonsteroidal anti-inflammatory drugs. Like alcohol, these analgesics irritate the lining of the stomach and may cause gastric bleeding. Combining the two intensifies the effect.

Insulin and oral hypoglycemics.   Alcohol lowers blood sugar and interferes with the metabolism of oral antidiabetics; the combination may cause severe hypoglycemia.

Sedatives and other central nervous system depressants (tranquilizers, sleeping pills, antidepressants, sinus and cold remedies, analgesics, and medication for motion sickness).   Alcohol intensifies the sedative effects of these medications and, depending on the dose, may cause drowsiness, sedation, respiratory depression, coma, or death.

Winter Squash

(Acorn, butternut, Hubbard, spaghetti squash)

See also Pumpkin.

Nutritional Profile

Energy value (calories per serving): *Low*
Protein: *Moderate*
Fat: *Low*
Saturated fat: *Low*
Cholesterol: *None*
Carbohydrates: *High*
Fiber: *High*
Sodium: *Low*
Major vitamin contribution: *Vitamin A, B vitamins, vitamin C*
Major mineral contribution: *Potassium*

About the Nutrients in This Food

Winter squash has sugar, some fiber (mostly gums and some pectins, with a bit of cellulose), a little protein and fat, and no cholesterol.

All winter squash are hard-skinned but they come in different shapes and colors. Acorn squash is round, ribbed, and green. Spaghetti squash is round and creamy. Hubbard is bumpy and orange. Butternut looks like a yellow-orange gourd, broad at the bottom, with a narrow neck.

An average one-half cup serving of orange/yellow baked winter squash cubes has 3 g dietary fiber, 5,354 IU vitamin A (2.3 times the RDA

The Vitamin A content of ½ Cup Baked Winter Squash

Squash	Vitamin A
Acorn	439 IU
Butternut	11,434 IU
Hubbard	6,186 IU
Spaghetti	85 IU

Source: USDA Nutrient Data Laboratory. National Nutrient Database for Standard Reference. Available online. URL: http://nal.usda.gov/fnic/foodcomp/search/

for a woman, 1.8 times the RDA for a man), 29 mcg folate (7 percent of the RDA), and 9.8 mg vitamin C (13 percent of the RDA for a woman, 11 percent of the RDA for a man). However, the vitamin A content of winter squash varies enormously depending on the variety of squash.

The Most Nutritious Way to Serve This Food

Ounce for ounce, baked winter squash has more vitamin A than boiled squash because in boiling the squash absorbs water that displaces some of the nutrients.

Diets That May Restrict or Exclude This Food

* * *

Buying This Food

Look for: Firm, heavy squash is smooth and unblemished skin. *Acorn squash* should have a wide-ribbed, dark green shell. The longer the squash is stored, the more orange it will become as its green chlorophyll pigments fade and the yellow carotenes underneath show through. *Butternut squash* should be a smooth, creamy brown or yellow. *Hubbard squash* has a ridged and bumpy orange red shell flecked with dark blue or gray. *Spaghetti squash* is smooth and yellow. If the squash is sliced, the flesh inside should be smooth and evenly colored.

Storing This Food

Store winter squash in a cool, dry cabinet to protect its vitamins A and C. Squash stores well. Hubbards, for example, may stay fresh for up to six months, acorn squash for three to six months.

Do not refrigerate winter squash. Winter squash stored at cold temperatures convert their starches to sugars.

Preparing This Food

Wash the squash and bake it whole, or cut it in half or in quarters (or smaller portions if it is very large), remove the stringy part and the seeds, and bake or boil. Baking is the more nutritious method since it preserves the most nutrients.

What Happens When You Cook This Food

When you bake a squash, the soluble food fibers in its cell walls dissolve and the squash gets softer. Baking also caramelizes and browns sugars on the cut surface of the squash, a process you can help along by dusting the squash with brown sugar. If you bake the squash long enough, the moisture inside its cells will begin to evaporate and the squash will shrink.

When you boil squash, its starch granules absorb water molecules that cling to the amylose and amylopectin, molecules inside, making the starch granules (and the squash) swell. If the granules absorb enough water they will rupture, releasing the moisture inside and once again the squash will shrink.

Neither baking nor boiling reduces the amount of vitamin A in squash since the carotenes that make squash yellow are impervious to the normal heat of cooking. Vitamin C, on the other hand, is heat-sensitive. Cooked squash has less vitamin C than raw squash does.

How Other Kinds of Processing Affect This Food

Canning. According to the USDA, canned "pumpkin" may be a mixture of pumpkin and other yellow-orange winter squash, all of which are similar in nutritional value.

Medical Uses and/or Benefits

Lower risk of some birth defects. As many as two of every 1,000 babies born in the United States each year may have cleft palate or a neural tube (spinal cord) defect due to their mothers' not having gotten adequate amounts of folate during pregnancy. The current RDA for folate is 180 mcg for a woman and 200 mcg for a man, but the FDA now recommends 400 mcg for a woman who is or may become pregnant. Taking folate supplements before becoming pregnant and continuing through the first two months of pregnancy reduces the risk of cleft palate; taking folate through the entire pregnancy reduces the risk of neural tube defects.

Possible lower risk of heart attack. In the spring of 1998, an analysis of data from the records for more than 80,000 women enrolled in the long-running Nurses' Health Study at Harvard School of Public Health/Brigham and Women's Hospital, in Boston, demonstrated that a diet providing more than 400 mcg folate and 3 mg vitamin B_6 daily either from food or supplements, might reduce a woman's risk of heart attack by almost 50 percent. Although men were not included in the study, the results were assumed to apply to them as well.

However, data from a meta-analysis published in the *Journal of the American Medical Association* in December 2006 called this theory into question. Researchers at Tulane University examined the results of 12 controlled studies in which 16,958 patients with preexisting cardiovascular disease were given either folic acid supplements or placebos ("look-alike" pills with no folic acid) for at least six months. The scientists, who found no reduction in the risk of further heart disease or overall death rates among those taking folic acid, concluded that further studies will be required to ascertain whether taking folic acid supplements reduces the risk of cardiovascular disease.

Adverse Effects Associated with This Food

* * *

Food/Drug Interactions

* * *

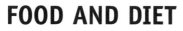

Appendix

FOOD AND DIET

The following charts list foods high in specific nutrients for specific diets. For more complete information regarding the food's effects, see the main listings.

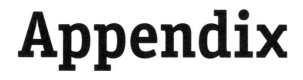

CONTROLLED CHOLESTEROL/CONTROLLED FAT DIET

The controlled cholesterol/low-fat diet restricts but does not eliminate either cholesterol, fat, or saturated fat. Instead it conforms to the USDA/Health and Human Services Dietary Guidelines for Americans recommendation that you consume no more than 300 mg cholesterol and get no more than 100 calories per day from saturated fat (nine calories per gram).

FOODS WITH 90 TO 150 MG CHOLESTEROL PER SERVING:

Beef	Game meat	Pork
Cheddar cheese	Lamb	Ricotta (whole milk)
Chicken	Lobsters	Shellfish
Crab	Oysters	Turkey Veal

FOODS WITH MORE THAN 150 MG CHOLESTEROL PER SERVING:

Beef brains	Eggs (whole)	Goose
Beef heart	Duck	Liver (all)
Beef tongue		

FOODS WITH MORE THAN TWO GRAMS (18 CALORIES) SATURATED FAT PER SERVING:

Avocado	Game Meat	Poultry
Beef	Lamb	Variety meats
Butter	Liver (all)	Veal
Chocolate	Pork	

HIGH-FIBER DIET

A high-fiber diet reduces your risk of heart disease, as well as some cancers. There is currently no RDA for dietary fiber; the Dietary Guidelines for Americans recommends 25 g per day.

FOODS WITH ONE TO TWO GRAMS FIBER PER SERVING:

Asparagus	Cherries	Plum
Beets	Chocolate (plain, sweet)	Quince
Blackberries	Currants	Raisins
Cabbage	Grapefruit	Rice
Celeriac	Peach	Spinach
Celery	Peppers	Tangerine

FOODS WITH TWO TO FIVE GRAMS DIETARY FIBER PER SERVING:

Apple	Banana	Coconut
Apricot	Bean sprouts	Corn
Artichoke (Jerusalem)	Carrot	Cranberries

Avocado (California)   Cauliflower   Green beans
Greens   Onions   Plantain
Guava   Orange   Potato
Kiwi fruit   Parsnip   Raspberries
Kohlrabi   Nectarine   Strawberries
Mango   Peanuts   Sweet Potato
Melon   Pear   Tomato
Mushrooms   Peas   Turnip
Oatmeal   Persimmon   Zucchini
Okra   Pineapple

FOODS WITH MORE THAN FIVE GRAMS DIETARY FIBER PER SERVING:

Avocado (Florida)   Eggplant   Prune
Barley   Fig   Pumpkin
Beans   Lentils   Raisins
Broccoli   Lima bean Soy beans
Cereals   Nuts   Winter squash
Dates   Papaya

HIGH-PROTEIN DIET

A high-protein diet encourages the growth of new tissue, including muscle tissue, and speeds wound healing. The RDA for proteins is 63 g for a man, 64 g for a woman. NOTE: The proteins in foods marked with an asterisk (*) are limited in some essential amino acids.

FOODS WITH FIVE TO 10 GRAMS PROTEIN PER SERVING:

Beans*   Gruyére   Egg (whole)
Broccoli*   Gorgonzola   Figs (dried)*
Cereals (bulgar)*   Leiderkranz   Lentils*
Cheese   Limburger   Milk*
  Blue   Monterey Jack   Pasta
  Brie   Mozzarella   Peas*
  Camembert Meunster   Potato*
  Cheddar Romano   Rice (enriched)*
  Edam   Swiss   Soy beans

FOODS WITH 10 TO 20 GRAMS PROTEIN PER SERVING:

Cheese   Tofu   Yogurt
  Cottage
  Ricotta

FOODS WITH MORE THAN 20 GRAMS PROTEIN PER SERVING:

Beef   Pork   Variety meat
Fish   Poultry   Veal
Game meat   Shellfish

HIGH-CAROTENOID DIET

Carotenes are plant pigments your body converts to a form of vitamin A. A diet high in carotenes, including beta-carotene, appears to lower the risk of some cancers.

FOODS WITH 20 TO 50 PERCENT RDA PER SERVING:

Brussels sprouts	Melon (watermelon)	Prunes
Butter	Nectarine	Spinach
Cabbage (bok choy)		

FOODS WITH 50 TO 100 PERCENT RDA PER SERVING:

Apricot	Greens (turnip)	Persimmon
Broccoli		

FOODS WITH MORE THAN 100 PERCENT RDA PER SERVING:

Carrot	Melon (cantaloupe)	Sweet potato
Mango	Peppers (red, bell)	Winter squash (butternut, Hubbard)

HIGH-FOLATE DIET

A high-folate diet before and during pregnancy reduces the risk of delivering a child with cleft palate or a neural tube (spinal cord) defect; a diet with adequate amounts of folate and vitamin B_6 reduces the risk of heart disease.

FOOD WITH 10 TO 50 PERCENT RDA PER SERVING:

Bean sprouts	Lettuces	Parsnips
Beans	Lima Beans	Peanuts
Beets	Melon (cantaloupe)	Soy beans
Broccoli	Nuts	Spinach
Brussels sprouts	Okra	Strawberries
Greens	Papaya	Winter squash

FOODS WITH MORE THAN 50 PERCENT RDA PER SERVING:

Asparagus	Lentils

FOODS HIGH IN VITAMIN B_6:

Beans	Game meat	Poultry
Beef	Grains (whole)	Shellfish
Cereal (whole)	Greens	Variety meats
Fish	Pork	Veal

HIGH–VITAMIN C DIET

Vitamin C, an antioxidant, reduce the risk of heart disease and cancer and speeds the healing of wounds.

FOOD WITH 20 TO 50 PERCENT RDA PER SERVING:

Artichoke (globe)	Greens	Pineapple
Avocado	Lemons	Potato
Blackberries	Mango	Quince
Red Cabbage	Okra	Raspberries
Cauliflower	Onions (green)	Sweet Potato
Currants	Persimmon	Tangerine

FOODS WITH 51 TO 100 PERCENT RDA PER SERVING:

Brussels sprouts	Kohlrabi	Tomato
Grapefruit	Strawberries	Watermelon

FOODS WITH MORE THAN 100 PERCENT RDA PER SERVING:

Broccoli	Guava	Orange
Cantaloupe	Kiwi fruit	Papaya

HIGH-CALCIUM DIET

A lifelong diet with adequate amounts of calcium protects bones density and reduces the risk of osteoporosis.

FOODS WITH MORE THAN 20 PERCENT RDA PER SERVING:

Cheese (1 oz.)	Mozzarella	Ricotta (cup)
Cheddar	(part skim)	Romano
Edam	Muenster	Swiss
Gruyère	Parmesan	Milk
Monterey Jack	Provolone	Yogurt

MOOD-ALTERING DIET

Many common foods provide natural chemicals that influence the brain's ability to use neurotransmitters, chemicals that enable cells to send messages back and forth. "Calming" foods increase the availability of the neurotransmitter serotonin. "Mood elevators" increase the availability of the neutrotransmitters dopamine and norepinephrine.

FOODS THAT CALM YOUR MOOD

Beans	Cereal	Pasta
Bread	Grains	

FOODS THAT ELEVATE YOUR MOOD

Beef (lean)	Fish	Shellfish
Chocolate	Pork (lean)	Tea
Coffee	Poultry (lean, no skin)	Veal (lean)

Bibliography/ Sources

Please note that older sources included here are considered classics in the field, groundbreaking works, or contain unique, valuable information unavailable in more recent publications.

INTERNET NUTRIENT DATABASES

Institute of Medicine. National Institutes of Health. Food and Nutrition. URL: http://www.iom.edu/CMS/3708.aspx.

U.S. Department of Agriculture, Agricultural Research Service. USDA Nutrient Data Laboratory. USDA National Nutrient Database for Standard Reference. URL: http://nal.usda.gov/fnic/foodcomp/search/.

BOOKS

American Dietetic Association. *Handbook of Clinical Dietetics.* New Haven, Conn.: Yale University Press, 1981.

Arkin, Freda. *Kitchen Wisdom.* New York: Holt, Rinehart and Winston, 1977.

Berkow, Robert, ed. *The Merck Manual.* 17th ed. Whitehouse Station, N.J.: Merck Research Laboratories, 2006.

———. *The Merck Manual.* 16th ed. Rahway, N.J.: Merck Research Laboratories, 1992.

———. *The Merck Manual.* 14th ed. Rahway, N.J.: Merck, Sharp & Dohme Research Laboratories, 1982.

Braun, Stephen. *Buzz.* New York: Oxford University Press, 1996.

Briggs, George M., and Doris Howe Calloway. *Nutrition and Physical Fitness.* 11th ed. New York: Holt, Rinehart and Winston, 1979.

Cook, L. Russell. *Chocolate Use and Production.* New York: Books for Industry, 1972.

Davidson, Alan. *The Oxford Companion to Food.* Oxford: The Oxford University Press, 1999.

DeVore, Sally, and Thelma White. *The Appetites of Man.* New York: Anchor Books, 1978.

Farb, Peter, and George Armelagos. *Consuming Passions.* Boston: Houghton Mifflin Company, 1980.

Griggs, Barbara. *Green Pharmacy.* New York: Viking, 1981.

Grosser, Arthur P. *The Cookbook Decoder.* New York: Warner Books, 1981.

Hampel, Clifford A., and Gessner G. Hawley. *Glossary of Chemical Terms.* New York: Van Nostrand Reinhold, 1976.

Handbook of Diagnostic Tests. 3rd ed. Philadelphia: Lippincott, Williams & Wilkins, 2003.

Harris, Marvin. *Good to Eat.* New York: Simon and Schuster, 1985.

Jacobs, Morris B., ed. *The Chemistry and Technology of Food and Food Products.* New York: Interscience, 1951.

Kasper, Dennis L., Eugene Braunwald, Anthony S. Fauci, Stephen L. Hauser, Dan L. Longo, and J. Larry Jameson, eds. *Harrison's Principles of Internal Medicine.* 16th ed. New York: McGraw-Hill, 2006.

Kiple, Kenneth F., and Kriemhild Coneè Ornelas, eds. *The Cambridge World History of Food.* 2 vols. Cambridge, England: Cambridge University Press, 2000.

Lewis, Walter H., and Memory P. F. Elvin-Lewis. *Medical Botany.* New York: Wiley, 1977.

Logue, A. W. *The Psychology of Eating and Drinking.* 2nd ed. New York: W.H. Freeman and Company, 1991.

McGee, Harold. *On Food and Cooking.* New York: Scribner, 1984.

———. *On Food and Cooking.* Rev. ed. New York: Scribner. 2004.

McPhee, Stephen J., and Maxine A. Papadakis. *Current Medical Diagnosis and Treatment 2008.* New York: McGraw-Hill Medical, 2008.

Merenstein, Gerald B., et al., eds. *Silver, Kempe, Bruyn & Fulginiti's Handbook of Pediatrics.* 16th ed. Norwalk, Conn.: Appleton & Lange, 1991.

Morris, Dan and Inez Morris. *The Complete Fish Cookbook.* Indianapolis: Bobbs-Merrill, 1972.

National Research Council. *Recommended Dietary Allowances.* 10th ed. Washington, D.C.: National Academy Press, 1939.

The New American Heart Association Cookbook. 7th ed. New York: Clarkson Potter, 2007.

Peckenpaugh, Nancy J., and Charlotte M. Poleman. *Nutrition Essentials and Diet Therapy.* 7th ed. Philadelphia: W.B. Saunders Company, 1995.

Quimme, Peter. *The Signet Book of Coffee and Tea.* New York: New American Library, 1976.

Rinzler, Carol Ann. *The Healing Power of Soy.* Rocklin, Calif.: Prima Publishing, 1998.

———. *Nutrition for Dummies.* 4th ed. Hoboken, N.J.: Wiley Publishing, 2006.

Rolfes, Sharon Rady, Kathryn Pinna, and Ellie Whitney. *Understanding Clinical Nutrition.* 7th ed. Belmont, Calif.: Thomson Higher Education, 2006.

Rombauer, Irma S., Marion Rombauer Becker, and Ethan Becker. *Joy of Cooking.* New York: Scribner, 1997.

Root, Waverly. *Food.* New York: Smithmark, 1996.

Rybacki, James J. *The Essential Guide to Prescription Drugs 2006.* New York: Collins, 2006.

Spock, Benjamin. *Baby and Child Care.* New York: Pocket Books, 1976.

Steiner, Richard P., ed. *Folk Medicine: The Art and Science.* Washington, D.C.: American Chemical Society, 1986.

Toxicants Occurring Naturally in Foods. 2nd ed. Washington, D.C.: National Academy of Sciences, 1973.

Tyler, Varro F. *Hoosier Home Remedies.* Lafayette, Ind.: Purdue University Press, 1985.

Waldo, Myra. *The Complete Round-the-World Meat Cookbook.* New York: Doubleday, 1967.

Whalen, Elizabeth M., and Frederick J. Stare. *Panic in the Pantry.* New York: Atheneum, 1975.

Winter, Ruth. *A Consumer's Dictionary of Food Additives.* New York: Crown, 1978.

Zapsalis, Charles, and R. Anderle Beck. *Food Chemistry and Nutritional Biochemistry.* New York: Wiley, 1985.

PERIODICALS

Adams, J. B. "Color Stability of Red Fruits." *Food Manufacture,* February 1973.

Angier, Natalie. "Benefits of Broccoli Confirmed as Chemical Blocks Tumors." *New York Times,* April 12, 1994.

"Another Reason to Drink Green Tea." *Science News,* April 13, 1992.

"Another Reason to Eat Your Broccoli Raw." *Science News,* June 9, 1997.

"Bacon Producers Permitted to Use Vitamin C Additives." *New York Times,* July 6, 1985.

Barnett, Robert. "Garlic, the Raw and the Cooked." *American Health,* January–February 1986.

Bazzano, Lydia A., Kristi Reynolds, Kevin N. Holder, and Jiang He. "Effect of Folic Acid Supplementation on Risk of Cardiovascular Diseases: A Meta-analysis of Randomized Controlled Trials." *Journal of the American Medical Association* 296, no. 22 (December 13, 2006): 2720–2726. Available online. URL: http://jama.ama-assn.org/cgi/content/abstract/296/22/2720. Accessed on April 9, 2008.

"Beet Fat Alert Lifted a Bit." *Tufts University Diet and Nutrition Letter,* January 1986.

"Berry Good Juices." *FDA Consumer,* May–June 1999.

Bock, S. Allan. "The Natural History of Food Sensitivity." *Journal of Allergy and Clinical Immunology* 69 (February 1982): 103.

"Broccoli Boosts the Aging Immune System." *Journal of Allergy and Clinical Immunology.* Available online. URL: http://www.redorbit.com/news/health/1284514/broccoli_boosts_the_aging_immune_system/#. Accessed on June 23, 2008.

Brody, Jane E. "Another Round in Drink-a-Day Debate." *New York Times,* January 2, 1999.

Burros, Marian. "Is It Pasteurized? Juice Labels Will Tell." *New York Times,* July 1, 1998.

———. "U.S. Eases Up on Irradiation, Antibiotics." *New York Times,* August 26, 1998.

———. "Value of a B-List Diet (as in Vitamin B)." *New York Times,* February 18, 1998.

———. "U.S.: National Study Finds High Levels of Mercury in Tuna." *New York Times,* January 25, 2008. Available online. URL: http://dinersjournal.blogs.nytimes.com/2008/01/24/national-study-finds-high-levels-of-mercury- in-tuna/?hp. Accessed on January 27, 2008.

"Canadian Consumers Gain Access to Omega-3 Pork." *Pork,* December 12, 2007. Available online. URL: http://www.porkmag.com/news_editorial.asp?pgID=678&ed_id=5609. Accessed on January 21, 2008.

"Can Plantains Prevent Ulcers?" *Hospital Tribune,* December 19, 1984.

Cenrofanti, M. "Much Ado over Brew: Linking Drink to Shape." *Science News,* December 2, 1995.

The Cherry Marketing Institute. "The Cherry Nutrition Report." Available online. URL: http://www.choosecherries.com/pdfs/CherryNutritionalReport.pdf. Accessed on December 20, 2007.

"Chicken Soup and the Common Cold." *Mayo Clinic Health Letter,* October 1984.

Christen, William G., Simm Liu, Robert J. Glynn, J. Michael Gaziano, and Julie E. Buring. "Dietary Carotenoids, Vitamins C and E, and Risk of Cataract in Women: A Prospective

Study." *Archives of Ophthalmology* 126, no. 1 (2008): 102–109. Available online. URL: http://archopht.ama-assn.org/cgi/content/abstract/126/1/102. Accessed on January 21, 2008.

"Coffee Boosts Pain-Free Walking Time for Patients with Chronic Stable Angina." *Medical World News,* March 12, 1984.

Collins, Karen. "Eggplant a Good Source of Antioxidants." *Daily Herald (Ill.),* April 2, 2008. Available online. URL: http://www.dailyherald.com/story/?id=164091. Accessed on July 21, 2008.

"Degenerative Diseases Such as Cancer May Be Combated by Consumption of Extra-Virgin Olive Oil." *Medical News Today.* Available online. URL: http://www.medicalnewstoday.com/articles/94348.php. Accessed on January 25, 2008.

"Diets High in Antioxidant Foods Appear to Protect the Brain Against Oxidative Damage, if Rat Tests Are Any Indication." *USDA Quarterly Report,* January–March 1997.

"Does Purple Juice Beat Red?" (letter). *Prevention,* December 1997.

"Drinking Coffee May Lower Ovarian Cancer Risk: Study." *Washington Post,* January 22, 2008. Available online. URL: http://www.washingtonpost.com/wp-dyn/content/article/2008/01/22/AR2008012200. Accessed on February 1, 2008.

"Drinking Tea May Offer Health Benefits, but Evidence Still Limited." *Mayo Clinic Health Letter,* April 2008. Available online. URL: http://www.newswise.com/articles/view/539358/?sc=mwtr. Accessed on July 21, 2008.

Duke, Jim. "Vegetarian Vitechart." *Quarterly Journal of Crude Drug Research* 15 (1977): 45–66.

Eckholm, Eric. "Warnings Issued on Eating Shellfish that Is Uncooked." *New York Times,* March 13, 1976.

"Eggplants Flavor Peaks at 42 Days." *Science News,* July 25, 1992.

Facklemann, K. A. "Cabbage Chemical May Bar Breast Cancer." *Science News,* June 16, 1990.

———. "Raspberry-Rich Diet Forestalls Cancer in Rats." *Science News,* April 11, 1998.

"Fish Oil May Ward Off 'Sudden Death.'" *Science News,* December 4, 1993.

"Food Safety." *FDA Consumer,* September–October 1998.

Fox, Nick. "Taking Worry Off the Plate." *New York Times,* January 30, 2008.

Franey, Pierre. "Step by Step: Squid without Tears." *New York Times,* July 2, 1986.

Fries, Joseph H. "Chocolate: A Review of Published Reports of Allergic and Other Deleterious Effects, Real or Presumed." *Annals of Allergy* 41, no. 4 (October 1978): 195–207.

Gilbert, Susan. "Fears Over Milk, Long Dismissed, Still Simmer." *New York Times,* January 19, 1999.

"Green Tea Boosts Antibiotic Effectiveness." United Press International, March 31, 2008. Available online. URL: http://www.upi.com/NewsTrack/Health/2008/03/31/green_tea_boosts_antibiotic_effectiveness/ UPI=15741207008521. Accessed on July 21, 2008.

Hall, Stephen S. "Deflating Beans." *Science 84,* July–August 1984.

"Health Claim for Oat Bran Approved." *Council for Responsible Nutrition News,* March 1997.

Henderson, Doug. "Cookware as a Source of Additives." *FDA Consumer,* March 1982.

Henkel, John. "Irradiation." *FDA Consumer,* May–June 1998.

"Here Is Why Some of Us Don't Drink Milk." *Mayo Clinic Health Letter,* July 1985.

"Hidden' Sodium and Fat in Cheese." *Tufts University Diet and Nutrition Letter,* March 1985.

Higdon, Jane. "Tea." Linus Pauling Institute, Oregon State University, January 2005. Available online. URL: http://lpi.oregonstate.edu/infocenter/phytochemicals/tea/. Accessed on May 8, 2008.

"High Risk Groups Warned: 'Don't Eat Alfalfa Sprouts." *FDA Consumer,* November–December 1998.

Hodgson, Jonathan M., Amanda Devine, Valerie Burke, Ian M. Dick, and Richard L. Prince. "Chocolate Consumption and Bone Density in Older Women." *American Journal of Clinical Nutrition* 87, no. 1 (January 2008): 175–180. Available online. URL: http://www.ajcn.org/cgi/content/abstract/87/1/175. Accessed on January 16, 2008.

"Honey and Infant Botulism." *Science News,* July 15, 1978.

"Honey Dressing Won't Speed Wound Healing." Reuters Health. Available online. URL: http://www.reutershealth.com/en/index.html. Accessed on January 21, 2008.

"Hot Prospects for Quelling Cluster Headaches." *Science News,* July 13, 1991.

"Hot Stuff: A Receptor for Spicy Foods." *Science News,* November 8, 1997.

"How Chili Peppers Deliver Their Fire." *New York Times,* October 28, 1997.

International Food Information Council Foundation. "Functional Foods Fact Sheet: Antioxidants." Available online. URL: http://www.ific.org/publications/factsheets/antioxidantfs.cfm. Accessed on June 24, 2008.

International Food Information Council Foundation. "Functional Foods Fact Sheet: Omega-3 Fatty Acids." Available online. URL: www.ific.org/publications/factsheets/omega3fs.cfm. Accessed on June 24, 2008.

"Irradiated Pork: Long-Awaited Arrival." *Tufts University Diet and Nutrition Letter,* October 1985.

"Irradiation of Pork Is Approved." *New York Times.* January 15, 1985.

"Is Olive Oil Right?" *Tufts University Diet and Nutrition Letter,* May 1986.

Jenkins, Nancy Harmon. "All Briny, All Tasty and All Oysters." *New York Times,* March 5, 1986.

Jensen, Elizabeth, D. M. Osborne, Abigail Pogrebin, and Ted Rose. "Consumer Alert." *Content,* October 1998.

Jull, A., et al. "Randomized Clinical Trial of Honey-Impregnated Dressings for Venous Leg Ulcers." *British Journal of Surgery 95,* no. 2 (February 2008): 175–182. Available online. URL: http://www.ncbi.nlm.nih.gov/pubmed/18161896. Accessed on March 16, 2008.

Kennedy, Cynthia Chandler. "New Light on Beans." *Diabetes Forecast,* March–April 1986.

Khashayar, Patricia. "Alternative Medicine: Walnut." *Press TV (Tehran).* Available online. URL: http://www.presstv.ir/detail.aspx?id=37135&sectionid=3510210. Accessed on January 3, 2008.

King, Dana E., Arch G. Mainous, III, and Mark E. Geesey. "Adopting Moderate Alcohol Consumption in Middle-Age: Subsequent Cardiovascular Events." *The American Journal of Medicine* 121, no. 3 (March 2008): 201–206. Available online. URL: http://www.galenicom.com/en/medline/article/18328303/Adopting+moderate+alcohol+consumption+in+middle+age:+subsequent+cardiovascular+events. Accessed on March 14, 2008.

Koopman, James S., et al. "Milk Fat and Gastrointestinal Illness." *American Journal of Public Health,* December 1984.

Kummer, Corhy. "Carried Away." *New York Times Magazine,* August 30, 1998.

Kurtzwell, Paula. "Questions Keep Sprouting about Sprouts." *FDA Consumer,* January–February 1999.

Lands, Lark. "Pulp Fiction . . . and Facts." *POZ,* September 1997.

Lehmann, Phyllis. "Food and Drug Interactions." *FDA Consumer,* March 1978.

Lynch, Darren M. "Cranberry for Prevention of Urinary Tract Infections." *American Family Physician* 70 (2004): 2175–2177. Available online. URL: http://www.aafp.org/afp/20041201/2175.html. Accessed on April 14, 2008.

Mahoney, C. Patrick, et al. "Chronic Vitamin A Intoxication in Infants Fed Chicken Liver. *Pediatrics* 65, No. 5 (May 1980): 893–896.

McCabe, Beverly, and Ming T. Tsuan. "Dietary Considerations in the MAO Inhibitor Regimens." *Journal of Clinical Psychiatry,* May 1982.

McGee, Harold. "Tainted Cheeses: How Dangerous?" *New York Times,* August 27, 1986.

———. "Frozen Foods: As Nutritious as Fresh?" *ACSH News and Views.* January–February 1984.

Miller, Brian. "Ban Asked on Sale of Raw Milk." *New York Times,* April 11, 1984.

Miller, Julius Sumner. "Physics in the Kitchen." *Science Digest,* August 1975.

"Miller Time." *MAMM,* August–September 1998.

Molotskv, Irvin. "U.S. Issues Ban on Sulfites' Use in Certain Foods." *New York Times,* July 9, 1986.

"Mumps Vaccine." *Morbidity and Mortality Weekly Report,* November 26, 1982.

"Mushroom Poisoning." *The Medical Letter,* July 20, 1984.

Nagle, Mary. "Cranberries." *Prevention,* November 1997.

"A Native American Grape Could Be a Source of New Health Food Products." *USDA Quarterly Report,* January–March 1998.

O'Brien, Denise, and Ann Ryan Haddad. "Counseling Patients on Drug-Food Interactions." *U.S. Pharmacist* 22, No. 6 (June 1997).

O'Neil, John. "Potassium-Rich Diet Linked to Lower Stroke Risk." *New York Times,* September 22, 1998.

"Ounce for Ounce, Blueberries, Concord Grape Juice, Strawberries, Kale and Spinach Had the Most Potent Antioxidant Activity of 40 Fruits, Juices, and Vegetables Measured in a 'Test Tube' Assay," *USDA Quarterly Report,* October–December 1996.

Park, Yikyung, et al. "Dietary Fiber Intake and Risk of Colorectal Cancer: A Pooled Analysis of Prospective Cohort Studies." *Journal of the American Medical Association* 294 (December 14, 2005): 2849–2857. Available online. URL: http://jama.ama-assn.org/cgi/content/full/294/22/2849. Accessed on April 13, 2008.

"A Peppery Preventive for Pain." *Science News,* November 14, 1992.

"Phytic Acid: Fiber's Double Agent." *American Health,* March 1986.

"Plans to Reduce Health Risk from Unpasteurized Juice." *FDA Consumer,* November–December 1997.

"Poisons May Lurk in the Parsnips." *Science News,* September 5, 1981.

Prial, Frank J. "Labeling Wine to Warn of Added Sulfite." *New York Times,* April 2, 1986.

Price, David P. "Beef and the Cholesterol Issue." *Beef Magazine,* March 1984.

"Q&A: Nightshade." *New York Times,* June 15, 1993.

"The Question of Milk Safety." *The Tufts University Diet and Nutrition Letter,* June 1985.

"Questions of Taste." *Food and Wine,* September 1984, June 1985, November 1985, February 1986.

Raloff, Janet. "Anticancer Agent Sprouts Up Unexpectedly." *Science News,* September 20, 1997.

———. "Coffee: Brewing's Link to Cholesterol." *Science News,* September 18, 1995.

———. "The Color of Honey." *Science News,* September 12, 1998.

———. "Coming: Drug Therapy for Chocoholics." *Science News,* June 17, 1995.

———. "Fish Oil Gets a Garlic Chaser for the Heart." *Science News,* February 15, 1997.

———. "The Heart Healthy Side of Lycopene." *Science News,* November 29, 1997.

———. "Heart Risks: This Is Nutty." *Science News,* July 25, 1992.

———. "Ka-Boom." *Science News,* June 6, 1998.

———. "New Heart Risk from Too Much Coffee?" *Science News,* January 14, 1997.

———. "Tallying Wheat Bran's Gutsy Benefits." *Science News,* May 9, 1998.

———. "Teasing Out Tea's Heart Benefits." *Science News,* November 29, 1997.

Raven, Karen. "Leafy Green Veggies Better for the Eyes." *Chicago Tribune,* January 29, 2008. Available online. URL: http://www.chicagotribune.com/features/chi-0129_health_antiox_rjan29,1,4357905.story?ctrack=3&cset=true. Accessed on February 2, 2008.

Rimm, E. B., et al. "Prospective Study of Alcohol Consumption and Risk of Coronary Disease in Men." *The Lancet,* August 24, 1991.

Robertson, Euggle. "A Nutty Idea for Protecting Your Heart." *Chillicothe (Ohio) Gazette,* April 1, 2008. Available online. URL: http://archives.foodsafety.ksu.edu./ffnet/2008/4-2008/ffnet_april_2.htm.

Ruben, Rita. "New Studies, Different Outcomes on Caffeine, Pregnancy." *USA Today,* January 21, 2008. Available online. URL: http://www.usatoday.com/news/health/2008-01-20-caffeine_N.htm. Accessed on January 23, 2008.

Schardt, David. "Just the Grapefruit Facts." *Nutrition Action Newsletter,* January–February 1997.

Segal, Marion. "Tonic in a Teapot?" *FDA Consumer,* March 1996.

Short, Robert. "Serum Potassium Level and Dietary Potassium Intake as Risk Factors for Stroke." *Neurology 59* (2002): 314–320. Available online. URL: http://www.docguide.com/news/content.nsf/NewsPrint/8525697700573E1885256C15006A8A50. Accessed on May 8, 2008.

"Some Ounces of Prevention that Lower Heart Risk." *New York Times,* August 31, 1986.

Stolberg, Sheryl Gay. "Fiber Does Not Help Colon Cancer, Study Finds." *New York Times,* January 21, 1999.

"Study Finds Calcium Can Limit Symptoms of Premenstrual Ills." *New York Times,* August 27, 1998.

"Sulfites as Food Ingredients." *Food Technology,* June 1986.

"Symposium Highlights More Potential Benefits from Tomatoes." *Food Insight,* March–April 1997.

"Testing for Trichinosis." *Science,* February 8, 1985.

Tucker, Marc O., and Chad R. Swan. "The Mango-Poison Connection" (letter). *New England Journal of Medicine,* July 23, 1998.

Turnbull, W. H., and A. R. Leeds. "Reduction of Total and LDL Cholesterol Plasma by Rolled Oats." *The Journal of Clinical Nutrition and Gastroenterology,* February 1987.

"Two Suspected Risk Factors in Breast Cancer." *USDA Quarterly Report.* April–June, 1993.

Villarosa, Linda. "Alcohol and Fertility." *New York Times,* August 25. 1998.

Waldecker, Marcus, Tanja Kautenburger, Heike Daumann, Selveraju Veeriah, and Frank Will. "Water Overload a Risk for People with Epilepsy." *Tufts University Diet and Nutrition Letter,* October 1985.

Waldecker, Marcus, Tanja Kautenburger, Heike Daumann, Selveraju Veeriah, Frank Will, Helmut Dietrich, and Beatrice Louise Pool-Zobel. "Histone-deacetylase inhibition and butyrate formation: Fecal slurry incubations with apple pectin and apple juice extracts." *Nutrition* 24 (April 2008): 366–374. Available online. URL: http://www.foodnavigator.com/news/ng. asp?n=84280-apple-pectin-butyrate-colorectal-cancer. Accessed on April 6, 2008.

Westphal, Sylvia Pagan. "Grapefruit Effect on Drug Levels Has Sweeter Side." *Wall Street Journal,* November 26, 2007. Available online. URL: http://online.wsj.com/article/ SP1196126136238047.html. Accessed on July 21, 2008.

Willensky, Diana. "Food to Chew On." *American Health,* September 1994.

Willett, William C., et al. "Moderate Alcohol Consumption and the Risk of Breast Cancer." *New England Journal of Medicine* 316, No. 19 (May 7, 1987): 1174–1180.

Williams, Linda. "Stalking the Dixie Kidney Stone: Collard Greens Are Prime Suspect." *Wall Street Journal,* April 1, 1985.

"Whole Grain Foods Might Reduce Diabetes Risk, but Evidence Weak." *Medical News Today,* January 23, 2008. Available online. URL: http://www.medicalnewstoday.com/articles/ 94808.php. Accessed on January 23, 2008.

Wu, C. "Putting the Squeeze on Grapefruit Juice." *Science News,* May 9, 1998.

Yuka, Tsuda, Fujine Toshaki, Tanaka Kiyotaka, Maeda Munenori, Hamada Tomoji, and Tsuboi Makoto. "Health Benefits of Cyanopicrin Contained in the Artichoke." *Journal of the Pharmaceutical Society of Japan* 126, Supplement 3 (2006): 88–89.

Zunft, H. J. F., W. Lüder, A. Harde, B. Haber, H. J. Graubaum. and J. Gruenwald. "Carob Pulp Preparation for Treatment of Hypercholesterolemia." *Advances in Therapy* 18, no. 5 (September 2001): 230–236. Available online. URL: http://www.springerlink.com/content/ rn3×64w37225655r/. Accessed on April 16, 2008.

BOOKLETS AND PRESS RELEASES

American Cancer Society. "Non-nutrient Compounds May Protect against Cancer." April 18, 1991.

Arthritis Foundation. "Fish Oils Show Promise for Rheumatoid Arthritis." February 3, 1995.

Chemical Congress of North America. "Studies Find Green Tea Inhibits Skin, Lung, Liver, and Digestive Tract Cancers in Animals," August 30, 1991.

Cornell University. "Finally: Microwave Directions for Blanching Vegetables." September 30, 1985.

———. "Nutritional Value of Microwave-Cooked Foods Is Higher than Other Methods." October 18, 1982.

———. "Sun Exposure May Affect Your Nutrition." April 14, 1986.

Division of Medical Devices, National Institute of Health Sciences. "Latex-Fruit Syndrome and Class 2 Food Allergy." N.d. Available online. URL: dmd.nihs.go.jp/latex/cross-e.html. Accessed July 24, 2008.

Federation of American Societies for Experimental Biology. "Occurrence of Resveratrol in Edible Peanuts." T. H. Sanders and R. W. McMichael, USDA Agricultural Research Service, Raleigh, N.C., April 20, 1998.

———. "High-Monounsaturated Fatty Acid Diets with Peanuts, Peanut Butter, or Peanut Oil Lower Total Cholesterol and LDL-C Identically to a Step 2 Diet but Eliminate the Triglyceride Increase." T. A. Pearson, T. D. Etherton, K. Moriarty, P. M. Kris-Etherton. April 20, 1998.

Institute of Food Technologists. "Health Claims on Oat Products Beat Caveats." January 22, 1997.

———. "Spices May Reduce *Escherichia coli* O157:H7 in Meat." July 20, 1998.

New York City Health Department. "One in Four NYC Adults Has Elevated Blood Mercury Levels." Press Release # 059-07, July 23, 2007. Available online. URL: http://www.home2.nyc.gov/html/doh/html/pr2007/pr059-07.shtml. Accessed on January 30, 2008.

Purdue University. "Cheeseburgers Rich in Cancer Fighting Compound." January 1996.

———. "Compound in Meat Prevents Diabetes, Study Says." January 1998.

———. "Purdue Research Shows Omega-3s Benefits Bone." November 1997.

———. "Researchers Discover How Green Tea May Prevent Cancer." January 1999.

United States Department of Agriculture. "Canning, Freezing, Storing Garden Produce." *Agriculture Information Bulletin* 410, 1977.

———. "Conserving the Nutritive Value in Foods." *Home and Garden Bulletin* 90, 1983.

———. "FSIS Facts: Safe Handling Tips for Meat and Poultry," FSIS 1981.

INTERNET

Associated Press. "Green Tea May Cut Prostate Cancer Risk," AetnaInteliHealth, December 20, 2007. Available online. URL: http://www.intelihealth.com/IH/ihtIH/WSIHW000/333/8015/651131.html. Accessed on December 20, 2007.

———. "Raw Milk Fans Oppose New Calif. Rules," AetnaIntelihealth, December 28, 2007. Available online. URL: http://www.intelihealth.com/IH/ihtIH/WSIHW000/333/8015/651269.html. Accessed on December 28, 2007.

Aston, Jonathan, Amy E. Lodoice, and Nancy L. Shapiro. "Interaction Between Warfarin and Cranberry Juice," Medscape, November 6, 2006. Available online. URL: http://www.medscape.com/viewarticle/545631. Accessed on April 23, 2008.

Bundy, Rafe, Ann F. Walker, Richard W. Middleton, Carol Wallis, and Hugh C. R. Simpson. "Artichoke Leaf Extract (Cynara Scolymus) Reduces Plasma Cholesterol in Otherwise Healthy Hypercholesterolemic Adults: A Randomised Double-Blind Placebo Controlled Trial," *Phytomedicine,* April 17, 2008. Available online. URL: 10.1016/j.phymed.2008.03.001. Accessed July 8, 2008.

Business Daily News. "Macadamia Nuts Are Heart-Healthy," January 3, 2008. Available online. URL: http://businessdailynews.org/health/macadamia-nuts-are-heart-healthy. Accessed on January 4, 2008.

Daniells, Stephen. "Berry Extracts Better than Whole Fruit for Obesity: Study," NutraIngredients USA, January 29, 2008. Available online. URL: http://www.nutraingredients-usa.com/news/ng.asp?n=82855-berries-obesity-anthocyanins. Accessed on February 6, 2008.

————. "Blueberry Compounds Linked to Colon Cancer Prevention," NutraIngredients Europe, March 26, 2007. Available online. URL: http://www.nutraingredients.com/news/print NewsBis.asp?id=75240. Accessed on April 11, 2008.

————. "Pomegranate Peel Could Be Edible Oil Antioxidant: Study," Food Navigator, January 22, 2008. Available online. URL: http://www.foodnavigator.com/news/ng.asp?n=82699-pomegranate-peel-antioxidant-edible-oil. Accessed on January 23, 2008.

————. "Potato Proteins Offer Blood Pressure Benefits," Food Navigator. March 12, 2008. Available online. URL: http://www.foodnavigator-usa.com/news/ng.asp?n =83904-potato-protein-ace-inhibitors-hypertension. Accessed on March 14, 2008.

————. "Soy Isoflavone Linked To Blood Pressure Improvements," NutraIngredients USA, January 30, 2008. Available online. URL: http://www.nutraingredients.com/news/ng.asp?n=82891-soy-isoflavones-genistein-hypertension. Accessed on February 5, 2008.

————. "Study Backs Isoflavones' Safety Rep for Blood Clotting," NutraIngredients USA. Available online. URL: http://www.nutraingredients.com/news/ng.asp?n=82006-iso flavones-soy-postmenopausal. Accessed on December 12, 2007.

————. "Tomatoes Better than Pure Lycopene for Health, Says Review," NutraIngredients Europe, August 18, 2006. Available online. URL: http://www.nutraingredients.com/news/printNewsBis.asp?id=69958. Accessed on May 7, 2008.

Decas Cranberry Products, Inc. "Research Shows Decas Sweetened Dried Cranberries Pack Twice the Proanthocyanidin Punch as Cranberry Juice Cocktail," Bio-Medicine, December 13, 2007. Available online. URL: http://www.bio-medicine.org/medicine-technology-1/Research-Shows-Decas-Sweetened-Dried-Cranberries-Pack-Twice-the-Proanthocyanidin-Punch-as-Cranberry-Juice-Cocktail-1058-1/. Accessed on December 14, 2007.

Fox, Maggie. "Meat Raises Lung Cancer Risk: Study," Reuters Health, December 11, 2007. Available online. URL: http://www.reutershealth.com/index.htm. Accessed on December 12, 2007.

Hitti, Miranda. "Whole-Grain Cereals Cut Heart Failure," WebMD, March 2, 2007. Available online. URL: http://www.medicinenet.com/script/main/art.asp?articlekey=79671. Accessed on April 16, 2008.

Hubbard, Sylvia. "Apple Juice Fights Disease," NewsMax, December 13, 2007. Available online. URL:http://www.newsmax.com/health/Apple_Juice_Disease/2007/12/13/56688.html. Accessed on December 14, 2007.

Johnson, Carla K. "Experts Change Advice on Kids' Allergies," Associated Press, January 7, 2008. Available online. URL: http://www.abcnews.go.com/Health/wireStory?id= 4095245. Accessed on January 9, 2008.

Kuntz, Lynn. "New Cherry Campaign Stresses Nutrition," FoodProductsDesign. Available online. URL: http://www.foodproductdesign.com/. Accessed on December 19, 2007.

Laino, Charlene. "Alcohol May Raise Breast Cancer Risk," WebMD, April 14, 2008. Available online. URL: http://www.webmd.com/breast-cancer/news/20080414/alcohol-may-raise-breast-cancer-risk. Accessed on April 20, 2008.

Medical News Today. "Apple Pectin, Apple Juice Extracts Shown to Have Anticarcinogenic Effects on Colon," March 27, 2008. Available online. URL: http://www.medicalnews today.com/articles/101856.php. Accessed on March 31, 2008.

———. "Artificial Sweeteners Could Make You Gain Weight, Study," February 11, 2008. Available online. URL: http://www.medicalnewstoday.com/articles/96849.php. Accessed on February 11, 2008.

———. "Blueberries May Hold the Key to Eradicating Forgetfulness," April 12, 2008. Available online. URL: http://www.medicalnewstoday.com/articles/103617.php. Accessed on April 14, 2008.

———. "The Health Risk of High-Fat Foods Could Be Reduced by New Discovery," January 3, 2008. Available online. URL: http://www.medicalnewstoday.com/articles/92956.php. Accessed January 4, 2008.

———. "Increase in Foodborne Outbreaks from Leafy Greens," March 18, 2008. Available online. URL: http://www.medicalnewstoday.com/articles/100938.php. Accessed on March 19, 2008.

———. "Marathon Runners Beware of Drinking Too Much Water," January 6, 2008. Available online. URL: http://www.medicalnewstoday.com/articles/93065.php. Accessed on January 9, 2008.

———. "Morning Jolt of Caffeine Might Mask Serious Sleep Problems," December 1, 2007. Available online. URL: http://www.medicalnewstoday.com/articles/91139.php. Accessed on December 6, 2007.

———. "Neuroprotection From Green Tea For Parkinson's Disease," Available online. URL: http://www.medicalnewstoday.com/articles/91851.php. Accessed on December 14, 2007.

———. "One Drink of Red Wine or Alcohol Is Relaxing to Circulation, But Two Drinks Are Stressful," February 13, 2008. Available online. URL: http://www.medicalnewstoday.com/articles/97111.php. Accessed on February 14, 2008.

———. "Overcoming Allergic Reactions to Soy," March 7, 2008. Available online. URL: http://www.medicalnewstoday.com/articles/99764.php. Accessed on March 7, 2008.

———. "Red Meat Consumption Linked to Colorectal Cancer: Experts Offer New Advice for Colorectal Cancer Awareness Month," March 4, 2006. Available online. URL: http://www.medicalnewstoday.com/articles/99293.php. Accessed on March 10, 2008.

———. "Resveratrol in Grape Skins Could Stop Diabetic Complications Such As Heart Disease, Retinopathy and Nephropathy," March 19, 2008. Available online. URL: http://www.medicalnewstoday.com/articles/101086.php. Accessed on March 20, 2008.

———. "Risk of Chronic Disease Lowered by Whole Grain Diets," February 6, 2008. Available online. URL: http://www.medicalnewstoday.com/articles/96374.php. Accessed on February 6, 2008.

———. "Routine Intake of Dairy Products Can Help Reduce Periodontal Disease," February 7, 2008. Available online. URL: http://www.medicalnewstoday.com/articles/96531.php. Posted on February 7, 2008.

———. "Soaking Potatoes in Water Before Frying Reduces Acrylamide," March 8, 2008. Available online. URL: http://www.medicalnewstoday.com/articles/99729.php. Accessed on March 12, 2008.

———. "Sugary Beverages May Increase Alzheimer's Risk," December 9, 2007. Available online. URL: http://www.medicalnewstoday.com/articles/91139.php. Accessed on December 12, 2007.

National Center for Alternative and Complementary Medicine. "Garlic." Available online. URL: nccam.nih.gov/health/garlic. Accessed on April 24, 2008.

Newswise. "Can Omega-3 Fatty Acids Help Depression?" December 17, 2007. Available online. URL: http://www.newswise.com/p/articles/view/536324/. Accessed on December 18, 2007.

———. "Compound Found in Soybeans Effective in Reducing Hot Flashes in Menopausal Women," January 9, 2008. Available online. URL: http://www.newswise.com/articles/view/536739/?sc=mwtr. Accessed on July 22, 2008.

———. "Cranberries Might Help Prevent Urinary Infections in Women," January 10, 2008. Available online. URL: http://www.newswise.com/articles/view/536794/?sc=mwtr. Accessed on January 12, 2008.

———. "Milk and Egg Allergies Harder to Outgrow." December 12, 2007. Available online. URL: http://www.newswise.com/articles/view/536213/?sc=mwtr. Accessed on December 12, 2007.

———. "Newer, Stronger Evidence Caffeine Increases Miscarriage Risk," January 16, 2008. Available online. URL: http://www.newswise.com/articles/view/536954/?sc=mwtr. Accessed on January 17, 2008.

———. "Research Links Diet, Gardening and Lung Cancer Risk," December 7, 2007. Available online. URL: http://www.newswise.com/articles/view/536043/?sc=mwtr. Accessed on December 7, 2007.

———. "Strawberries May Help Reduce Risk of Having Elevated Inflammation in Blood Vessels," January 11, 2008. Available online. URL: http://www.newswise.com/articles/view/536803/?sc=sptr. Accessed on January 16, 2008.

———. "Why Fish Oil Is Good for You," December 21, 2007. Available online. URL: http://www.newswise.com/articles/view/536485/?sc=mwtr. Accessed on December 25, 2007.

NutraIngredients Europe. "Pilot Study Supports Raspberry Potential for Oesophageal Cancer," December 10, 2007. Available online. URL: http://www.nutraingredients.com/news/printNewsBis.asp?id=81928. Accessed on December 12, 2007.

NutraIngredients USA. "Broccoli Compound May Protect Against AMD," July 15, 2004. Available online. URL: http://www.nutraingredients-usa.com/news/ng.asp?n=53549-broccoli-compound-may. Accessed on April 25, 2008.

Office of Dietary Supplements, National Institutes of Health. "Dietary Supplement Fact Sheet: Folate." Updated August 22, 2005. Available online. URL: http://dietary-supplements.info.nih.gov/factsheets/folate.asp. Accessed on April 9, 2008.

Rauscher, Megan. "Green Tea May Protect against Colon Cancer," Reuters Health, December 12, 2007. Available online. URL: http://www.reutershealth.com/en/index.html. Accessed on December 13, 2007.

Reuters. "Drinking May Raise Breast Cancer Risk," April 14, 2008. Available online. URL: http://www.healthday.com/Article.asp?AID=614432. Accessed on July 21, 2008.

———. "Sweet Tidings for Pregnant Chocoholics," April 30, 2008. Available online. URL: http://www.theage.com.au/news/world/sweet-tidings-for-pregnant-chocoholics/2008/04/29/1209234861933.html. Accessed on May 4, 2008.

Reuters Health. "Sugar Promotes Alzheimer's-Like Disease in Mice," updated December 17, 2007. Available online. URL: http://www.reutershealth.com/en/index.html. Accessed on December 18, 2007.

ScienceDaily. "Artichoke Leaf Extract Lowers Cholesterol," July 7, 2008. Available online. URL: www.sciencedaily. com/releases/2008/07/080702170607.htm. Accessed July 8, 2008.

Vann, Madeline. "Blackberries, Broccoli Sprouts Battle Cancer," Yahoo News, December 6, 2007. Available online. URL: http://news.yahoo.com/s/hsn/20071207/hl_hsn/blackberriesbroccolisproutsbattlecancer. Accessed on December 12, 2007.

World Poultry. "Poultry Workers Carry Antibiotic-Resistant Germs," December 19, 2007. Available online. URL: http://www.worldpoultry.net/home/id2205-37650/poultry_workers_carry_antibiotic-resistant_germs.html. Accessed on December 20, 2007.

Index